Dermal Fillers for Facial Harmony

Dedication

This book is dedicated to my father and mother. Along the way, I have been missing them, but all that I learned from both of them always brings light to the path. To my beloved sister, Marya, an angel of kindness and strength, always teaching me. To my brother, Antônio, with whom I learned how to write. To my beloved wife, Cláudia, the one who makes dreams come true. To Gabriel, my son, my best friend—the one who has overcome all difficulties without losing his joy. To Ana Sofia, my daughter, you make me believe that anything is possible. To Jesus Christ, my Lord, the only one who gave his life to save us. Nothing would be enough to pay for your sacrifice. Thank you, Father!

Library of Congress Control Number:2019943798

QUINTESSENCE PUBLISHING
USA

Quintessence Publishing Co, Inc
411 N Raddant Road
Batavia, IL 60510
www.quintpub.com

5 4 3 2 1

Editor: Leah Huffman
Design: Sue Zubek
Production: Sue Robinson

Printed in China

Dermal Fillers *for* Facial Harmony

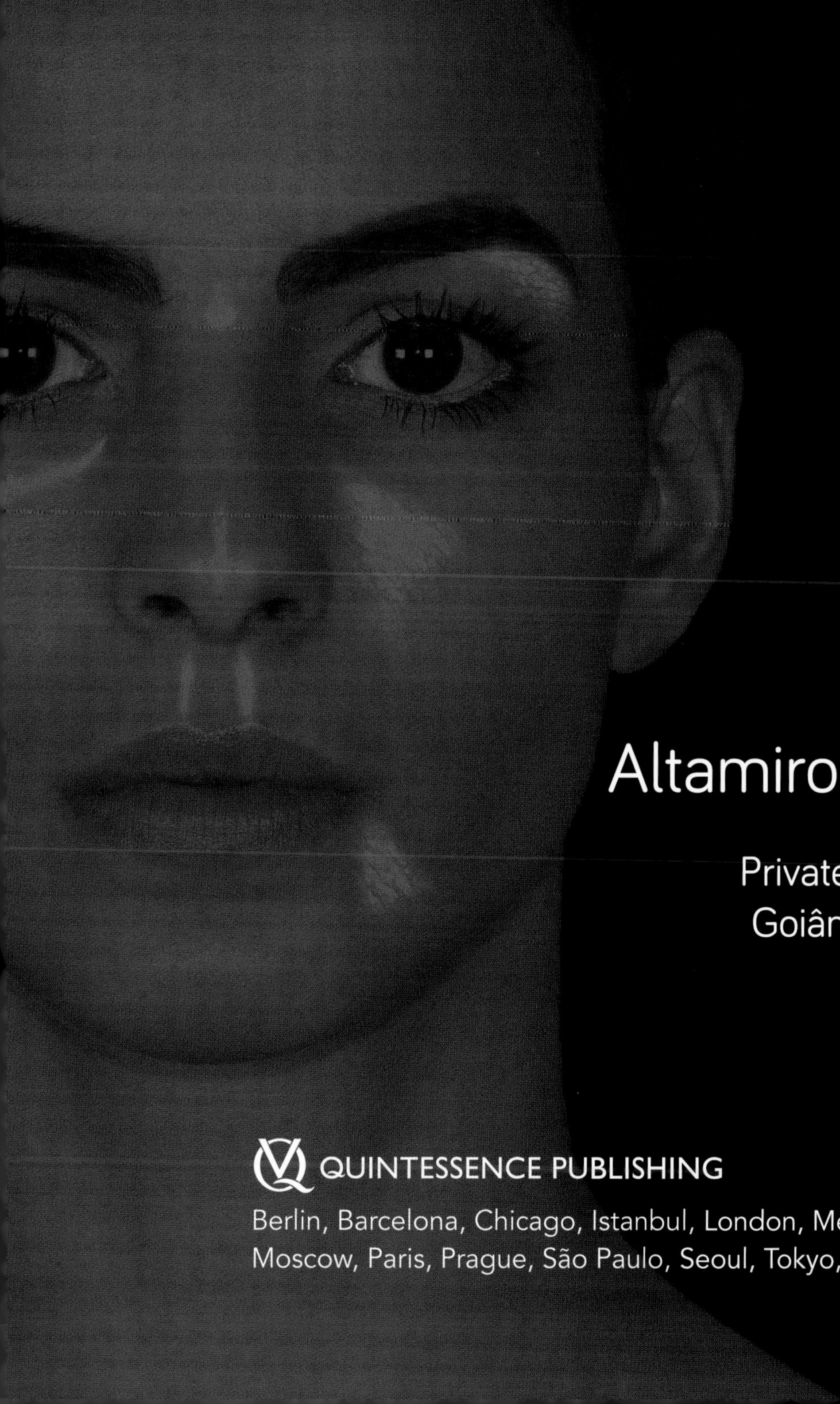

Altamiro Flávio, DDS

Private Practice
Goiânia, Brazil

QUINTESSENCE PUBLISHING

Berlin, Barcelona, Chicago, Istanbul, London, Mexico City, Milan,
Moscow, Paris, Prague, São Paulo, Seoul, Tokyo, Warsaw

contents

Extra content
Extra content is available online. QR codes throughout the book link to files and videos that can be used by the professional to facilitate better treatment planning and delivery of care. Scan the QR code here to access this supplementary information. The full list of links may also be found at www.quintpub.com/fillers.

foreword

Over the years, I have been following Professor Altamiro Flávio's career, and it is an honor to write this preface as one of his former students in esthetic procedures and facial harmonization courses. Currently, I am a researcher and professor at a dental school, and without a doubt I can state that Dr Altamiro has strong and important skills as an expert clinician, opinion leader, dental photographer, and speaker. Now he shares new knowledge about dermal fillers for esthetic and functional treatments in this wonderful book. The sequence of chapters and clinical cases show how contemporary dentistry can help patients achieve a wonderful smile and nice facial esthetics, and how dentists can develop this type of procedure with safe clinical protocols. Readers will find concepts, principles, evidence-based case reports, and important clinical hints to elaborate planning and treatment protocols with several types of products. Every student and all dental professionals performing esthetic procedures need to read this book to understand injectable materials, techniques, and principles of facial esthetics and the smile. All professionals in the area of esthetic dentistry will find something to enjoy and learn in this book.

Paulo Vinícius Soares, DDS, MS, PhD
Federal University of Uberlândia, Brazil

preface

The title of professor is not 100% acquired. In part, the individual is born with this gift, while the other part comes on a daily basis after hours and hours of dedication to professional growth and sharing all our acquired knowledge with our students. When teaching, we share in a few hours what was learned from years of study and dedication. We donate the best of us to people who are sometimes unknown. Thus, our work is mainly a donation, whose reward is the satisfaction of others. This is how we share a lot of what has been given to us by God. Being a teacher is an honor to which I have tried every moment to do justice while working on this book. I tried to condense all the knowledge necessary so that students could be able to safely develop their practice.

The second step is to practice everything that was learned. I believe that all injectable facial procedures should be initially practiced in a cadaver. The procedures described herein can be practiced by attending our course of anatomy applied to facial fillers at the Miami Anatomical Research Center, where we use fresh cadavers. To train as much as possible before helping a patient should be the main rule.

This book contains a lot of information that will be useful to dedicated readers who strive to fulfill their mission to treat well their patients, who are children of God and therefore our brothers.

Enjoy the reading!

Acknowledgments

I would like to express my gratitude to my friends at the Miami Anatomical Research Center—Dr Eduardo Sadao, Heloíse Peixoto, Justin Fraioli, Steve Canona, Sheila Herrera, Jorge Carrasco, and Maylin Peres Carrasco—for their effort in keeping up with our courses that help educate so many professionals. A special thanks to Mr Al Weinstein, the great entrepreneur, who once told me "if you are always by the book, you will never be on the book." Thanks for your unique view. Dear Dr Paulo Vinícius Soares, you were the first one to believe in this book, and now it is a reality. Thank you Dr Christian Coachman, who linked facial aspects to the smile, and Dr Rubelisa Cândido Gomes de Oliveira, who once again has assisted me with the scientific format of the book, contributing much to its success. My appreciation to Denise Riley, who has spent so many hours dealing with words that will spread knowledge, you are great my sister. I also wish to acknowledge my assistant professors—Márcia Viotti, Rogério Zambonato, Dr Francisco Célio Dantas, Luciana Rezende, Maria Geovânia, Danielle Dias, and Rosa Amaoedo—for the amazing support they have given me during so many courses. I wish to thank my secretary, Walquiria, for her dedication to our courses. My greatest respect and gratitude for all those who have selflessly given their precious bodies to Science. To my dear patients who allowed me to use their photographs and clinical history to improve the knowledge of so many health professionals through this book, I cannot thank you enough. I would like to acknowledge the important role of so many teachers I have had throughout my lifetime. I will always carry with me their teachings. Finally, my eternal gratitude to the greatest teacher of all, Jesus, for the daily blessings.

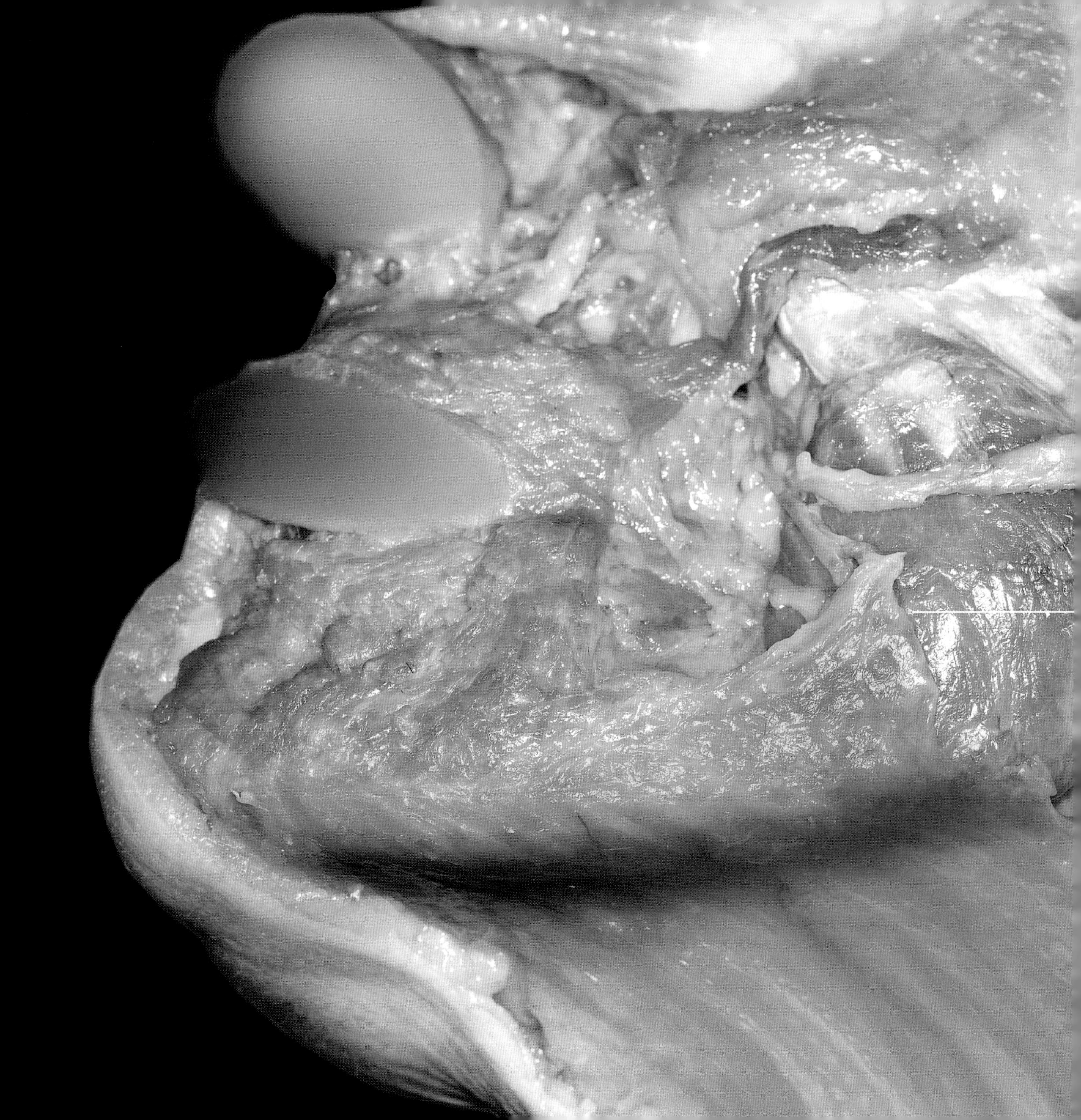

CHAPTER

01

Facial Anatomy

The search for beauty seems to be a natural human instinct—beauty in nature, beauty in art, beauty in manmade design, and perhaps above all else, beauty in our own physical esthetics. For many centuries, humans have sought to enhance natural beauty and slow aging. The recent discovery of safe dermal fillers has ushered in an era of minimally invasive treatment for wrinkles, depressions, grooves, and volume deficiencies, revolutionizing the way patients perceive aging and their ability to control its physical consequences.

Understanding the basic anatomy of the face and the natural aging process is central to effective treatment with dermal fillers. This chapter details the facial manifestations of the aging process and describes the tissue layers and blood supply of the face. Chapter 2 introduces dermal fillers, and chapter 3 illustrates their various injection techniques.

Facial Aging

Skin, like many other organs, undergoes deleterious changes with the passage of time and the associated hormonal and dietary variations. Unlike most other organs, however, skin is also directly affected by exposure to the environment, especially ultraviolet (UV) irradiation from the sun. Chronic exposure to UV irradiation causes an aged phenotype (photoaging) that is superimposed with aging caused by the passage of time (chronologic aging). As a result, areas of the body that are frequently exposed to the sun, such as the face, neck, forearms, or back of the hands, acquire visible signs of aging more rapidly than other areas of the body. Evidently, photoaging is a cumulative process and, as such, is more severe in older individuals. The passage of time and repeated exposure to harmful aspects of the environment alter both the epidermal and dermal compartments of the skin.[1]

Aging of the face is characterized by different phenomena happening at more or less the same time (Fig 1-1). Flattening of the dermal-epidermal junction is thought to reduce the exchange surface between the epidermis and dermis, thereby reducing the nutrient flux; as a result, this flattening might have a role in reducing keratinocyte proliferation.[2] Flattening of the dermal-epidermal junction also reduces epidermal resistance to shearing forces and thereby makes the epidermis more fragile.[2] The thickness of the stratum corneum remains unaltered with advanced age,[2,3] and stratum corneum hydration is modestly lowered or unchanged in aged versus young individuals.[4,5] Accordingly, transepidermal water loss (a measure of stratum corneum integrity) is unaltered with chronologic aging.[5] However, surface lipid production decreases significantly with age on some areas of the skin,[4,5] increasing the incidence of xerosis (dry skin), pruritus (itchy skin), and skin irritation in elderly populations.[6] These modifications lead to the following:

- Variable skin atrophic changes and wrinkle formation caused by genetic, actinic, and environmental factors
- Bone volume and facial fat loss primarily in the bony skeleton and fat compartments with predictable patterns
- Skin sagging

With aging, the bony layer undergoes a reabsorption of the skeleton, mostly in the orbital, periorbital, malar, submalar, and mandibular areas,[7,8] and the fat compartments follow a rather predictable pattern of depletion. In the deep supraperiosteal layer, most of the volume loss takes place in the lateral and medial suborbicularis oculi fat, the deep medial cheek compartment, and the chin fat compartments. In the superficial subcutaneous layer, most of the volume loss takes place in the lateral compartments, both in their temporal and preauricular districts and to a lesser extent in the middle and medial fat compartments of the superficial cheek fat pad.[9,10] It is remarkable that both the superficial nasolabial compartment and the superior and inferior jowl compartments are not greatly affected by volume loss and tend to move medially due to a lack of lateral support caused by volume depletion in the lateral fat areas and a lack of fibrous fixation points.[11] All the areas of fat reabsorption are confined in between the ligaments,[9,12] so on the surface of the skin, several grooves become identifiable with this volume deflation: the tear trough and the palpebromalar groove (tear trough ligament and orbital retaining ligaments), the midcheek groove (zygomaticocutaneous ligament), the nasolabial fold (nasolabial ligament), the buccal fat groove (parotidomasseteric ligament), and the marionette line (labiomandibular ligament).[10,12,13] All these ligaments tend to keep their strength in the central area of the face, where a strong fixation point exists, and become looser laterally.[14]

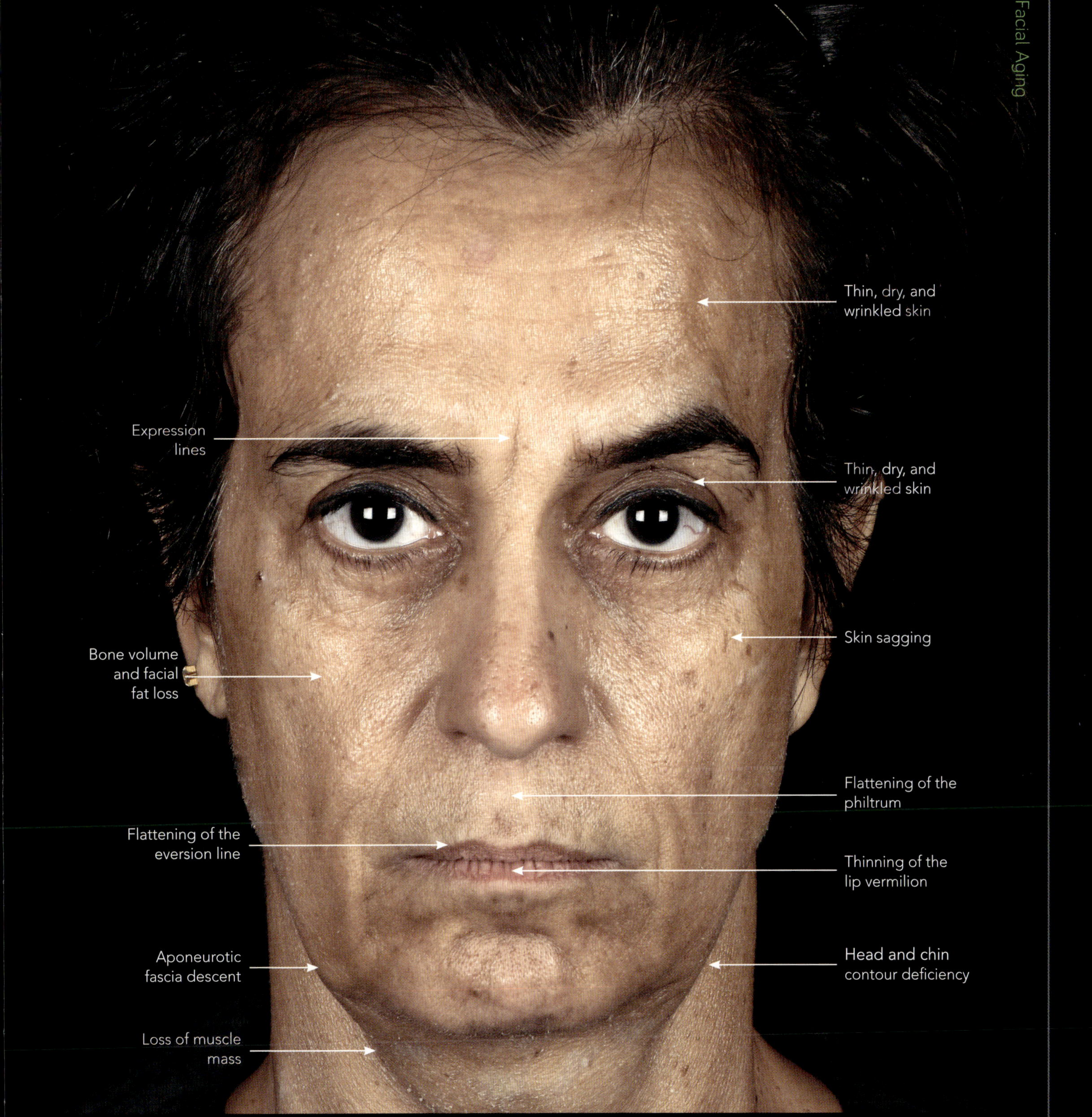

Fig 1-1 Various manifestations of facial aging.

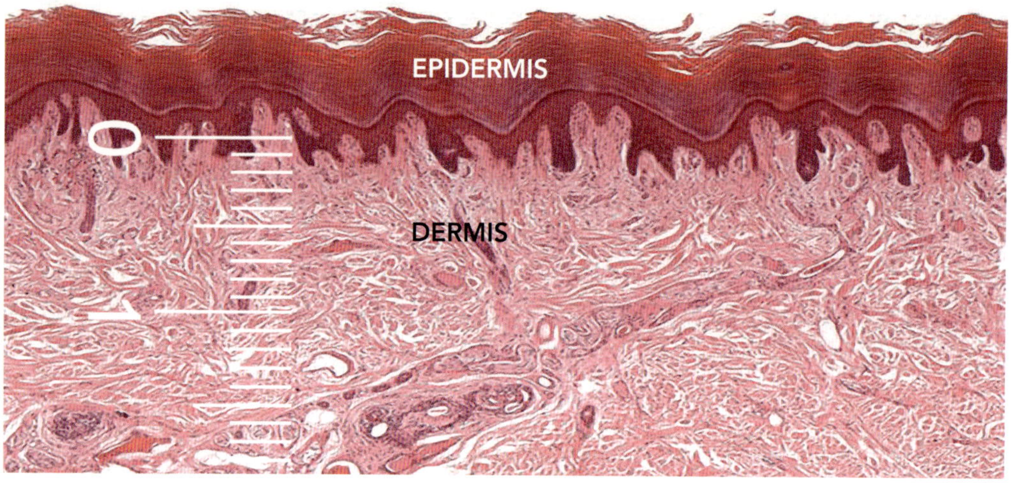

Fig 1-2 Layers of the skin. The dermal thickness varies from 1.04 to 1.86 mm.

Skin and Connective Tissue

The skin is the largest organ of the human body, and it has several functions. It acts as a physical, chemical, and bacteriological barrier; it prevents dehydration; it regulates body temperature; it mediates the sense of touch; and it plays a role in immune surveillance, hormone production, and social communication.[1]

The skin has two layers: the epidermis and the dermis (Fig 1-2). The epidermis is the outermost layer of the skin. It contains no blood vessels and relies exclusively on the underlying dermis for nutrients. The epidermis is primarily made up of keratinocytes organized in a stratified epithelium.[1] The dermis consists of connective tissue with a variable amount of elastic fibers and several nerves, blood vessels, and lymphatic vessels. Its thickness varies from 1.04 to 1.86 mm.[15] This connective tissue is composed of two different layers: a deep or reticular layer and a superficial or papillary layer. The reticular layer is made up of fibroelastic connective tissue and mainly collagen fibers. The cells in this layer are mainly fibroblasts and histiocytes. Sebaceous and sweat glands, hair follicles, and small groups of cells are also found in deeper layers of the reticular dermis.[1,15] The hypodermis or subcutaneous tissue is a layer of loose connective tissue immediately below the dermis.

Superficial Muscular Aponeurotic System

Beneath the dermis lies the superficial muscular aponeurotic system (SMAS), a layer composed of superficial aponeuroses blended with muscles and fat (top right in Fig 1-3). Contrary to the other skeletal muscles, the muscles of facial expression are not surrounded by a fascia because they originate and/or are inserted in the skin. Unlike botulinum toxin, **fillers should not be injected in the muscles**. The SMAS in the face is composed of several muscles of facial expression, and therefore the operator should carefully watch the depth of this layer to prevent fillers from being injected in this muscle layer.

Figure 1-3 illustrates the tissue layers of the human face, and Fig 1-4 illustrates how different anatomical areas can support different volumes of fillers. In most cases, the target layer for fillers is the superficial fat layer.

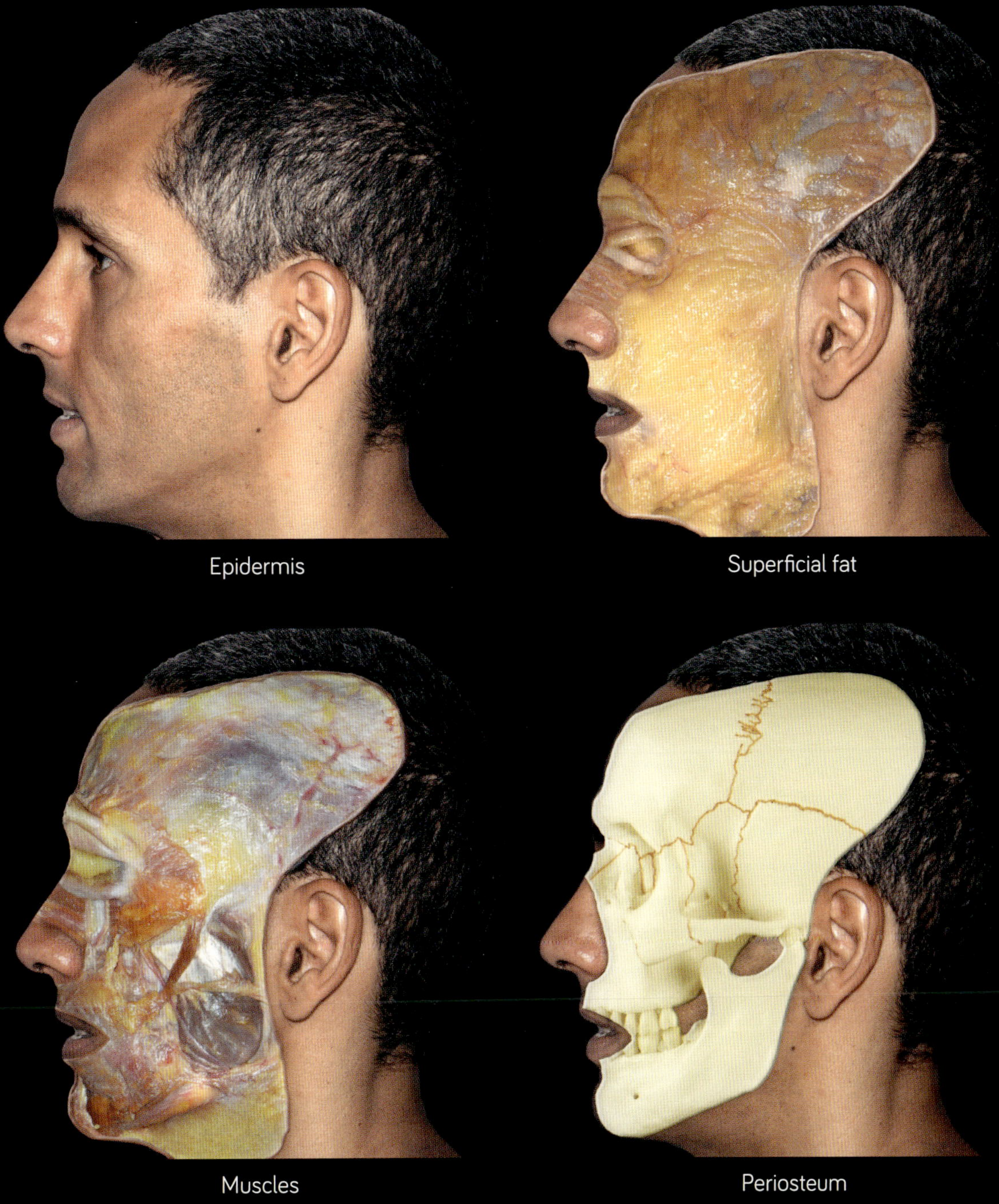

Fig 1-3 Layers of facial tissues.

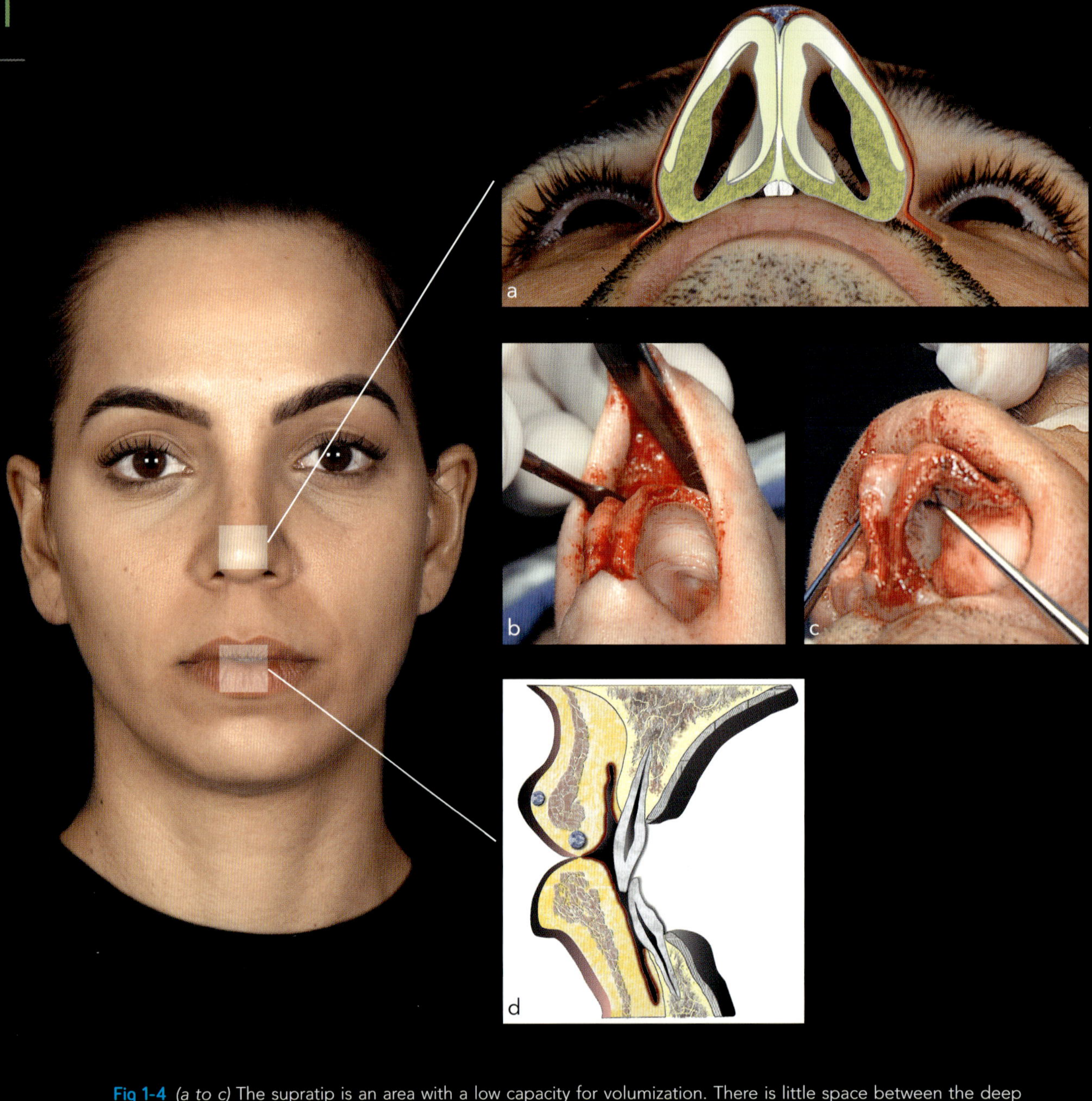

Fig 1-4 *(a to c)* The supratip is an area with a low capacity for volumization. There is little space between the deep dermis and the cartilage. Therefore, this region only supports a very small amount of fillers. *(d)* The lip vermilion is a region that shows elasticity and malleability, allowing it a good capacity for volumization. It can accommodate various volumes of fillers.

Blood Supply to the Face

Areas with minimal soft tissue coverage over the blood supply are at a risk for necrosis with dermal filler injection. The injected volume applies pressure on the vessels, decreasing blood flow and causing tissue ischemia. For this reason, it is essential that any practicing clinician know the locations of blood vessels in the face.[16]

The external carotid artery is the main artery that supplies blood to the face. Its most studied branch is the facial artery and its branches. This artery runs in the outer surface of the mandible under the platysma and up to the inner corner of the eye. It crosses the buccinator muscle and the maxilla deep to the zygomaticus major and levator labii superioris muscles. Branches of the facial artery supply the lips and lateral aspect of the nose.

Blood supply to the lips

The anatomical topography of the lips is not generally well known by clinicians.[17] However, the popularity of lip injection treatments underscores the importance of understanding the blood supply to this area of the face.

The arteries that supply the lips are the superior and inferior labial arteries (branches of the facial artery), which are connected by anastomoses with those on the opposite side of the face, forming an arterial circle around the vermilion border.[18] The superior and inferior labial arteries are located exactly where dermal fillers are injected: between the upper and lower lip's wet and dry mucous membrane line and in the internal part of the upper lip. There are also terminal infraorbital artery branches (inferior palpebral, superior, and nasal labial) that arise from the infraorbital foramen.[19]

In most cases, the superior labial artery (SLA) originates above the labial commissure and follows a route from the horizontal to medial plane, along the upper lip. In fewer than 25% of cases, its origin coincides with the labial commissure. The mean distance from the SLA's origin to the labial commissure ranges from 5 to 9 mm. The diameter is approximately 1.5 mm at its origin, and it goes deep into the orbicular oris muscle, emitting perforating branches to reach the skin, vermilion, and oral mucosa. It is located at an average depth of 4.5 mm in the skin, 2.6 mm from the oral mucosa, and 5.6 mm from the inferior border of the upper lip. Compression of the SLA at about 1 cm above the oral commissure, a point at which it passes near the oral angle, is recommended during the injection of fillers to decrease its caliber and therefore minimize the risk of perforation.

The philtrum's arterial supply is carried out by the central artery of the philtrum, the left and right lateral ascendant arteries of the philtrum, and the left and right accessory arteries of the philtrum (branches of the SLA).[16] These arteries ensure the main contribution to the ascendant columellar arteries.[20] It is important to note that the arteries that make up this arch in the philtrum are located above the orbicularis oris muscle.

The inferior labial artery (ILA) originates near the labial commissure following a route from the horizontal to medial plane, along the lower lip. Most of the time it originates below the oral commissure. The ILA's path runs close to the alveolar border, outside the lower lip's vermilion. Most labial branches cross into the vermilion perpendicularly, and the marginal arteries that connect with these terminal branches in the vermilion are of a very small caliber. The veins are tributaries of the facial, temporal, superficial, pterygoid plexus, and the superoexternal portion. The maxilla region has a deep venous compound that must be avoided when injecting fillers,[21] especially for injections close to the infraorbital foramen.

Blood supply to the nose

The angular artery is a terminal branch of the facial artery that runs along the nose to the inner angle of the eye to supply the eyelids. It supplies the lateral region of the dorsum of the nose, close to the root, and crosses the levator muscle of the upper lip and the wing of the nose. Due to its characteristics and the size of the area it supplies, the angular artery plays a very important role when we consider the consequences of its occlusion. Because of the injection, there may be spasm or compression that can lead to necrosis, ischemia, and scarring throughout the area.[21] In the inner corner of the eye, it joins the supra- and infratrochlear arteries and the infraorbital artery (maxillary branch). Thus, it also supplies part of the frontal region.[18]

The columella and lateral nasal artery branches (branches of the angular artery) irrigate the ala, dorsum, and tip of the nose. The lateral nasal and columellar arteries form an anastomosis over the dome, forming an alar arcade.[22] On the other hand, the dorsal nasal artery (a branch of the ophthalmic artery) supplies the root and dorsum of the nose. One of its branches joins the angular artery in the root of the nose while the other descends, anastomosing with the external nasal artery, which is a branch of the infraorbital artery. The lateral nasal veins are located 2 to 3 mm from the alar crease. They appear deeply in the nasal base with the columella artery and end in the tip of the subdermal plexus.[21]

Blood supply to the temporal region

The superficial temporal artery is a terminal branch of the external carotid artery. It originates at the parotid gland and ascends in a superficial plane to the posterior part of the zygomatic process of the temporal bone up to neck of the mandible. It ascends and crosses anteriorly to the external acoustic pore, giving off the terminal branches 2 to 3 cm above the zygomatic arch. In this region, it runs between the cutis and the epicranial aponeuoris.[23] It supplies the temporal, frontal, and parietal regions and the parotid gland with its duct through branches with similar names. When filling the pretragal region, injections should be delicate and slow in the subcutaneous deep plane, perpendicular to the superficial temporal artery. To prevent serious traumas, the needle must not be introduced repeatedly in the same place. Moreover, the pressure of injecting large volumes into this area can cause paresthesia and thus must be avoided.

Blood supply to the middle third of the face

The infraorbital artery originates in the pterygomaxillary fissure (close to the maxillary tuberosity) and penetrates the orbit, exiting the face through the infraorbital foramen.[23] For safety reasons, deeper filler procedures close to the foramen should be avoided because of the blood supply net in this area. The terminal branches of the infraorbital artery irrigate the soft tissues in the middle third of the face (lower eyelid), external nose, and upper lip.

Blood supply to other regions of the face

In the mentum, the most important arteries are the submental and mental. The submental arteries originate from the facial artery in the submandibular region, pass by the mandible's base up to the mentum, and irrigate the mylohyoid muscle, the digastric muscle's anterior belly, and adjacent structures. At the mandibular symphysis, it makes an ascending path that bypasses the edge of the mandible and anastomoses with the inferior labial artery. Because of this, any preparations for a chin augmentation must be made with a cannula so that the chances of embolization are smaller.

The mentum is also supplied by the mental artery, a branch of the inferior alveolar artery that emerges through the mental foramen.[23] The venous drainage corresponds to the arterial supply. The mandible is supplied by the facial and inferior alveolar arteries.[21]

In the side of the mouth, the facial artery gives off the superior and inferior labial branches and then, in its ascendant path, goes along the border of the nose to become the angular artery. At the glabella, it becomes the supratrochlear artery, supplying the medial frontal region. The frontal region above the eyes is supplied by the supraorbital artery, which is a branch of the ophthalmic artery.[18]

The orbital region concentrates some points of anastomosis of the external carotid system with the internal carotid system. One of the most important is the anastomosis of the dorsal nasal artery with the angular artery. The facial artery, a branch of the external carotid artery, leads into the angular artery after superficially crossing the medial canthal tendon, where it forms an anastomosis with the dorsal nasal branch of the ophthalmic artery, which in turn is a branch of the internal carotid artery. One of its branches joins the angular artery at the root of the nose, and the other runs downward, being joined by an anastomosis with the external nasal artery, a branch of the infraorbital artery.[19]

The supraorbital artery forms anastomosis with the superficial temporal artery and establishes limits between the central region of the forehead and the temporal region. A reference in terms of the route of the superficial temporal artery is that it passes under the preauricular crease.[17] Thus, it is important not to insert the cannula or needle in this crease when injecting fillers at the zygomatic arch. Facial fillers injected with the purpose of making the face look more masculine and highlighting the border between the forehead and temple should be avoided because the superficial temporal artery and its anastomosis with the supraorbital artery are right below the fat layer and above the temporal muscle. It is also superficial to the occipitofrontalis muscle in the forehead. This is a region of high risk of vascular injury because there is little space between the surface of the skin and the bone.

Facial Lymphatic System

In practice, in cosmetic dermatology, and in physiotherapy and esthetics studies, drainage problems in the periocular region are very frequent. For instance, patient complaints about "swelling" in the eyes following the application of botulinum toxin are very common. When large volumes of fillers are injected in the tear trough or when a periocular sculpture is carried out—or even in surgeries in that area—the appearance of edema is also common. In fact, the palpebral lymphatic system is very delicate and not prepared for traumas or procedures like these.

The alteration of pressure due to a variation in volume also leads to the occlusion of the ducts, which are very delicate and sensitive. Although lymphatic drainage is usually described within a regional context, advanced studies show that massage (manual or with the aid of equipment) in the medial direction (toward the nasal region's drainage system) and lateral direction (toward the parotid gland) can help patients with lymphatic drainage problems in the eyelid area.[19]

References

1. Rittie L, Fisher GJ. Natural and sun-induced aging of human skin. Cold Spring Harb Perspect Med 2015;5:a015370.
2. Lavker RM, Zheng PS, Dong G. Morphology of aged skin. Clin Geriatr Med 1989;5:53–67.
3. Lavker RM. Cutaneous aging: Chronologic versus photoaging. In: Gilchrest BA (ed). Photodamage. Cambridge, MA: Blackwell, 1995:123–135.
4. Man MQ, Xin SJ, Song SP, et al. Variation of skin surface pH, sebum content and stratum corneum hydration with age and gender in a large Chinese population. Skin Pharmacol Physiol 2009;22:190–199.
5. Luebberding S, Krueger N, Kerscher M. Age-related changes in skin barrier function—Quantitative evaluation of 150 female subjects. Int J Cosmet Sci 2013;35:183–190.
6. Kligman AM. Perspectives and problems in cutaneous gerontology. J Invest Dermatol 1979;73:39–46.
7. Shaw RB Jr, Kahn DM. Aging of the midface bony elements: A three dimensional computed tomographic study. Plast Reconstr Surg 2007;119:675–683.
8. Mendelson B, Wong CH. Changes in the facial skeleton with aging: Implications and clinical applications in facial rejuvenation. Aesthet Plast Surg 2012;36:753–760.
9. Rohrich RJ, Pessa JE. The fat compartments of the face: Anatomy and clinical implications for cosmetic surgery. Plast Reconstr Surg 2007;119:2219–2231.
10. Sandoval SE, Cox JA, Koshy JC, Hatef DA, Hollier LH. Facial fat compartments: A guide for filler placement. Semin Plast Surg 2009;23:283–287.
11. Ozdemir R, Kilinç H, Unlü RE, Uysal AC, Sensöz O, Baran CN. Anatomico-histologic study of the retaining ligaments of the face and use in face lift: Retaining ligament correction and SMAS plication. Plast Reconstr Surg 2002;110:1134–1149.
12. Russo PR, Fundarò PS. Florence: The Invisible Lifting. Florence: OEO, 2014:109–157.
13. Haddock NT, Saadeh PB, Boutros S, Thorne CH. The tear trough and lid-cheek junction: Anatomy and implications for surgical correction. Plast Reconstr Surg 2009;123:1332–1342.
14. Salti G, Rauso R. Facial rejuvenation with fillers: The dual plane technique. J Cutan Aesthet Surg 2015;8:127–133.
15. Payne Dessinioti CMER, Verner I. Fillers and soft tissue augmentation. In: Katsambas AD, Lotti TM, C, D'Erme AM (eds). European Handbook of Dermatological Treatments. Berlin: Springer, 2015.
16. Paixão P, Conheço M. A anatomia labial? Implicações para o bom preenchimento. Surg Cosmet Dermatol 2015;7:10–15.
17. Pessa JE, Rohrich RJ. Topografia facial—Anatomia clínica da face. Rio de Janeiro: Editora Dilivros, 2014.
18. Radlanski RJ, Wesker KH. The Face—Pictorial Atlas of Clinical Anatomy, ed 2. Berlin: Quintessence, 2016.
19. Palermo EC. Anatomy of the periorbital region. Surg Cosmet Dermatol 2013;5:245–256.
20. Warren RJ. Cirurgia plástica estética, vol 2. Centro, Brazil: Editora Elsevier, 2015.
21. Tamura BM. Facial anatomy and the application of fillers and botulinum toxin—Part II. Surg Cosmet Dermatol 2010;2:291–303.
22. Filho LA, Cândido PL, Larosa PRR, Cardoso AC. Anatomia topográfica da cabeça e do pescoço. São Paulo: Editora Manole Ltda, 2005
23. Madeira MC. Anatomia da face—Bases anatomo-funcionais para prática odontológica. São Paulo: Editora Sarvier, 2013.

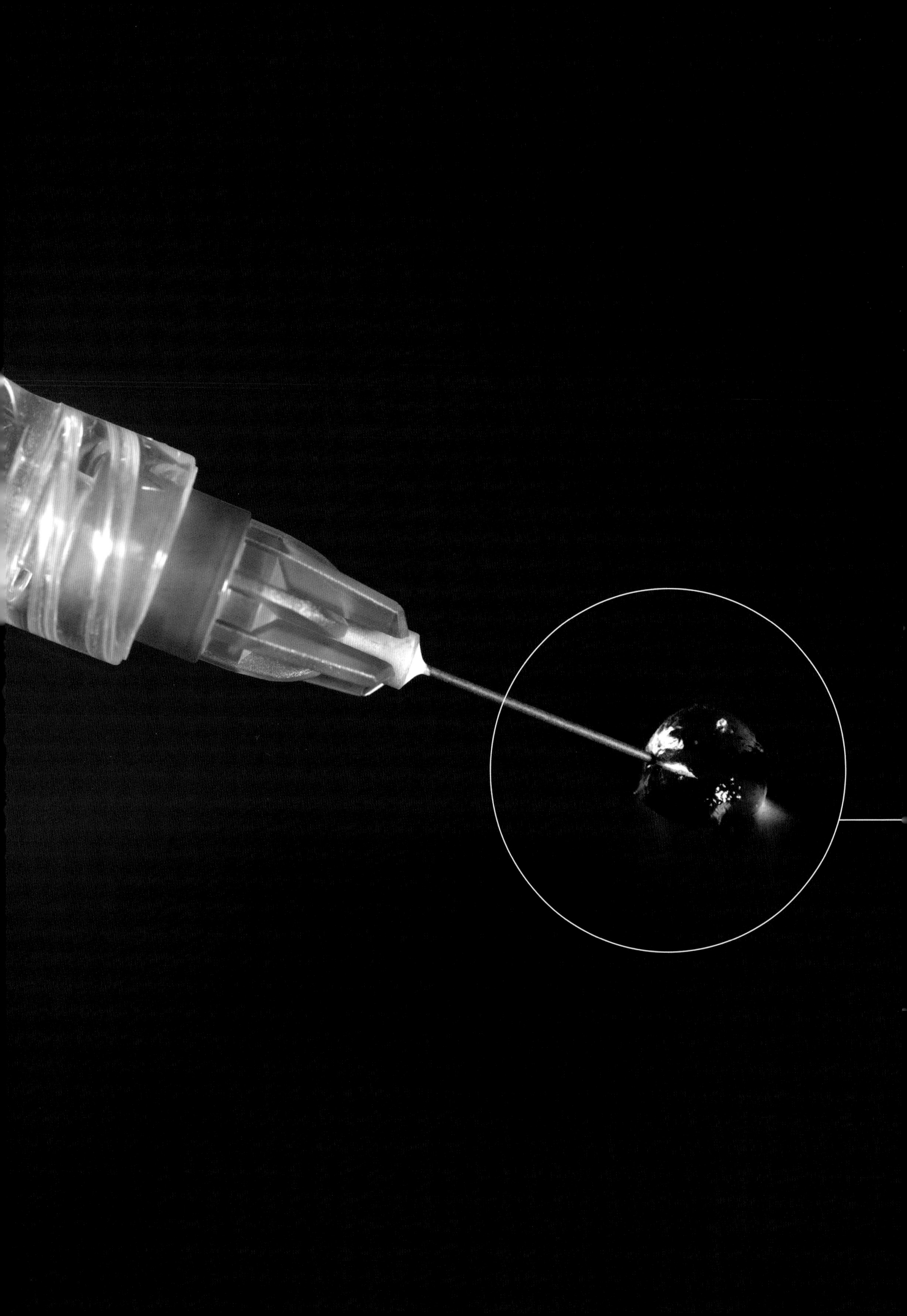

CHAPTER

02

History, Classification, and Characteristics of Fillers

02

History of Fillers

The development of biocompatible and safe fillers required many years of study and research. Table 2-1 illustrates the historical evolution of fillers. With the development of local anesthesia and surgical techniques toward the end of the 19th century, more invasive cosmetic procedures became available, including soft tissue fillers. Fat was one of the first soft tissue fillers to be used after trauma and is still widely used today. However, autologous fat transplantation is considered a relatively major procedure, as it requires the transplantation of fat from another site, and its results may be variable. Prior to the introduction of autologous fat grafting, paraffin oil had been used for the restoration of volume and symmetry. However, its use was accompanied by a high incidence of inflammatory foreign body granulomatous nodules (paraffinomas), with consequent facial distortion and occasionally life-threatening pulmonary emboli. Hence, the use of paraffin oil was discontinued.[3]

In the mid-20th century, a shift was seen toward purified synthetic polymers in the form of injectable silicone. Although seemingly promising at first, the US Food and Drug Administration (FDA) eventually banned this material because of its similar complications of granuloma formation.[8] However, microdroplet injection of limited amounts of silicone material is still used today as an off-label use for silicone that is FDA approved for ocular injections.[9–11] Teflon, a synthetic polytetrafluoroethylene polymer, was next tested as a soft tissue filler, but it was quickly abandoned because of the resultant inflammatory reaction and the difficulty of injection.[12]

The first facial filler to receive FDA approval was bovine collagen, under the trade name Zyderm (Inamed, now Allergan), in 1981. The approval of Zyderm led to widespread research and development of other fillers, including alloplastic and implantable materials, as well as a renewed interest in and use of autologous fat.[13] Despite this added research, bovine collagen remained the only FDA-approved filler until 2003, when the FDA approved the first hyaluronic acid (HA) dermal

Table 2-1 History of facial fillers

YEAR	FILLER	DESCRIPTION
1863	Paraffin	Used during and after the Civil War. Complications included migration, foreign body granuloma, and pulmonary embolism.[1,2]
1923	Autologous fat	Used to fill volumes after trauma or to treat diseases such as lipoatrophy, scars, lipodystrophy (aging), and gluteal augmentation.[1,2]
1950	Silicone	At first, the same silicone used to manufacture flexible catheters to correct urethral strictures was employed as a filler.[1,2]
1961	Liquid silicone	Liquid injectable silicone used for breast augmentation and facial surgeries. It was banned by the US Food and Drug Administration (FDA).[3]
1962	Polydimethylsiloxane (PDMS)	Pasty, noninjectable silicone for industrial use. Because it is an alloplastic material, it tends to be encapsulated.[1,2]
1981	Bovine collagen	The first agent to be approved by the FDA for cosmetic injection. Because it caused allergies, an allergy test was necessary before injection into the patient. In addition, its effect was short.[1,2]
1989	Polymethyl methacrylate (PMMA)	Nonresorbable and provides a permanent result.[4]
2003	Hyaluronic acid (HA)	First HA dermal filler to be approved by the FDA (Restylane, Galderma).[5] It is the most popular dermal filler.[4]
2003	Calcium hydroxyapatite (CaHA)	Semisolid, cohesive subdermal product; its main component is the synthetic CaHA.[6]
2004	Poly-L-lactic acid (PLLA)	Biodegradable and bioresorbable polymer used in areas of high loss of tissue volume; not suitable for filling individual wrinkles.[7]

Table 2-2 **Injectable fillers listed by date of FDA approval**

YEAR OF FDA APPROVAL	TRADE NAME (MANUFACTURER)	DESCRIPTION
1981	Zyderm 1 (Inamed/Allergan)	Bovine collagen (35 mg/mL)
1983	Zyderm 2 (Inamed/Allergan)	Bovine collagen (65 mg/mL)
1985	Zyplast (Inamed/Allergan)	Bovine collagen (35-mg/mL collagen crosslinked with glutaraldehyde)
2003	Cosmoderm (Inamed/Allergan)	Human collagen
	Cosmoplast (Inamed/Allergan)	Human collagen
	Restylane (Galderma)	HA
2004	Hylaform (Inamed/Allergan)	Animal-derived HA
	Captique (Genzyme)	Non–animal-derived HA
	Sculptra (Valeant)	PLLA
2005	Cosmoderm 2 (Inamed/Allergan)	Human collagen
2006	**Juvéderm Ultra** (Allergan)	Non–animal-derived HA
	Juvéderm Ultra Plus (Allergan)	Non–animal-derived HA
	Artefill (Suneva Medical)	PMMA
	Radiesse (Merz)	CaHA
2007	**Perlane** (Medicis)	Non–animal-derived HA
	Elevess (Anika)	Non–animal-derived HA
2008	Prevelle Silk (Mentor)	Non–animal-derived HA
	Evolence (ColBar LifeScience)	Porcine collagen
2009	Hydrelle (formerly Elevess) (Anika)	Non–animal-derived HA
	Sculptra Aesthetic (Valeant)	PLLA
2010	**Juvéderm XC** (Allergan)	Non–animal-derived HA with lidocaine
	Restylane-L (Galderma)	Non–animal-derived HA with lidocaine
	Perlane-L (Medicis)	Non–animal-derived HA with lidocaine
2011	**Belotero** (Merz)	Non–animal-derived HA
	LaViv (Fibrocell)	Autologous fibroblasts
2013	**Juvéderm Voluma-XC** (Allergan)	Non–animal-derived HA with lidocaine
2017	**Juvéderm Vollure-XC** (Allergan)	Non–animal-derived HA

Products in **boldface** are currently available. The FDA is aware that unapproved versions of Juvéderm, such as Juvéderm Ultra 2, 3, and 4, are being sold and distributed in the US, including by online retailers.
(Data from Kontis.[8])

Box 2-1 **FDA-approved indications for dermal fillers**

- Mid to deep dermis to treat facial wrinkles and folds
- Perioral rhytids
- Dorsum of the hands
- Lips for lip augmentation
- Contour deficiencies
- Acne scars

filler, under the trade name Restylane (Galderma), for temporary soft tissue augmentation.[14] Since then, numerous fillers have received FDA approval in response to the growing popularity of minimally invasive facial rejuvenation procedures[5] (Table 2-2 and Box 2-1). Further investigations and research have continued, and more long-lasting synthetic fillers have become available, including calcium hydroxyapatite (CaHA) and poly-L-lactic acid (PLLA).[15]

Classification of Fillers

Dermal fillers can be classified according to their material properties, biodegradability, and duration of effect:

Material properties

- Autologous: Derived from the same individual (eg, autologous fibroblasts)
- Heterologous: Derived from a different species (eg, bovine collagen)
- Alloplastic: Nonbiologic material such as metal, ceramic, or plastic (eg, polymethyl methacrylate [PMMA])

Biodegradability

- Biodegradable: Capable of being broken down, especially into innocuous products (eg, HA, PLLA)
- Nonbiodegradable: Substance or chemical that cannot be changed to a natural state (eg, PMMA)

Duration of effect

- Temporary: Effective for less than 6 months (eg, collagen)
- Long-lasting: Effective for 6 to 24 months (eg, HA [12–24 months], CaHA [18–24 months])
- Semipermanent: Effective for 2 to 5 years (eg, PLLA [2–3 years])
- Permanent: Nonfading results (eg, PMMA)

HA is a naturally occurring polysaccharide found in the skin dermis, umbilical cord, synovial joint fluid, hyaline cartilage, and connective tissues. Because it is biodegradable, biocompatible, and nonimmunogenic, it is an ideal filling agent.[8]

Characteristics of Fillers

Fillers are materials used to add volume to soft tissues. Characteristics of an ideal soft tissue filler include the following[16,17]:

- Adds volume
- Easy to use, giving an opportunity to shape the tissues
- Has reversible results
- Durable and good duration of effect
- Safe to use, giving satisfaction to the patient and the physician
- Has a natural effect
- Does not cause the patient discomfort
- Requires no time for recovery
- Predictable
- Does not cause allergic reactions or irritation

The two most important characteristics for any soft tissue filler are its viscoelasticity and cohesivity.[18] *Viscoelasticity* describes the hardness or softness of a gel and is defined by its elasticity (elastic modulus, G')—that is, how the filler is able to retain its shape when a force is applied—and its viscosity (viscous modulus, G")—that is, how the filler resists gradual deformation by shear stress. These accumulated values identify the viscoelastic modulus (G*). The higher the G*, the higher the resistance to deformation and the greater capacity to keep its shape and, hence, a major lifting effect. *Cohesivity* describes the property of the gel to stick together when an external force is applied. Gels with higher cohesivity tend to uniformly infiltrate the tissues and are not fractionated by movements.[17]

For reasons of cost and patient comfort, a filler should also have good durability. However, it is known that facial topography changes over time; therefore, the use of permanent fillers will result in an unnatural facial appearance because the filler will not undergo changes in contrast to the surrounding tissues.[16]

> It is important to understand that soft tissue fillers work using two main mechanisms: The filler material occupies space in the tissue and stimulates fibroblasts to synthesize collagen, resulting in tissue volume.[19]

Table 2-3 lists the characteristics of currently available dermal fillers.[20–22]

Table 2-3 **Characteristics of currently available dermal fillers**

AGENT	CONTENTS	MECHANISM OF ACTION	INDICATIONS
Restylane Lyft with lidocaine (1,4-BDDE*)	HA chemically crosslinked with BDDE and formulated to a concentration of 20 mg/mL and suspended in a physiologic buffer at a pH of 7.0. The largest fraction of gel particles are 940–1090 μm in size.	Adds natural volume as it integrates into the deep dermal tissue or subcutis, then attracts and binds water molecules to help maintain volume.	Implantation into the deep dermis to the superficial subcutis for correction of moderate to severe facial folds and wrinkles, such as nasolabial folds, or in patients older than 21 years who have age-related volume loss.
Radiesse (CaHA)	Sterile, nonpyrogenic, semisolid, cohesive implant whose principal component is synthetic CaHA suspended in a gel carrier of sterile water for injection, glycerin, and sodium carboxymethylcellulose. Radiesse (1.5 mL, 0.8 mL) has a CaHA particle size range of 25–45 μm and should be injected with a 25G to 27G needle.	Stimulates formation of new collagen (collagenesis) in the skin, adding volume over time.	Subdermal implantation for restoration or correction of signs of facial fat loss (lipoatrophy) in people with HIV infection. Also for subdermal implantation for correction of moderate to severe facial wrinkles and folds, such as nasolabial folds.
Restylane and Restylane-L (HA)	Medium-sized particles of stabilized HA generated by streptococcal bacteria and formulated to a concentration of 20 mg/mL and suspended in a physiologic buffer at a pH of 7.0.	It adds natural volume as it integrates into the dermal tissue, then attracts and binds water molecules to help maintain volume.	Mid to deep dermal implantation for correction of moderate to severe facial wrinkles and folds, such as nasolabial folds; submucosal implantation for lip augmentation in patients older than 21 years.
Sculptra (PLLA)	Synthetic, biodegradable, biocompatible, immunologically inert polymer from the alphahydroxy-acid family. Must be reconstituted with at least 3–5 mL of sterile water for injection, and must stand for at least 2 hours to ensure hydration prior to treatment.	Particles of PLLA stimulate the formation of new collagen (collagen neosynthesis) in the skin, adding volume over time.	Intended for the restoration and/or correction of the signs of facial fat loss (lipoatrophy) in people with HIV infection; in immunocompetent people, it is used as a single regimen for correction of shallow to deep nasolabial fold contour deficiencies and other facial wrinkles for which a deep dermal grid pattern (crosshatch) injection technique is appropriate.
Bellafill (previously Artefill; PMMA)	Composed of PMMA microspheres (diameter 30–50 μm) suspended in a water-based gel carrier containing 3.5% purified bovine collagen, 92.6% buffered isotonic water for injection, 0.3% lidocaine hydrochloride, 2.7% phosphate buffer, and 0.9% sodium chloride.	Microspheres provide permanent volume for wrinkle correction.	FDA approved for correction of nasolabial folds. Lip volumizing contraindicated.
Serial microdroplet silicone (SMDS; liquid silicone)	Synthetic polymer of dimethylsiloxane	It elicits a fibrosis-granuloma tissue response with new collagen formatting around the injected silicone, such that tiny collagen pearls develop around each microdroplet.	Liquid injectable silicone (LIS) has been utilized for soft tissue augmentation for more than five decades. Currently, only two LIS products (AdatoSil and Silikon 1000) are FDA approved and only for the treatment of retinal detachment. Therefore, any cosmetic injection of these products is off-label.

*BDDE = 1,4-butanediol diglycidyl ether, the crosslinking agent used in the majority of the market-leading HA fillers.

INJECTION	DURATION	LIMITS
Supplied in 1-mL glass syringes for injection; injected into the mid to deep dermis.	Approximately 6–12 months.	20 mL/60 kg (130 lb) body mass per year.
Supplied as a 1.5-mL or 0.8-mL syringe. Insert the needle with the bevel down at approximately a 30-degree angle to the skin; the needle should slide under the dermis to the point where the injection should begin. Advance the needle into the subdermis to the starting location; slowly inject the material in linear threads, while withdrawing the needle, until the desired level of correction is achieved.	Approximately 1 year, although the gel carrier is lost by 6 months, causing depreciation of initial gain.	Amount injected varies depending on the site and extent of restoration or augmentation desired. Use a 1:1 correction factor. No overcorrection needed.
Supplied in a disposable glass syringe; each syringe contains 0.4 mL, 1 mL, or 2 mL of gel for injection into the mid dermis.	Approximately 6 months.	20 mL/60 kg (130 lb) body mass per year.
Supplied as a sterile, freeze-dried preparation for injection in a clear glass vial; to be injected into the deep dermis or subcutaneous layer.	Approximately 1 year.	Volume should be limited to approximately 0.1–0.2 mL per each individual injection; the volume of product injected per treatment area varies depending on the surface area to be treated.
Aseptic product that has an opaque, off-white appearance and is supplied in a sealed tray containing five syringes (three with 0.8 mL, two with 0.4 mL). Must be brought to room temperature prior to use. A 26G needle is used, and the best cosmetic result is achieved by moving the needle back and forth two to three times beneath each skin fold being treated, while maintaining constant pressure throughout the implantation procedure. Do not overcorrect because the result is considered permanent.	Permanent support structure for wrinkle correction.	The safety of injecting more than 3.5 mL per treatment site or 8.2 mL overall has not been established.
When used in the dermis, 0.005–0.01 mL of microdroplets of silicone are injected at 1- to 2-mm intervals along the length of a rhytid.	To achieve the desired result, a series of at least four or five sessions of injections, at 4- to 6-week intervals, is needed.	Not for use in cosmetic injections.

02

Hyaluronic Acid

The techniques and clinical cases described in this book use HA fillers because of their practicality and biosafety. HA is a natural polymer biologically synthesized by cells in the body via an enzymatic process. It is produced and secreted by cells including fibroblasts, keratinocytes, and chondrocytes.[23] It has a linear structure, composed of fragments of polysaccharides of D-glucuronic acid and N-acetyl-D-glucosamine arranged alternately.

HA was first discovered in the vitreous humor of the eye in 1934 and subsequently synthesized in vitro in 1964. It is one of the major elements in the extracellular matrix (ECM) of vertebrate tissues, including the connective tissue (eg, dermis), synovial fluid, vitreous and aqueous humor of the eyeball, umbilical cord, and hyaline cartilage.[24–27] It shows no species or tissue specificity, in contrast to collagen.[7]

The HA biopolymer functions as a scaffold binding other matrix molecules[3] and is involved in several important biologic functions:

- *Regulation of cell adhesion and motility:* Several cell surface receptors such as CD44, RHAMM, and ICAM-1 have been shown to interact with HA, influencing cellular processes including morphogenesis, wound repair, inflammation, and metastasis.[28,29]
- *Manipulation of cell differentiation and proliferation:* See previous point.
- *Provision of mechanical properties to tissues*[17]*:* Viscoelasticity of synovial fluid and vitreous humor of the eye and control of tissue hydration and water transport.[30]
- *Stimulation of gene expression in macrophages, endothelial cells, eosinophils, and certain epithelial cells:* Wound healing and scar formation.[31]
- *Activation or suppression of inflammation (repair process after damage):* Cell infiltration and proliferation of proinflammatory cytokines.[31,32]

The degradation byproducts of HA seem to have properties that actively affect wound healing and cellular kinetics.[33] In addition, HA has been found during embryonic development in the umbilical cord, suggesting that materials composed of HA may persuade favorable conditions for tissue regeneration and growth.[34,35]

As mentioned above, HA performs several structural tasks in the ECM as it binds with cells and other biologic components through specific and nonspecific interactions. Several ECM proteins are stabilized upon binding to HA. Specific molecules and receptors that interact with HA are involved in cellular signal transduction. Molecules such as aggrecan, versican, and neurocan and receptors including CD44 (cell surface glycoprotein), RHAMM (receptor for HA-mediated motility), TSG6 (35-kDa glycoprotein with a link module in the N-terminus), GHAP (glial hyaluronate-binding protein), ICAM-1 (intracellular adhesion molecule-1) and LYVE-1 (lymphatic vessel endothelial HA receptor) are examples of cell components that bind to HA.[30] New receptors for HA have been identified recently, and the functions of some HA receptors have also been recently described. RHAMM, for example, has been found on cell surfaces as well as in the cytosol and nucleus. It regulates cellular responses to growth factors and plays a role in cell migration, particularly for fibroblasts and smooth cells.[30,36,37]

Hyaluronic acid as a filler

HAs work well as fillers because of their low potential for allergic reactions, their consistency across species, and their viscoelastic and hygroscopic (swelling by the absorption of water) properties (Box 2-2). Some early HA fillers were derived from rooster combs; however, residual avian proteins caused allergic reactions in some patients.[8] Non–animal-derived stabilized HAs were developed by the fermentation of *Streptococcus equi* bacterium and are currently the only class of HA fillers used today for cosmetic purposes.[38]

HA fillers can differ from one another by their degree of crosslinking, gel consistency properties, and concentration. Crosslinking is required to stabilize the HA and prevent degradation when injected into the skin. The degree of crosslinking determines the durability and biocompatibility of the formulation. In addition, HAs can be classified as either monophasic or biphasic gels.[39] Biphasic gels such as Restylane and Perlane (Medicis) are particles of crosslinked HA suspended in a liquid. They differ by particle size: Restylane particles are roughly 250 μm in diameter, while Perlane particles are about 550 μm in diameter, with concentrations of 100,000 particles/mL and

Box 2-2 Properties of hyaluronic acid

- Low allergenicity
- Crosslinking provides stability
- Effective
- Viscoelastic
- Consistent across species
- Hygroscopic
- Biocompatible
- Good safety profile

Box 2-3 Adverse events related to HA fillers

- Bruising
- Swelling
- Tenderness
- Redness
- Pain
- Itching

8,000–10,000 particles/mL, respectively. Monophasic gels such as Juvéderm Ultra and Juvéderm Ultra Plus (Allergan) are crosslinked in one process (Hylacross technology, Allergan), producing an entirely stabilized smooth gel without particles. Belotero (Merz) is also a monophasic gel crosslinked by cohesive polydensified matrix technology, which produces increased elastic and viscous properties.[39]

HAs have a high molecular weight (50 kDa) and connect a large amount of water (one molecule is able to join a weight 1,000 times larger than itself). The content of HA in the skin decreases with age, leading to its dehydration and wrinkle occurrence. Due to the stabilizing, hydrating, and cushioning properties and high biocompatibility of HA, it is an ideal material for soft tissue filling.[40]

The concentration of the gel is reduced during its resorption, but the volume remains high until the last molecules of HA are subject to degradation. Depending on the concentration and crosslinking, HA fillers can be applied to the superficial layers of the dermis, the middle layers of the dermis, the lower layers of the dermis, and subcutaneously.[19]

Since their introduction in 2003, HA fillers have been shown to have excellent effectiveness and acceptable safety profiles. They have been used on-label to improve the nasolabial folds and lips as well as off-label to correct lines and wrinkles and to volumize the aging face.[8] They have been found to provide a longer-lasting improvement over both collagen-based products and animal-derived HA. Safety was reviewed from worldwide data of 144,000 patients treated with HA (Restylane and Perlane) in 1999 and 262,000 patients treated in 2000.[41]

In regard to total adverse events, they decreased from 0.15% to 0.06% after the introduction of a more purified HA raw material. The most common adverse event is a hypersensitivity reaction, seen in 1 of every 5,000 patients treated. Temporary events include redness, swelling, localized granulomas, and bacterial infections[21] (Box 2-3).

As the most widely used filler substance currently on the market, HA has a number of advantages over its predecessors. Crosslinked HA fillers have been used for longer than 15 years and are considered to be generally well tolerated. They have structural properties similar to those of native tissue, excellent biocompatibility, and good tissue integration. They have a tunable duration of action spanning the entire range of the temporary filler category (6–24 months), and because of

Table 2-4 Indications for HA fillers based on consistency

FILLER	INDICATION	CONSISTENCY
Restylane Volyme	Loss of malar, mentum, or mandibular volume	High
Restylane Defyne	General volume loss and deep creases	
Restylane Kysse	Lip shape and texture	
Restylane Refyne	Moderate wrinkles like marionette lines	
Restylane Fynesse	Fine wrinkles like perioral rhytids	
Restylane Skinbooster	Deep moisturizing of the skin	Low

their relatively stable molecular composition, they can be stored without refrigeration for up to 2 years. Because of the hydrophilic nature of HA, these fillers also serve to hydrate the skin, and uniquely among other filler substances, HA can be reversed using hyaluronidase. In most commercial products, HA is crosslinked to increase its longevity, and the crosslinking agent used has an important effect on the properties of the final product; 1,4-butanediol diglycidyl ether (BDDE) is the crosslinking agent used in the majority of the market-leading HA fillers, and its stability, biodegradability, and long safety record spanning more than 15 years are what make it the industry standard, ahead of other crosslinkers such as divinyl sulfone and 2,7,8-diepoxyoctane.[21]

Table 2-4 illustrates the indications for HA fillers based on consistency.

References

1. Kontis TC, Rivkin A. The history of injectable facial fillers. Facial Plast Surg 2009;25:67–72.
2. Chacon AH. Fillers in dermatology: From past to present. Cutis 2015;96:E17–E19.
3. Payne Dessinioti CMER, Verner I. Fillers and soft tissue augmentation. In: Katsambas AD, Lotti TM, C, D'Erme AM (eds). European Handbook of Dermatological Treatments. Berlin: Springer, 2015.
4. Chuang J, Barners C, Wong BJF. Overview of facial plastic surgery and current developments. Surg J (N Y) 2016;2:e17–e28.
5. Attenello NH, Maas CS. Injectable fillers: Review of material and properties. Facial Plast Surg 2015;31:29–34.
6. Jacovella PF. Use of calcium hydroxylapatite (Radiesse) for facial augmentation. Clin Interven Aging 2008;3:161–174.
7. Macierzyńska A, Pierzchała E, Placek W. Volumetric techniques: Three-dimensional midface modeling. Postepy Derm Alergol 2014;31:388–391.
8. Kontis TC. Contemporary review of injectable facial fillers. JAMA Facial Plast Surg 2013;15:58–64.
9. Benedetto AV, Lewis AT. Injecting 1000 centistoke liquid silicone with ease and precision. Dermatol Surg 2003;29:211–214.
10. Orentreich DS. Liquid injectable silicone: Techniques for soft tissue augmentation. Clin Plast Surg 2000;27:595–612.
11. Webster RC, Gaunt JM, Hamdan US, Fuleihan NS, Smith RC. Injectable silicone for facial soft-tissue augmentation. Arch Otolaryngol Head Neck Surg 1986;112:290–296.
12. Landman MD, Strahan RW, Ward PH. Chin augmentation with polytef paste injection. Arch Otolaryngol 1972;95:72–75.
13. Miller PJ, Levine J, Ahn MS, Maas CS, Constantinides M. Softform for facial rejuvenation: Historical review, operative techniques, and recent advances. Facial Plast Surg 2000;16:23–28.
14. Dermal Fillers Approved by the Center for Devices and Radiological Health. https://www.fda.gov/MedicalDevices/ProductsandMedicalProcedures/CosmeticDevices/ucm619846.htm. Updated 27 July 2015. Accessed 16 November 2015.
15. Rohrich RJ, Ghavami A, Crosby MA. The role of hyaluronic acid fillers (Restylane) in facial cosmetic surgery: Review and technical considerations. Plast Reconstr Surg 2007;120(suppl 6):S41–S54.
16. Muhn C, Rosen N, Solish N, et al. The evolving role of hyaluronic acid fillers for facial volume restoration and contouring: A Canadian overview. Clin Cosmet Investig Dermatol 2012;5:147–158.
17. Sundaram H, Cassuto D. Biophysical characteristics of hyaluronic acid soft-tissue fillers and their relevance to aesthetic applications. Plast Reconstr Surg 2013;132(suppl 2):5S–21S.

18. Carruthers J, Carruthers A. Soft Tissue Augmentation. Philadelphia: Saunders, 2013:91–94.
19. Burges CM. Principles of soft tissue augmentation for the aging face. Clin Investig Aging 2006;1:49–55.
20. Dermal fillers Medscape. http://www.med-pdf.com/82w/26210-silicone-the-queen-of-fillers.html. Accessed 4 December 2018.
21. De Boulle K, Glogau R, Kono T, et al. A review of the metabolism of 1,4-butanediol diglycidyl ether–crosslinked hyaluronic acid dermal fillers. Dermatol Surg 2013;39:1758–1766.
22. Fabbrocini G, Annunziata MC, D'Arco V, et al. Acne scars: Pathogenesis, classification and treatment. Derm Res Practice 2010;2010.
23. Fakhari A, Berkland C. Applications and emerging trends of hyaluronic acid in tissue engineering, as a dermal filler, and in osteoarthritis treatment. Acta Biomater 2013;9:7081–7092.
24. Falcone S, Palmeri D, Berg R. Biomedical applications of hyaluronic acid. ACS Symposium Series 2006;94: 155–174.
25. Zheng SX, Liu Y, Palumbo F, Luo Y, Prestwich G. In situ crosslinkable hyaluronan hydrogels for tissue engineering. Biomaterials 2004;25:1339–1348.
26. Vejlens L. Glycosaminoglycans of human bone tissue. Calcified Tissue Int 1971;7:175–190.
27. Dumitriu S. Polymeric Biomaterials. New York: Marcel Dekker, 2002.
28. Segura T, Anderson B, Chung P, Webber R, Shull K, Shea L. Crosslinked hyaluronic acid hydrogels: A strategy to functionalize and pattern. Biomaterials 2005;26:359–371.
29. Underhill C. CD44: The hyaluronan receptor. J Cell Sci 1992;103:293.
30. Necas J, Bartosikova L, Brauner P, Kolar J. Hyaluronic acid (hyaluronan): A review. Veterinarni Medicina 2008;53:397–411.
31. Brecht M, Mayer U, Schlosser E, Prehm P. Increased hyaluronate synthesis is required for fibroblast detachment and mitosis. Biochem J 1986;239:445.
32. Mian N. Analysis of cell-growth-phase-related variations in hyaluronate synthase activity of isolated plasma-membrane fractions of cultured human skin fibroblasts. Biochem J 1986;237:333.
33. Chen WYJ, Abatangelo G. Functions of hyaluronan in wound repair. Wound Rep Regen 1999;7:79–89.
34. Eng D, Caplan M, Preul M, Panitch A. Hyaluronan scaffolds: A balance between backbone functionalization and bioactivity. Acta Biomaterialia 2010;6:2407–2414.
35. Kim J, Kim I, Cho T, et al. Bone regeneration using hyaluronic acid-based hydrogel with bone morphogenic protein-2 and human mesenchymal stem cells. Biomaterials 2007;28:1830–1837.
36. Turley EA, Noble PW, Bourguignon LY. Signaling properties of hyaluronan receptors. J Biol Chem 2002;277: 4589–4592.
37. Christofori G. Changing neighbours, changing behaviour: Cell adhesion molecule-mediated signalling during tumour progression. EMBO J 2003;22:2318–2323.
38. Monheit GD, Coleman KM. Hyaluronic acid fillers. Dermatol Ther 2006;19:141–150.
39. Flynn TC, Sarazin D, Bezzola A, Terrani C, Micheels P. Comparative histology of intradermal implantation of mono and biphasic hyaluronic acid fillers. Dermatol Surg 2011;37:637–643.
40. Greco TM, Antunes MB, Yellin SA. Injectable fillers for volume replacement in the aging face. Facial Plast Surg 2012;28:8–20.
41. Friedman PM, Mafong EA, Kauvar ANB, Geronemus RG. Safety data of injectable nonanimal stabilized hyaluronic acid gel for soft tissue augmentation. Dermatol Surg 2002;28:491–494.

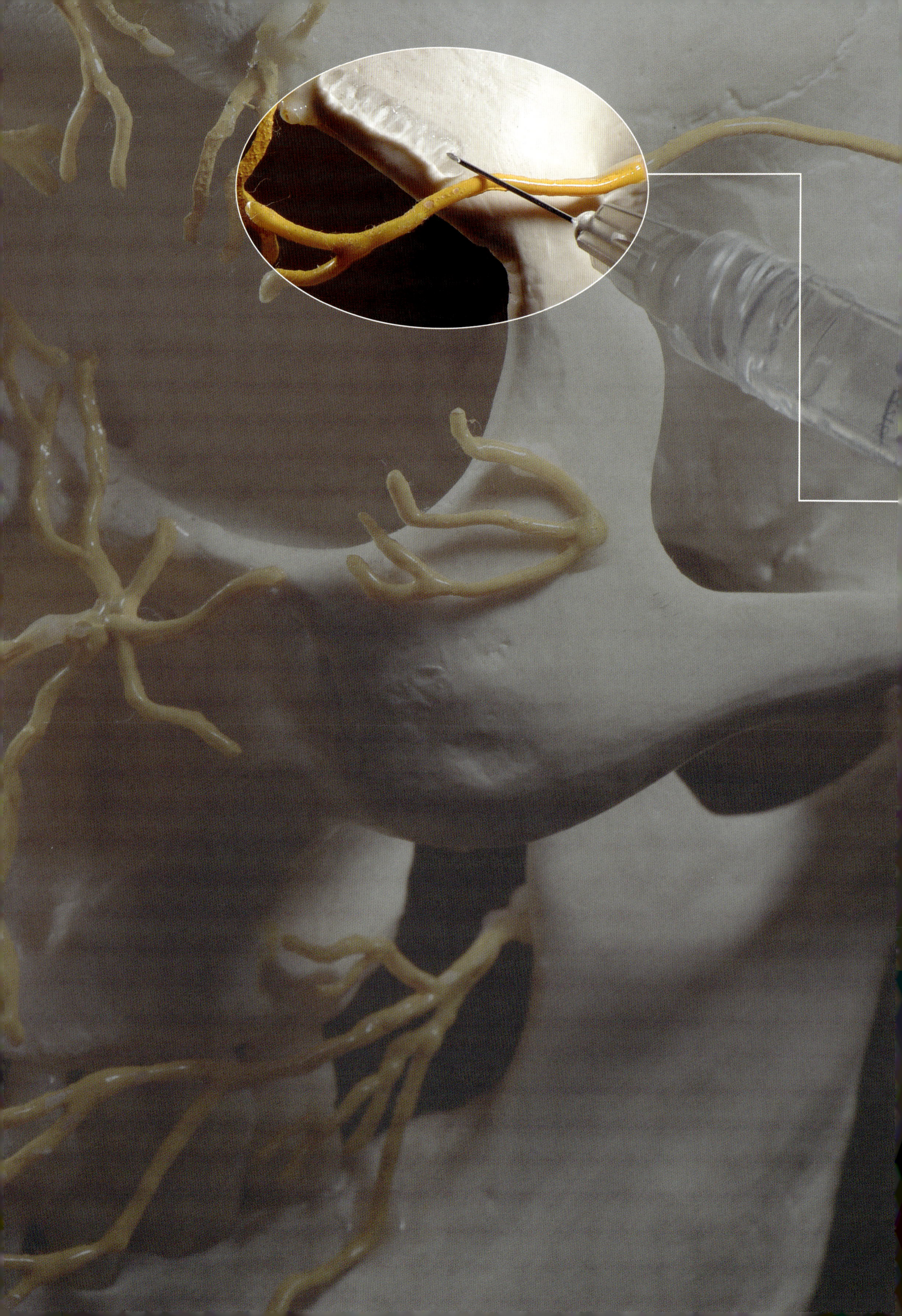

Table 3-1 Injection planes and their characteristics

CHARACTERISTIC	SUPERFICIAL FAT	DEEP FAT
Duration	Long	Short
Injected volume	Small	Large
Depth	3 mm	Bone plate
Instrument	Needle or cannula	Needle or cannula
Regions	All	Tear trough
Result	Concentrated	Diffuse
Layers to elevate	Two	Four

Planes of Injection for Fillers

While botulinum toxin should be injected intramuscularly, *fillers should not be*. The separation of muscle fibers caused by the filler injection would result in damage and inflammation. The ideal injection plane for dermal fillers is the fat area. In terms of anatomy, fat works as a natural filler, so it stands to reason that fatty areas are good sites to inject fillers.

Facial mimetic muscles do not have a fascia that separates and envelops them. Instead, a layer of fat is responsible for separating the muscles from each other and from bone. The fat located in the face also has the function of filling and smoothing the facial anatomy and is distributed into two planes: shallow and deep. The shallow plane lies just underneath the skin, while the deep plane is beneath the muscle layer. Different results can be achieved when fillers are injected into these two planes.

Injections in the deep layer of fat demand a larger amount of filler for a noticeable result in the skin of the face. This can be explained by the fact that the product physically would have to elevate the muscle layer and the skin. On the other hand, applications made in the superficial fat demand a smaller amount of the filler to obtain a similar result, because the filler has fewer layers to physically elevate (ie, only the superficial layer of fat and the skin).

Because the deep fat layer is beneath the muscle plane, injections in this area might have a shorter duration in that the repeated contraction of the muscle could flatten the enhanced volume. Therefore, *the ideal technique is to inject facial fillers in the superficial fat layer*. A notable exception is the tear trough. This is the only area in the skin that is exceptionally thin, with a tendency to make the filler too evident when deposited in this region. The solution for this undesirable effect is a deep injection of the filler, that is, at the deep fat layer between the orbital bone and the orbicularis oculi muscle. When depositing the filler under the orbicularis oculi muscle, it works as a shield to disguise the filler volume under the muscle, resulting in a natural appearance.

In order to find the correct injection plane, the clinician should take into consideration the depth required. For instance, if the plane is the superficial fat, the depth should be approximately 3 mm under the epidermis. In the deep fat, the plane of reference is the contact between the needle or cannula and the bone plane (Table 3-1). Fillers should be injected at the right depth not only to achieve the desired results but also to prevent damage to the patient. Clinicians who have not been trained in fresh cadavers might find it more difficult to perceive these planes. Figures 3-1 and 3-2 illustrate these distinct planes as well as their indications.[1,2]

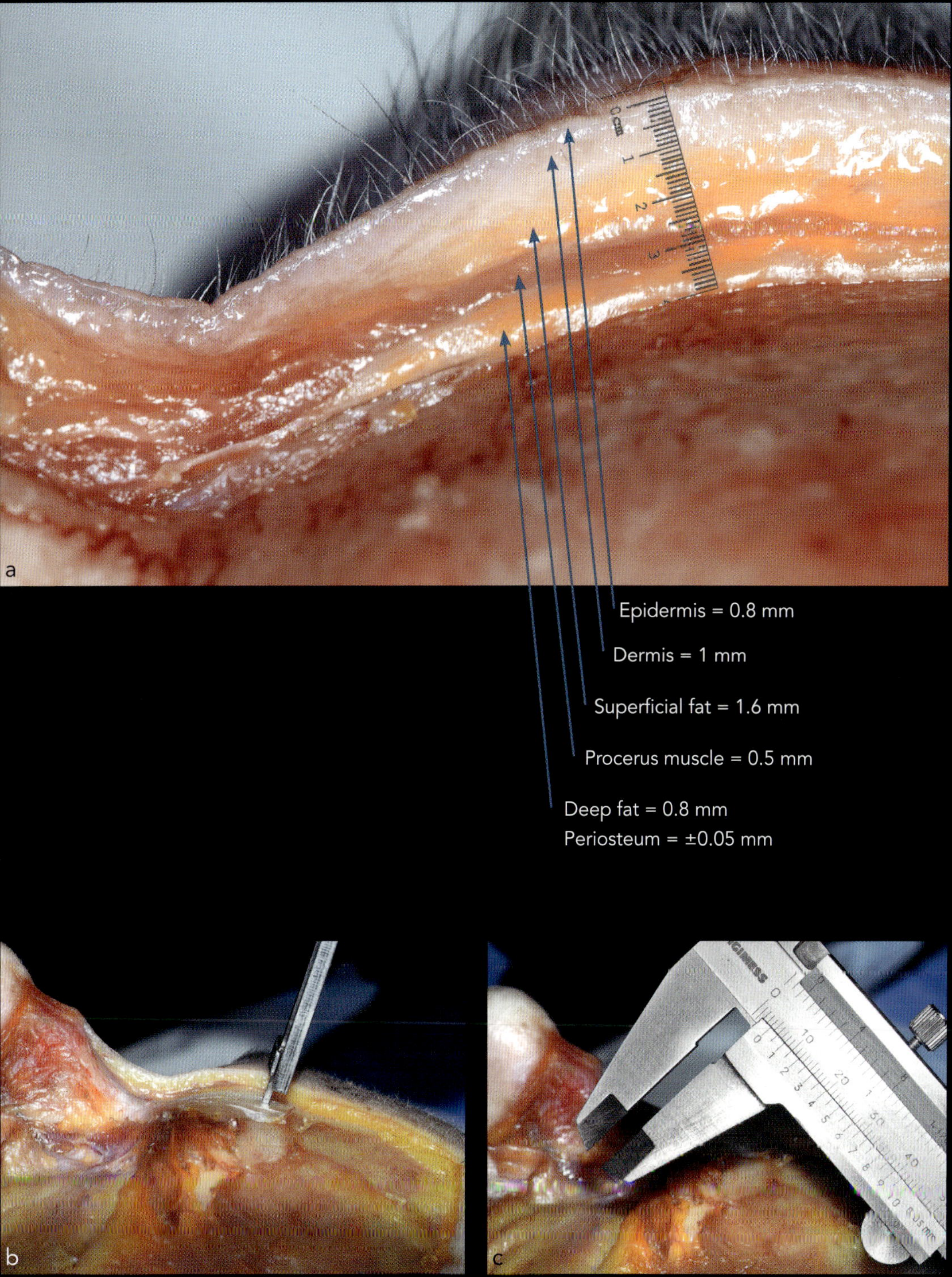

Fig 3-1 Tissue layers of the forehead. *(a)* The total thickness of the glabella is 4 mm. These measurements of thickness are different for distinct areas and individuals.[1] *(b)* A caliper being used to measure the depth. *(c)* Caliper showing the depth measurement.

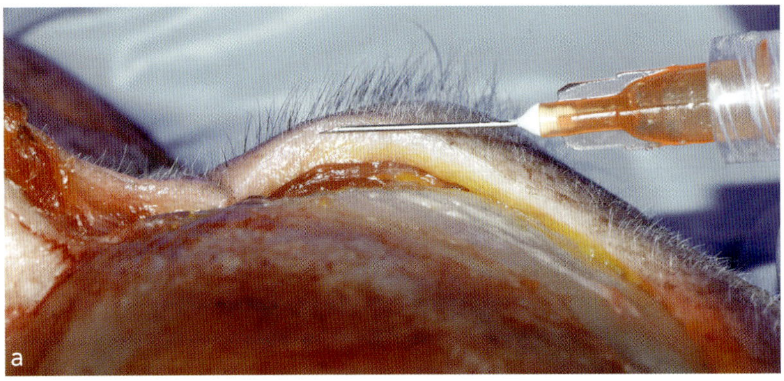

DEEP DERMAL FILLING

Purpose: It is not used for volume enhancement. Instead it is only used for subcutaneous hydration because the dermis is not expandable.

Instrument: Needle. Cannulas are not able to divulse the dermis because it is firm.

Product: Skin booster or thin fillers.

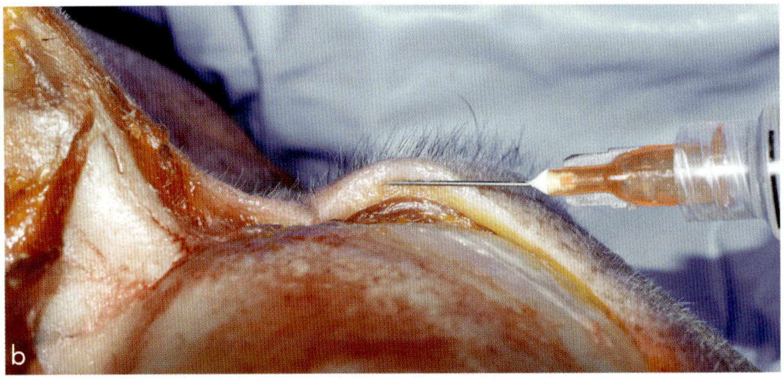

SUPERFICIAL FAT FILLING

Purpose: Volumization with or without defining the sculpt.

Instrument: Needle or cannula. Cannulas easily divulse this layer of fat.

Product: Filler of an average consistency.

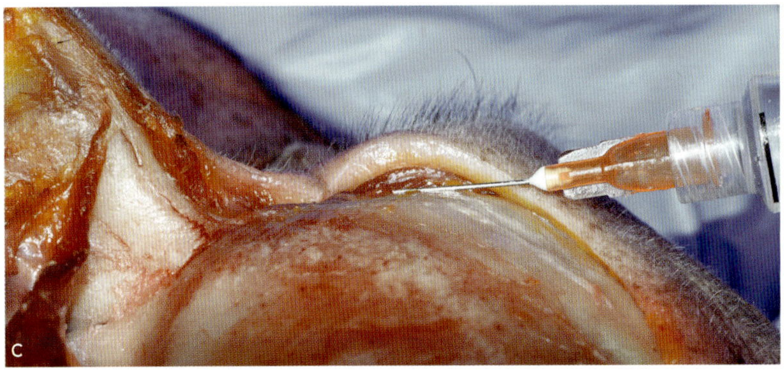

SUPRAPERIOSTEAL FILLING

Purpose: Volumization without defining the sculpt.

Instrument: Needle or cannula. Because they are blunt, cannulas slide over the periosteum, decreasing the possibility of damaging the muscles.

Product: Thick fillers.

Fig 3-2 The glabellar region of a fresh cadaver with the three possible injection planes to deposit the filler. The clinician might choose one, two (dual-plane technique involves injections in the supraperiosteal layer and the superficial fat layer),[2] or three planes in the same region in a single session. *(a)* Deep dermal filling. *(b)* Superficial fat filling. *(c)* Supraperiosteal filling.

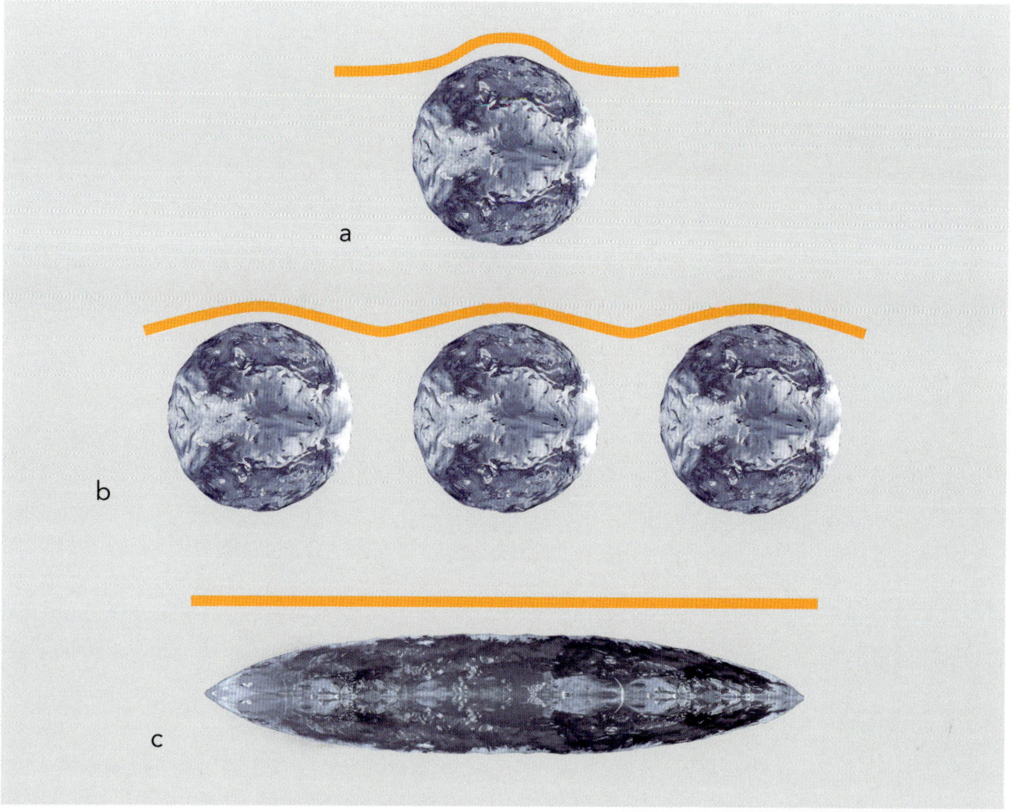

Fig 3-3 Effects of different injection techniques on the superficial anatomy of the skin: *(a)* Puncture. *(b)* Serial puncture. *(c)* Linear threading.

Injection Techniques

The different injection techniques affect the superficial anatomy of the skin in several ways (Fig 3-3):

- *Puncture:* If superficially injected, the filler causes a noticeable elevation in the skin surface. When deeply injected, it only makes the punctual flaws uniform without lifting the skin beyond surrounding areas. It is used in punctual depressions and/or to sculpt a visible volume such as the upper lip stomion, acne scars, malar region, nasolabial angle, glabella, and lateral depression of the chin region.
- *Serial puncture:* If injected superficially, the filler might cause a lump in the skin surface. Although this is an easy technique, it tends to produce irregularities, and for this reason it is not recommended. The results using this technique are poorly predictable.
- *Linear threading:* If superficially injected, the filler causes a linear elevation noticeable in the surface of the skin. When deeply injected, it only levels the depressions. Sites include the philtrum of the upper lip, eversion area of the lip vermilion, malar region, lateral depression of the chin region, marionette lines, jawline, supratip, bone structure of the orbit and zygomatic bone, infrapalpebral depression, and sulcus in general.

The techniques described in Fig 3-4 can be used with needles or cannulas. The clinician should choose the technique according to the desired final result.

Because fillers come in the form of a gel, they demand a stronger manual pressure on the plunger when using needles and cannulas. For this reason, filler syringes are like the Luer-Lok (BD Medical) type and require that the needle or cannula is strongly screwed to the tip of the syringe to avoid the extrusion of gel in the side of the hub during injection (Fig 3-5).

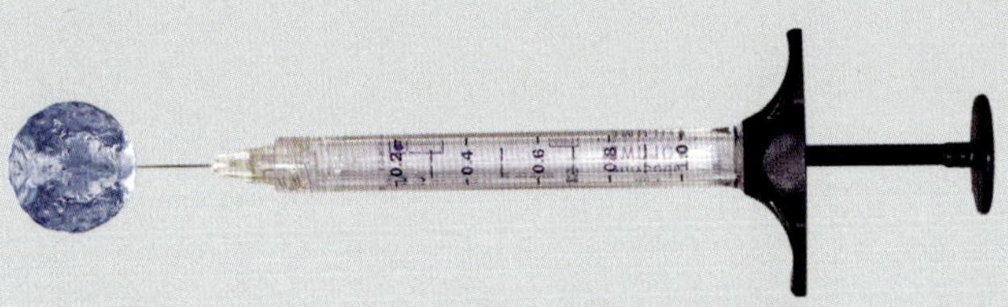

PUNCTURE

Technique:

1. Insert the needle to the desired depth.
2. Apply pressure to the plunger and keep the syringe steady.

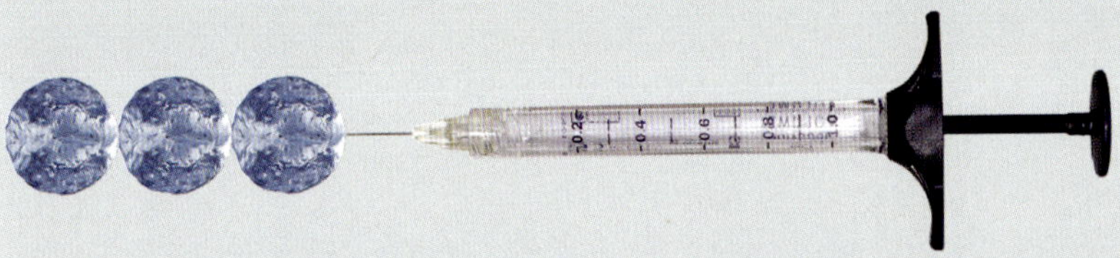

SERIAL PUNCTURE

Technique:

1. Insert the needle to the desired depth.
2. Apply pressure to the plunger and keep the syringe steady.
3. Repeat the same procedure throughout the area to be sculpted.
4. Massage the site to make the surface uniform.

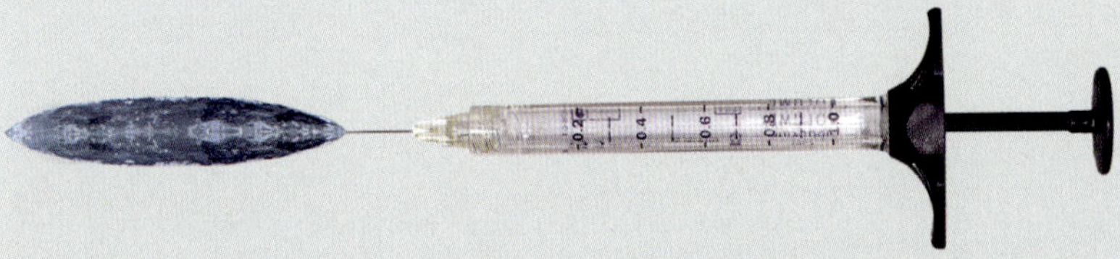

LINEAR THREADING

Technique:

1. Insert the needle to the desired depth.
2. Apply pressure to the plunger and simultaneously pull the syringe in order to make a regular thread.
3. Massage if necessary.

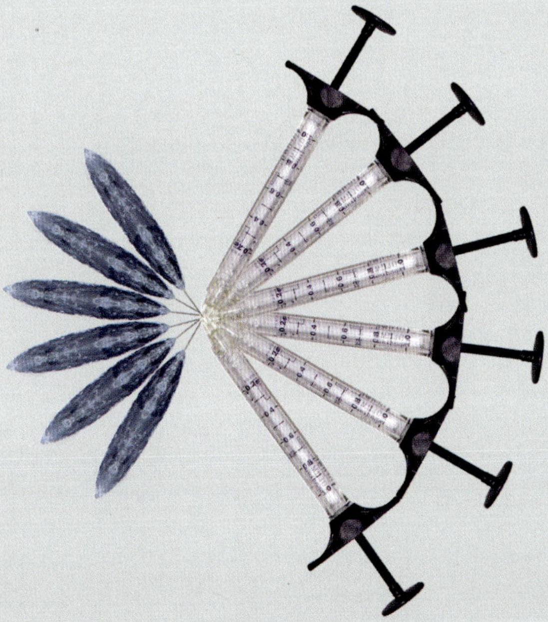

FANNING

Technique: It consists of multiple injections with a retrograde insertion using the same entrance point. The needle or cannula is not completely withdrawn between the retrograde injections.

Sites: Areas of depression (wider than the sulcus)—eg, marionette lines.

Characteristics: It produces a regular surface and natural appearance.

Fig 3-4 Different injection techniques.

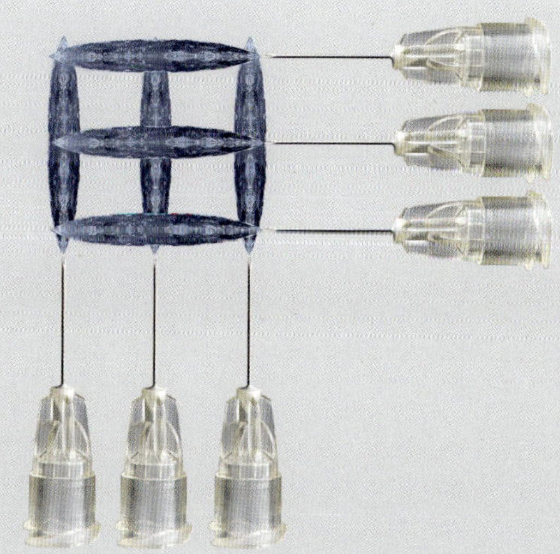

CROSSHATCHING

Technique: It consists of a series of parallel linear injections in a grid pattern.

Sites: Broad areas of the depression and/or for subcutaneous hydration—eg, side of the face.

Characteristics: It produces a regular surface and a natural appearance.

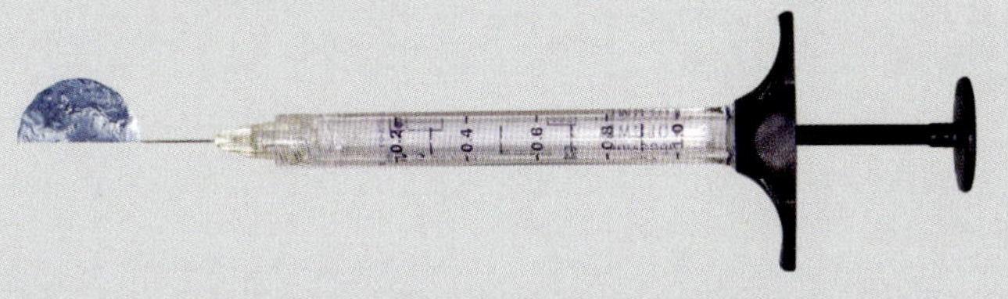

SUPRAPERIOSTEAL BOLUS

Technique: It consists of a puncture application in contact with the periosteum.

Sites: Depressions caused by bone losses and deficiencies—eg, the malar and chin region.

Characteristics: It simulates the support provided by the bone tissue to the skin.

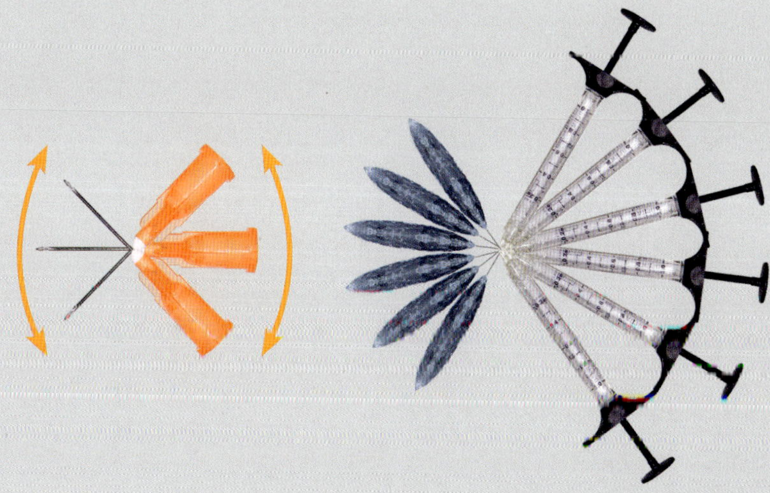

SUBCISION

Technique:

1. Using a conventional needle or Nokor needle (BD Medical), insert the needle in only one entry point following the length of the area to be filled.
2. At the same time the syringe is removed, shake it upward to remove the adherence. The undulations should not be larger than the area to be filled.
3. Deposit the filler in the same extension of the area to be filled to prevent the formation of new adhesion of the skin.

Areas: Areas of adhesion of skin—eg, scars.

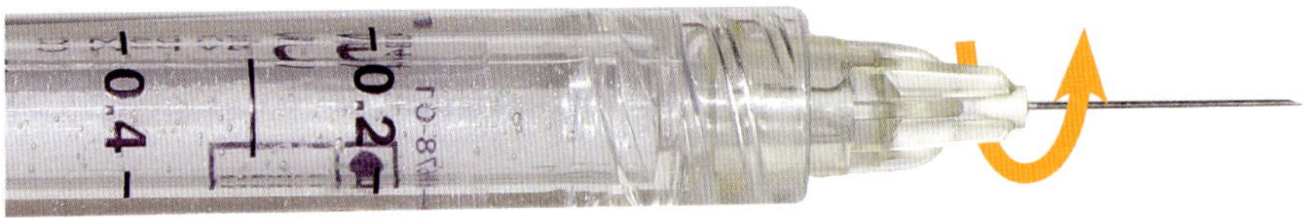

Fig 3-5 The needle or cannula must be strongly screwed to the tip of the syringe to avoid gel extrusion during injection.

Needles and Cannulas

Dermal filler syringes can be used with needles or cannulas.

Needles

The manufacturers of gel fillers provide syringes along with the needle appropriate for each type of filler (Fig 3-6). Smaller needles (around 0.3 mm) are included in the packaging for thinner fillers and bigger needles (around 0.4 mm) for thicker ones. The advantages of needles are that they are provided by the manufacturer, and self-piercing, and can be used for intradermal filling. However, because of the cutting bevel, they might puncture a blood vessel and cause embolism. Because they are short, they require a larger number of perforations to reach broader areas. They can also cause bruises, tear the skin, and traumatize the tissues.

Cannulas

Cannulas are sold separately and are not provided by the manufacturer (Fig 3-7). The clinician might choose the length according to the size of the area to be filled. The gauge can be chosen based on the filler density. The primary advantages of cannulas are that they do not cause trauma and divulse the tissue instead of cutting it, which prevents bruises and possible embolization. They are also long, thereby demanding fewer piercings, and are able to make uniform threads. They can also be curved, enabling them to adjust and be pressed against the internal surface of the skin without tearing it when the goal is a superficial filling.

Cannulas smaller than 25G are sharp and do not offer the safety profile of the other sizes. Because they are so thin, they effectively function as needles. This type of cannula might cause embolism in the vessels and result in necrosis. For this reason, 25G, 22G, and 18G cannulas are recommended. Some brands of cannulas include a needle for the entry point. The needle should have the same gauge as the cannula. Different cannula gauges are indicated by different colors (Fig 3-8).

References

1. Payne Dessinioti CMER, Verner I. Fillers and soft tissue augmentation. In: Katsambas AD, Lotti TM, C, D'Erme AM (eds). European Handbook of Dermatological Treatments. Berlin: Springer, 2015.
2. Salti G, Rauso R. Facial rejuvenation with fillers: The dual plane technique. J Cutan Aesthet Surg 2015;8: 127–133.

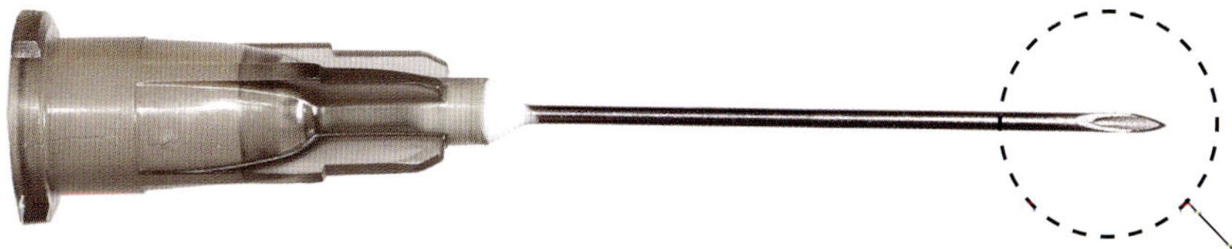

a

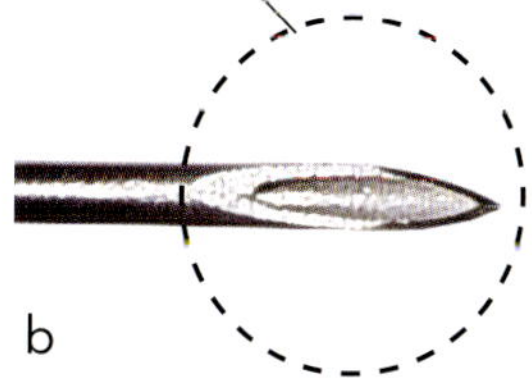

b

Fig 3-6 *(a)* Example of a needle provided by the manufacturer. The needle shown here is 13 mm long with a 0.3-mm gauge. *(b)* Magnification of the bevel.

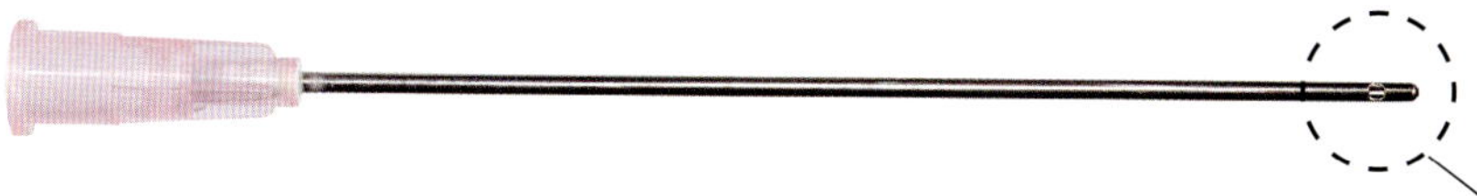

a

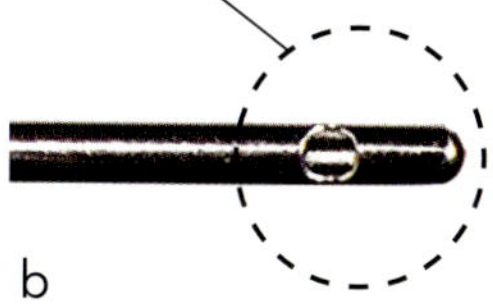

b

Fig 3-7 *(a)* Example of a cannula. The cannula shown here is 30 mm long and 18G. *(b)* Magnification of the atraumatic tip.

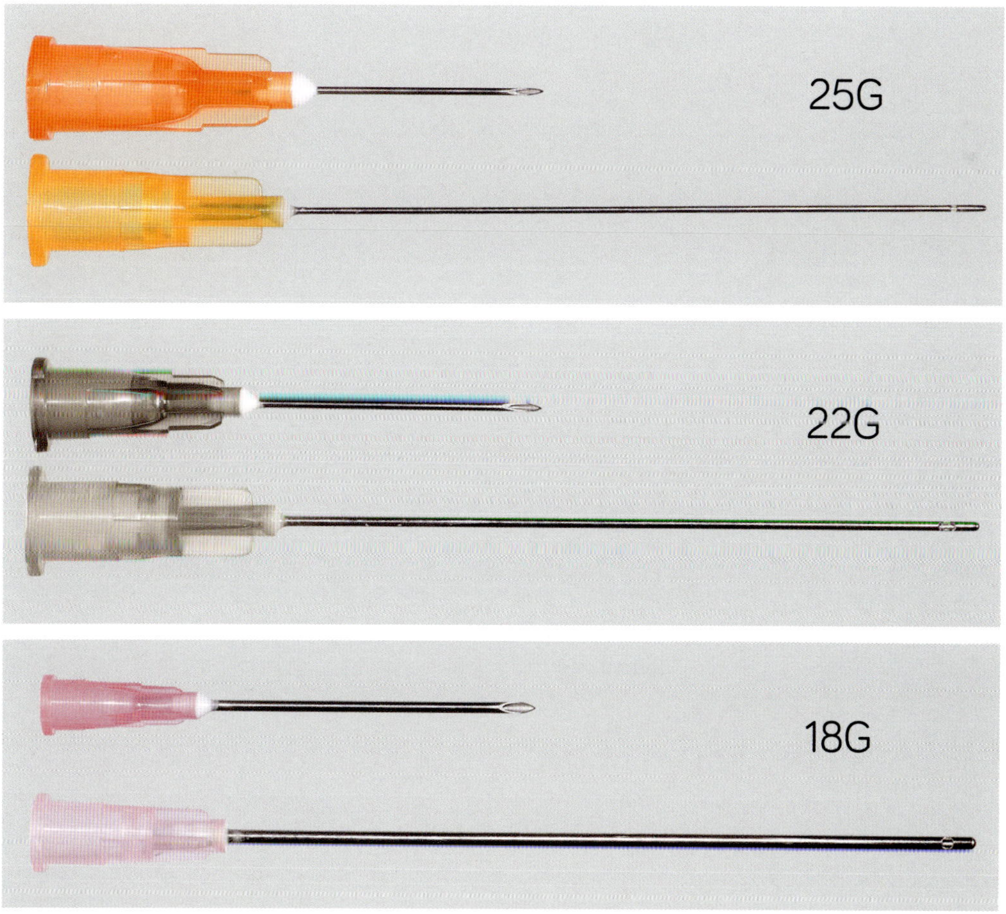

Fig 3-8 Different cannula gauges.

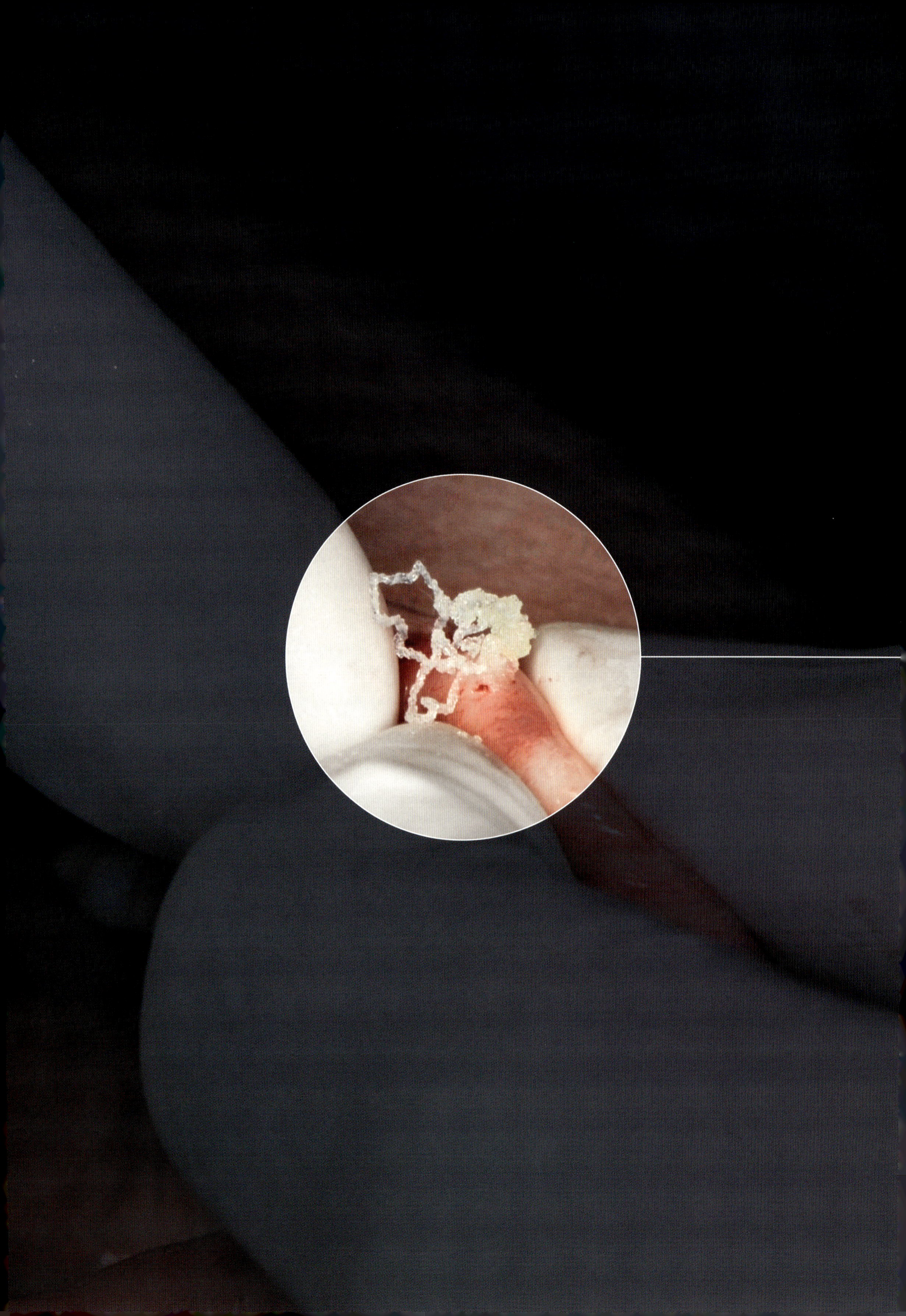

CHAPTER

04

Complications

Box 4-1 Classification of soft tissue filler complications by onset of adverse event[4]

EARLY REACTIONS	LATE REACTIONS
• Vascular infarction/soft tissue necrosis	• Infection
• Inflammatory reactions (acute/chronic)	• Granuloma (typically chronic)
• Allergic reactions/hypersensitivity	• Nodules
• Injection-related events	• Dyspigmentation
• Pain	• Displacement of hyaluronic acid filler material
• Ecchymosis	
• Erythema	
• Bruising	
• Bleeding	
• Inappropriate/superficial placement	
• Distant spread	

Dermal fillers vary in their composition, duration of effect, palpability, ease of administration, potential complications, and other factors, all of which affect the therapeutic results.[1,2] Hence, achieving desirable outcomes with dermal fillers depends critically on understanding their different characteristics, capabilities, methods of injection, risks, and limitations. In addition, there is a learning curve associated with the administration of dermal fillers; it requires practice to achieve consistently desirable results. Perhaps the most important guideline for preventing complications with dermal fillers, more so than selecting the appropriate patients, is not to treat inappropriate ones.[3]

Box 4-1 classifies soft tissue filler complications according to onset.[4] Some anatomical areas, such as the glabella, alar base, nose, and temple, are known to be associated with higher risks of vascular complications.[5–8] In addition, patient history may be a pertinent factor in the emergence of adverse reactions. Insufficient operator experience is also a contributory factor to the development of complications.[9] Clinicians should select products appropriately and practice proper techniques to minimize adverse reactions. Clinicians performing injections should have a thorough knowledge of injection-related anatomy as well as a full patient history of previous cosmetic procedures to determine whether relative or absolute contraindications exist. Specifically, the clinician should query the patient regarding previous complications with dermal fillers, significant allergy, or other significant medical conditions.

With hyaluronic acid (HA) in particular, the following guidelines will help clinicians minimize the risk of adverse reactions[4]:

- Understand the anatomy of the injection site.
- Beware of "danger" areas.
- Aspirate before injecting.
- Slowly inject with the least amount of pressure possible.
- Incrementally inject 0.1 to 0.2 mL of product.
- Use blunt microcannulas.
- Carefully consider the patient's medical history.
- Stop injecting if resistance is encountered or if the patient experiences pain/discomfort.
- Always monitor the patient.

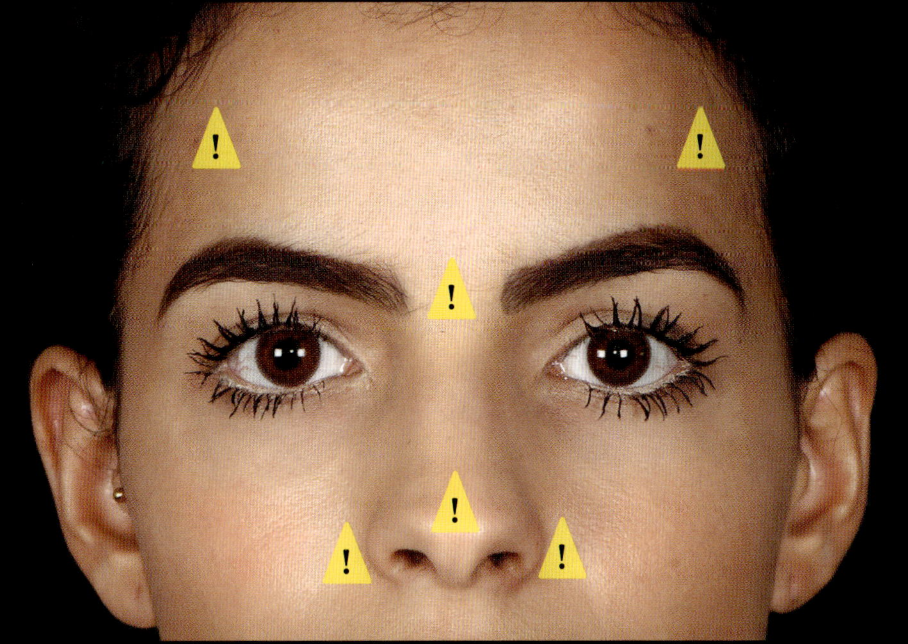

Fig 4-1 Highest areas of risk for tissue ischemia.

Vascular Obstruction and Skin Necrosis

One uncommon but potentially serious complication of HA filler injection is skin necrosis.[10] It has been proposed that ischemia may occur secondary to compression of the vasculature by extravascular filler material after the HA hydrates and expands, or through inadvertent intra-arterial HA injection or intravascular embolism[11–13] (Fig 4-1). There are also reports of skin necrosis in areas distant from the injection site, suggesting embolization after introduction of intra-arterial filler material.[11,14] One particularly ominous complication is the potential for visual impairment secondary to intra-arterial injection and obstruction of branches of the retinal or ophthalmic arteries,[15,16] which has most commonly been reported after filler injection into the glabella or nasolabial folds.[13] Similarly, the glabella and nasal ala are the injection sites most commonly associated with skin necrosis[11,15] (Fig 4-2), as these regions have limited collateral blood supply.[11] Skin necrosis generally presents with blanching and dusky discoloration, along with pain in the affected area.[10,11] Venous occlusion has also been described, presenting with the delayed onset of vague discomfort and ecchymotic-appearing lesions.[15]

Management of ischemic complications may include the promotion of vasodilation through warm compresses, 2% nitroglycerine paste, or sildenafil, as well as systemic corticosteroids, anticoagulation with aspirin or low–molecular weight heparin, and intralesional hyaluronidase injection.[13] The key to preventing the skin ischemia from progressing to necrosis is to identify and treat it as early as possible. There is no consensus on the ideal treatment in these cases, but it is important to maintain good local hygiene, use warm compresses and 2% nitroglycerine paste, and massage the area to dissolve the embolus.[17] In cases of tissue necrosis, hyaluronidase injection is recommended as soon as possible (ie, within 24 hours) to reduce damage caused by the necrosis.[11] In case of embolization, full heparin therapy might also be necessary.[18] In this context, the hyaluronidase should be given in doses ranging from 30 to 75 units in normal saline or lidocaine.[13,17]

When managing a case of intra-arterial HA injection, studies suggest that direct intravascular administration of hyaluronidase is not typically required, as hyaluronidase readily diffuses into the vascular lumen.[1,2] Therefore, hyaluronidase may be injected into the region of a suspected obstruction rather than directly into the vasculature.[19,20]

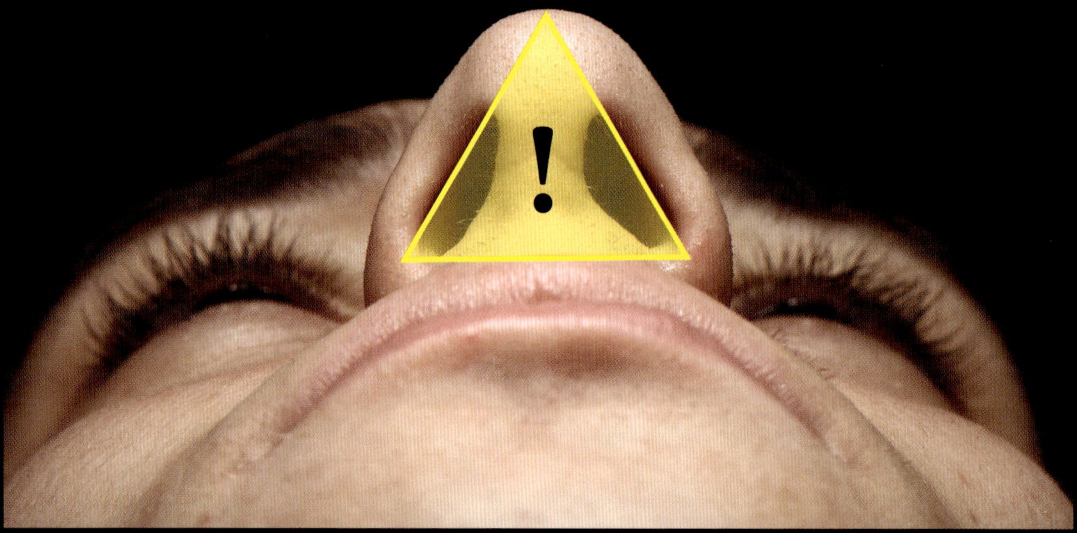

At supratip, the amount to be injected at the filament located at the midline should not exceed 0.1 mL (10% of the syringe). Lateral filaments tend to block blood supply at the midline.

A greater blood vessel compression occurs when using high-density fillers, increasing the risk of necrosis.

The use of needles at supratip increases the chance of vascular embolization and necrosis.

The amount to be injected at the region of the anterior nasal spine should not exceed 0.3 mL.

The base of the alar cartilage is located at the danger triangle of the face, described as such because of its proximity to the facial vein. Its embolization may flow back to the cavernous sinus as a result of a thrombophlebitis, which, if infected, may progress to a meningitis (through the propagation inside the intracranial venous system) and even death. On the other hand, the thrombosis may affect the central retinal vein, leading to an irreversible vision loss. Another complication that may occur at the same area is a retrograde embolism of the angular artery at the end of the nasolabial fold that presents anastomosis with the ophthalmic artery; this can result in irreversible blindness. Avoid this area.

The use of Nexcare micropore tapes or similar tapes as well as nasal decongestants are not recommended within 20 days after the surgery. Many of these products contain benzalkonium chloride (BKZ, quaternary ammonia-based disinfectants), a bactericide ineffective against spore-forming bacteria, fungi, and viruses. BKZ causes histomorphologic alterations at the cells of the nasal mucosa and decreases local immunity (reducing phagocytic activity of neutrophils). Consequently, it can increase the risk of opportunistic infections.

Nasal decongestants cause local vasoconstriction, which can lead to necrosis.

Previous rhinoplasties increase the risk of necrosis.

Fig 4-2 The delicacy of the nose's vascularization increases the potential for complications after filler injections.

Noninflamed Lesions

Excessive quantities or misplacement of HA may result in the development of subcutaneous nodules.[7,20,21] Given that HA is resorbable, uncomplicated nodules will eventually self-resolve over time.[21] However, if a nodule is painful or if the patient is bothered by its appearance, hyaluronidase can be injected to resolve the nodule.[13]

Lumps, asymmetries, or contour deformities occurring in the early posttreatment period may respond to massage. Needle aspiration or minimal stab wound incision with evacuation may be an option. A benefit of HA fillers is that irregularities can be reversed with hyaluronidase, a feature that other fillers do not share.[4,8,10,22] Products with a higher elastic modulus (G′) are not recommended in delicate areas such as the tear trough.

Inflammatory Nodules

The development of inflammatory nodules has also been described after HA injection and may occur due to infection and development of an active biofilm in the region of application.[20,22] If infection is suspected, initial management may include oral antibiotics, incision and drainage if the lesion is fluctuant, and intralesional corticosteroids.[18,20] Steroids should be administered after antibiotic treatment has been initiated.[20] Hyaluronidase injection has also been described in the management of painful inflammatory nodules. Hyaluronidase has been demonstrated in vitro to effectively break down bacterial biofilms[23] and has been shown to have a clinical role in the management of infections related to filler injections.[24] Concurrent management with oral antibiotics is recommended because the administration of hyaluronidase may disseminate the injection by breaking up the collection.[25]

Inflamed nodules may also occur due to granulomatous reactions associated with HA gel or contaminating proteins.[13] The following empiric antibiotic regimen is recommended: clarithromycin 500 mg plus moxifloxacin 400 mg twice daily for 10 days, or ciprofloxacin 500 to 750 mg twice daily for 2 to 4 weeks, or minocycline 100 mg once daily for 6 months.[4]

Undesired Volume

A potential complication of filler treatment is undesirable volume, and effective treatment relies on appropriate diagnosis. Table 4-1 illustrates the common diagnoses for undesirable volume and their therapies.

Table 4-1 **Diagnoses for undesirable volume and their appropriate treatment**

DIAGNOSIS	CHARACTERISTICS	THERAPIES
Low-quality HA	Relevant product-related factors include the concentration and rheologic properties of the filler and the manufacturing processes (eg, purification). After the procedure = regular volume. Postsurgery = palpable nodules of a stable size.	1. Massage. Proceed to step 2 if not resolved. 2. If located at the lip vermilion, apply pressure, make a puncture using an 18G needle, and squeeze the nodule. In areas under the skin, an incision in the area will not be effective. Hyaluronidase will not dissolve a low-quality HA because it is not made only of HA.
Excessive HA	Appropriate injection techniques as well as appropriate dosage help to limit the risk of adverse reactions and contour irregularities. After the procedure = excessive volume. Postsurgery = excessive and stable volume.	If located at the lip vermilion, apply pressure with the fingers, puncture the nodule with an 18G needle, and squeeze it. In areas covered by dermis, the nodules cannot be punctured or squeezed. In these situations, hyaluronidase is required.
Allergy	After the procedure = progressive volume. Postsurgery = volume rapidly increases and redness develops.	Wait 48 hours for a spontaneous resolution or prescribe an oral antihistamine for 2 days to make the patient more comfortable.
Infection	Effective skin asepsis using 2% chlorhexidine gluconate in 70% isopropyl alcohol can reduce the risk of infection. Disposable sterile gloves and sterile dressing trays and drapes should be used. After the procedure = normal volume. Postsurgery = volume slowly increases and pain and redness develop. Noticeable after 2 days.	Prescribe antibiotics according to the clinical history of the patient. Prescribe anti-inflammatory agents in case of excessive edema. Prescribe analgesics in case of pain.
Acute/chronic inflammation (occurs with alloplastic material)	After the procedure = normal volume and redness. Postsurgery = volume presents oscillations from normal and is slightly increased with palpable nodules and redness. **HA does not present this adverse effect because it is bioidentical**.	Prescribe oral anti-inflammatory and/or local infiltrations (eg, triamcinolone) and/or topical anti-inflammatory agents (eg, betamethasone).
Compression over lymphatic vessels resulting from excessive product injected superficially	After the procedure = normal volume. Postsurgery = volume ranges from normal to excessive. The most common site for this adverse reaction is the tear trough. The volume is high in the first hours of the day and decreases after noon.	Inject hyaluronidase.

Hyaluronidases

In the uncommon event that an undesirable outcome occurs with HA, correction is possible with the injection of commercially available hyaluronidase, an enzyme that breaks down the unwanted HA dermal filler.

Hyaluronidases are a family of injectable enzymes that act as dispersion agents. These help speed up the natural breakdown of HA through hydrolysis.[26] Licensed for therapeutic indications, such as increasing tissue permeability to enhance the delivery of drugs or to increase the uptake of subcutaneous fluids, in esthetics it is widely used off-label.[27] *Off-label* does not necessarily mean that it is unsafe to use but rather that it is being prescribed and administered in a way that is different from its licensed use.[28]

In addition to humans, hyaluronidases have been found in a variety of venoms from snakes, lizards, and insects. In this capacity, they contribute to the local damage and accelerate the spread of toxins at the bite site and affect the local integrity of the extracellular matrix due to degradation of HA.[29] Moreover, various species of gram-positive bacteria (eg, *Staphylococcus aureus*) are capable of producing bacterial HA lyases as a potential virulence factor to promote tissue penetration.[30,31]

Hyaluronidase treatment and application is generally well tolerated, and adverse events are rare.[32] Allergy tests must be performed before its application as a precaution, because side effects such as temporary postinjection pruritus or allergic reactions have been reported.[31,33] Wohlrab et al[31] investigated the influence of adjuvant hyaluronidase on wound healing using the suction blister method in a prospective, single-center, placebo-controlled, double-blind, intraindividual comparison study of 20 participants, and no retardation of wound healing or other relevant risks were observed. These clinical results are in line with the author's in vitro wound healing analyses using primary human structural skin cells (primary human keratinocytes and dermal fibroblasts, unpublished data).

Based on the literature, Buhren et al[34] propose the following recommendations for the use of hyaluronidase in esthetic medicine:

- When working with dermal HA filler, hyaluronidase should always be immediately available.
- For esthetic indications, hyaluronidase (Hylase, Dessau) should be dissolved in 1.0 mL saline solution (0.9% NaCl).
- Severe complications of vascular necrosis following accidental intravascular HA filler injection should be immediately treated with infiltrations of large volumes of hyaluronidase in the entire area (ideally less than 4 hours after filler injection).
- For the correction of HA overfill, the applied volume of hyaluronidase should not exceed the estimated volume of the overcorrection in order to avoid complete degradation of the effect of HA augmentation. Ideally, hyaluronidase should be injected gradually in small volumes and, when necessary, over multiple sessions in order to achieve the desired extent of correction and to prevent overtreatment.
- For the treatment of lower eyelid edema following HA augmentation of the tear trough, only a small volume of hyaluronidase should be applied at a time in order to gradually dissolve excessive HA and to avoid complete reversal of the effect of HA augmentation.
- The efficacy of hyaluronidase treatment in the management of lower eyelid edema following HA augmentation of the tear trough is more effective when applied early (within weeks of the first appearance of edema).

The use of hyaluronidase for esthetic purposes is not approved by the US Food and Drug Administration and is considered an off-label use. In many cases, 10 to 30 units of unpreserved hyaluronidase is sufficient to achieve the desired correction. Local site reactions may occur in up to 25% of patients, but they are typically transient and mild. Initial treatment with as little as 5 to 10 units of hyaluronidase is commonly recommended and is often effective, although some clinicians treat with as much as 75 units with few adverse effects. Additional corrections can be performed, although full correction may take up to 4 weeks to fully appreciate. Some preparations are bovine derived, and skin testing should be considered prior to treatment with these dermal fillers.[35,36]

Hyaluronidase preparations are clear, concentrated liquids that are stored in a refrigerated vial (Table 4-2). To reconstitute these dermal fillers, physicians typically add normal saline or lidocaine (with or without epinephrine). When using Amphadase (Amphastar), reconstitution in 3 mL of 1% lidocaine with 1:100,000 epinephrine has been commonly used with great success. After mixing, the vial is gently swirled. Prior to treatment, a skin test can be performed by injecting 3 to 5 units (0.06–0.1 mL) of the reconstituted solution into the superficial dermis at the antecubital fossa. A positive hypersensitivity reaction consists of a wheal appearing within 5 minutes and lasting 20 to 30 minutes, accompanied by local itching.[37]

Table 4-2 Commercially available hyaluronidase products

TRADE NAME	SOURCE	PRODUCT DETAILS	DOSAGE
Amphadase (Amphastar)	Bovine derived	150 USP units per mL in 2-mL vial. Contains edetate disodium, calcium chloride, monosodium basic buffer, and thimerosal.	**Vascular/tissue compromise:** 30–75 units of hyaluronidase reconstituted in normal saline[a] **Noninflamed nodule or overcorrection:** 5–15 units of hyaluronidase reconstituted in normal saline[b]; 1.5–3 units for eyelid area[c] **Inflamed or painful nodule:** 5–15 units of hyaluronidase reconstituted in normal saline[b]
Hydase (PrimaPharm)	Bovine derived	150 USP units per mL in 2-mL vial. Contains edetate disodium, calcium chloride, sodium chloride, and monosodium basic buffer.	
Hylenex (Halozyme)	Human recombinant source (significantly reduced risk of hypersensitivity)	150 USP units per mL in 2-mL vial. Contains human albumin, edetate disodium, and polysorbate 80.	
Vitrase (Bausch and Lomb)	Ovine derived	200 USP units per mL in 2-mL vial. Contains lactose, potassium phosphate dibasic buffer, and potassium phosphate monobasic buffer.	

[a] Reconstitute 0.5 mL of a 150 IU hyaluronidase vile in 1 mL of normal saline (75 units total). Inject 0.06 to 0.2 mL (equivalent to 30–75 units).
[b] Reconstitute a 150 IU hyaluronidase vile in 1 mL of normal saline. Inject 0.2 to 0.5 mL (equivalent to 5–15 units).
[c] Reconstitute 0.1 mL of a 150 IU hyaluronidase vile in 1 mL of normal saline (15 units total). Inject 0.1 to 0.2 mL volume (equivalent to 1.5–3 units).
(Data from Cohen et al.[13])

Case Report: Ischemia

A patient presented to the office after having another professional inject a dermal filler in the base and tip of her nose. Four hours after the procedure, the patient noticed a "whitish area" at the injection site and felt a "slight pain" in the filled area (Figs 4-3a and 4-3b). She also complained of a numbness in the area under her nose.

Signs and symptoms

Change in color

Redness after the filling might occur and is considered normal as a result of trauma from the injection. This redness appears up to 12 hours after filling and tends to resolve within 3 days. However, in cases of ischemia, the color observed is not exactly red but rather bluish-red (see Fig 4-3a). At first, the distribution is not homogenous but intermittent, similar to the aspect of small vessels. On palpation, these areas feel cold and painful to the touch compared to other areas of the face.

Pain at the injected site

Pain at the injected site might result from trauma caused by the cannula, needle, or even the filler itself, which causes the divulsion of tissues. This type of pain is a normal occurrence after filling procedures. However, in this case the pain increased in the first 3 days, which is not considered normal.

Prolonged numbness

If anesthesia is administered before the filling and/or if the filler has an anesthetic in its composition, the patient will immediately feel numbness in the area. The numbness will fade with time,

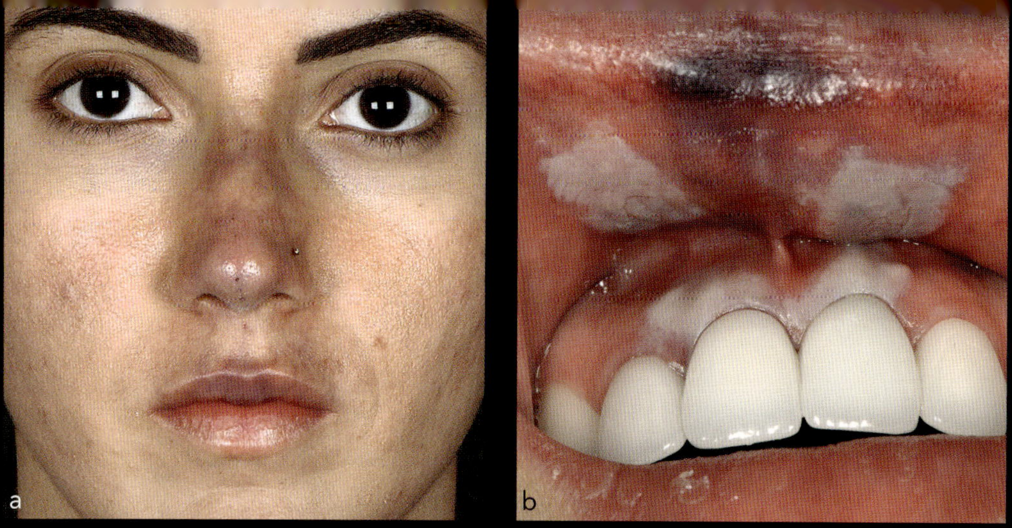

Fig 4-3 Case report of ischemia after filling. *(a)* Frontal view of the patient 12 hours after the filling. Note a bluish-red color of the skin in the nose and upper lip. *(b)* Intraoral view showing that the filler injected at the base of the nose affected the blood supply in the upper lip and anterior upper gingiva.

eventually disappearing entirely. However, when numbness is felt after the procedure and lasts longer than normal, it can be considered a sign of ischemia. Necrosis might occur when an excessive amount of filler compresses a blood vessel or nerve.

Diagnosis

The combination of bluish-red color, progressive pain, numbness, and cold tissue led to a diagnosis of necrosis.

Not all patients with necrosis show the signs and symptoms described above. Therefore, it is crucial that all information about the products used, injection planes, instruments, and data are available and correctly recorded.

Therapeutics

Most clinicians simply wait for the spontaneous resolution of ischemia. However, this is a dangerous practice. As soon as the diagnosis is made, the patient should be immediately treated while the tissue still shows some integrity. When the therapeutic procedure is delayed, tissues become fragile and might be easily traumatized during procedures such as massage.

1. Allergy test

Before injecting hyaluronidase to eliminate unwanted or problematic HA, an allergy test on the inside of the forearm is necessary (Figs 4-3c and 4-3d). The skin test is performed as follows:

1. An anesthetic cream is applied to the area.
2. Once anesthesia is confirmed, chlorhexidine is applied to disinfect the skin.
3. One unit of diluted hyaluronidase (as recommended by the manufacturer) is injected immediately under the epidermis.
4. A pen is used to mark the injection site. Do not use a red pen because it can stain the skin when in contact with sweat or humidity, resulting in a false-positive result.
5. Wait 20 minutes to read the result.

If the test is negative, the patient is ready for the corrective hyaluronidase injection.

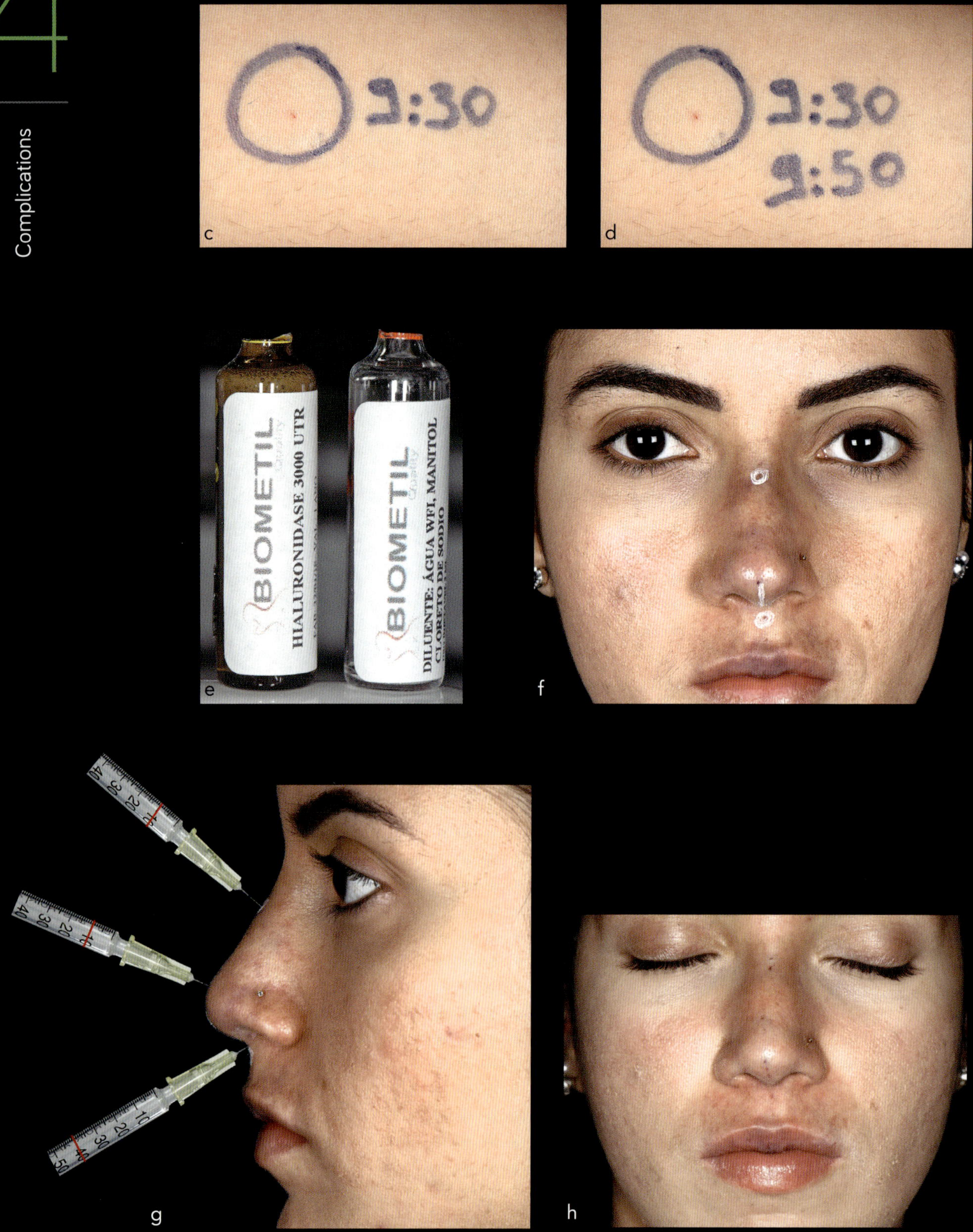

c d e f g h

Fig 4-3 *(cont)* *(c)* Allergy test showing the inside of the patient's forearm immediately after the injection of hyaluronidase (0.01 mL). *(d)* Result 20 minutes later, showing the absence of an allergic reaction (petechiae, papules, erythema, and itching). *(e)* Example of the hyaluronidase and diluent. *(f)* The hyaluronidase should be injected exactly at the same sites and depths as the HA. *(g)* A 100U syringe was used to inject the hyaluronidase at the same places as the filler but using half the amount of the filler previously injected. *(h)* Right after the procedure. Note that the amount injected did not create a volume in the skin, which would have resulted in a vascular compression.

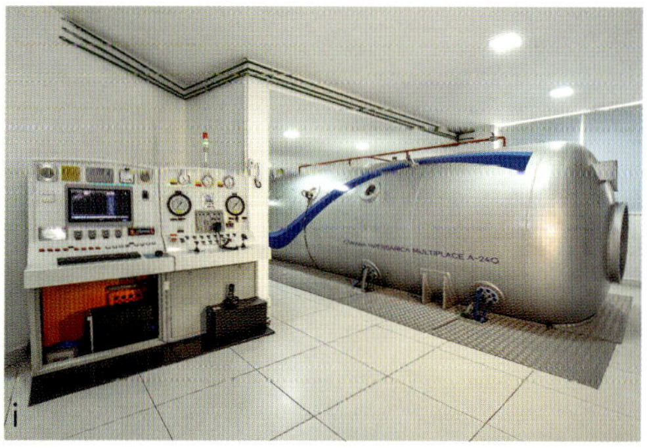
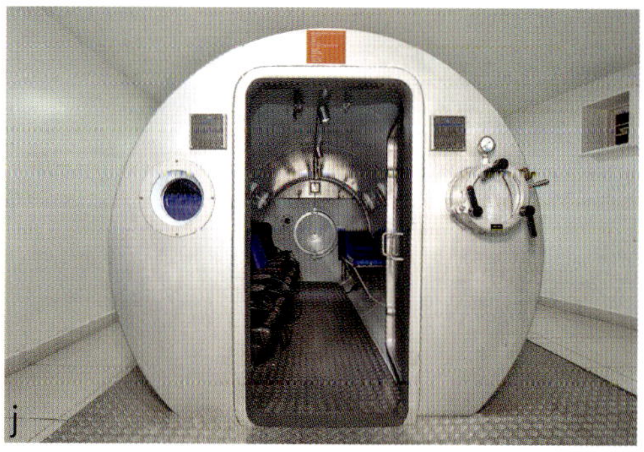
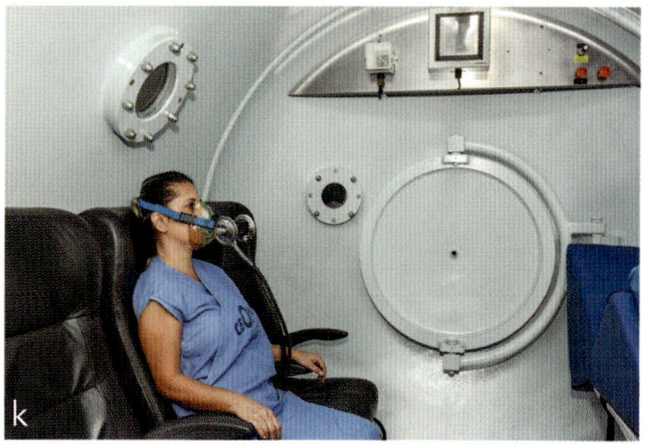
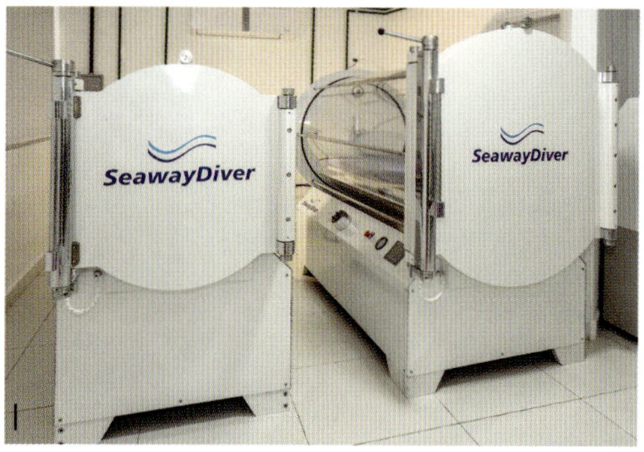

Fig 4-3 *(cont) (i to k)* Views of a multipatient chamber, showing a patient positioned for a hyperbaric oxygen therapy session. *(l and m)* Views of monopatient chambers, showing a patient in the proper position for a hyperbaric oxygen therapy session. The blue bracelet with a spiral cable withdraws the static energy from the patient.

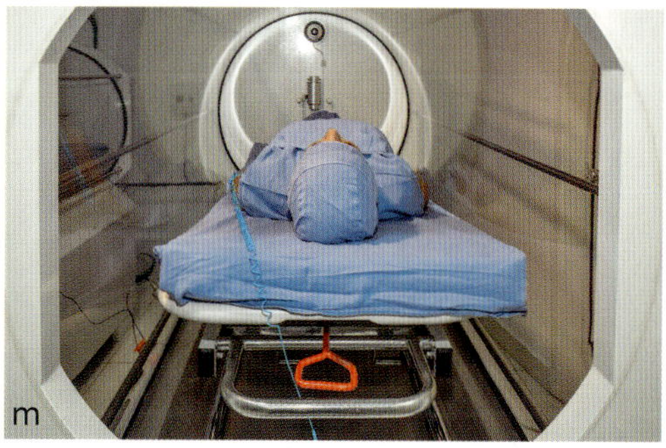

2. Hyaluronidase injection

Prior to injection, anesthetic must be delivered (see chapter 6). Next, the hyaluronidase is diluted according to the manufacturer's instructions in the product packaging (Fig 4-3e). The same type of instrument used for the filler (cannula or needle) should be used for hyaluronidase injection. Half the quantity of HA that was previously used to fill the target area is injected (Figs 4-3f to 4-3h).

Do not massage the area to avoid migration to other regions. If the area is massaged before the hyaluronidase injection, the filler can be spread everywhere, making the enzyme action difficult. Thus, the affected area can only be massaged after the effect of the hyaluronidase is complete.

3. Massage

Massage should be postponed until after the hyaluronidase starts its effects (ie, at least 6 hours after the procedure). Because the massage is very vigorous, anesthesia is necessary. An anesthetic without a vasoconstrictor should be used to avoid vasoconstriction. The massage should be vigorous enough that the area will not need to be massaged again, as it would damage the fragile tissue resulting from the ischemia. The area is massaged to reduce the filler volume in order to alleviate a possible pressure over the blood vessels.

4. Hyperbaric chamber

A hyperbaric chamber can be used to increase oxygen in the ischemic tissue. As soon as the patient is diagnosed with ischemia, the hyperbaric oxygen treatment should start. Patients should be treated with hyperbaric oxygen until the signs and symptoms disappear.

The hyperbaric chamber is a sealed pressure-resistant chamber, generally in the shape of a cylinder, made of steel or acrylic. It can be pressurized with compressed air or pure oxygen. It can be large and able to hold several patients simultaneously (multipatient chamber; Figs 4-3i to 4-3k) or smaller for one individual only (monopatient chamber; Figs 4-3l and 4-3m). Oxygen is provided

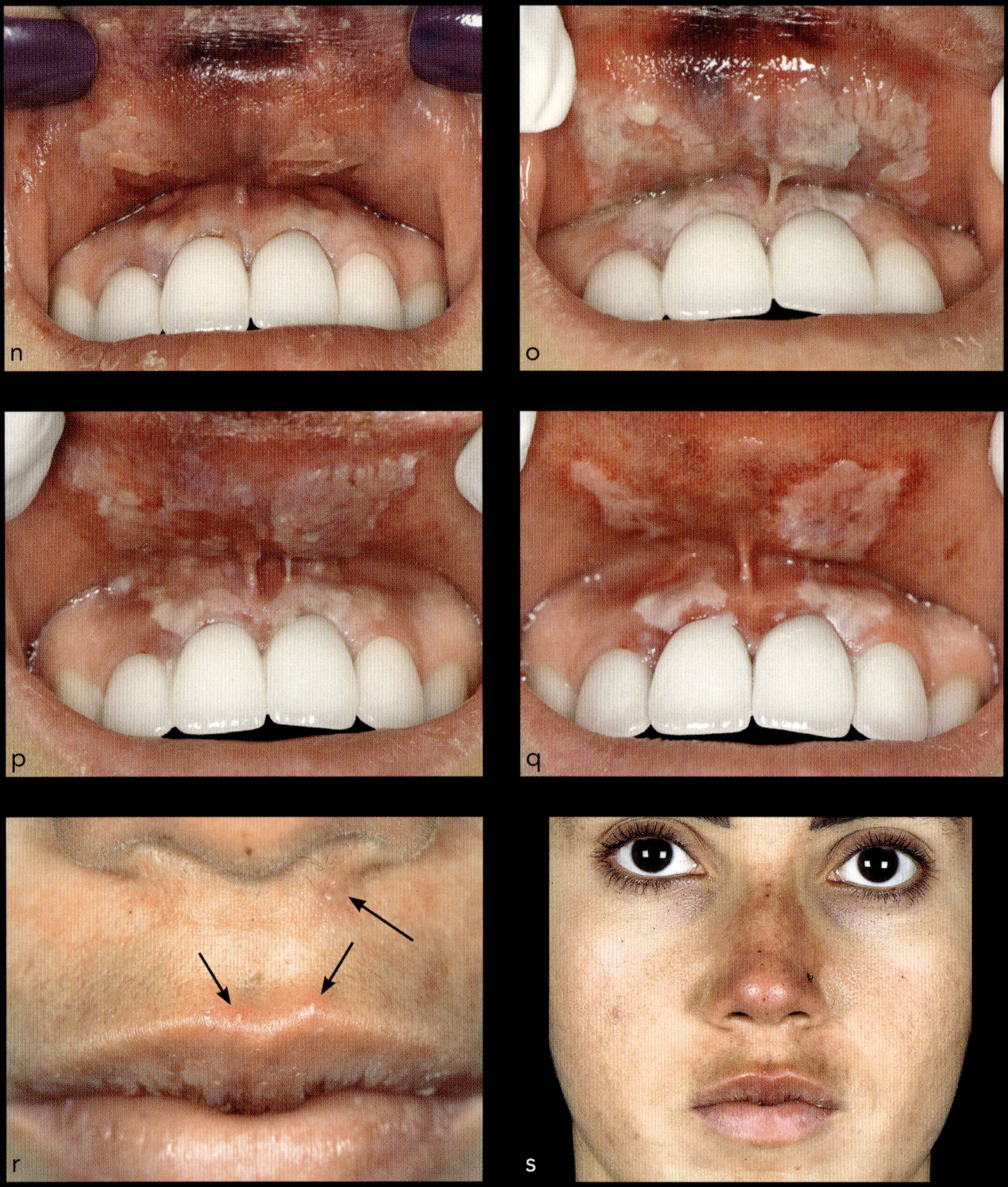

Fig 4-3 *(cont) (n)* One day after the initial filling, immediately after massage. Note that the white scab was removed because of the mechanical trauma caused by the massage. *(o)* Two days after the filling, the white scab is back. *(p)* Three days after the filling. The scab is still located in the same area, but it already shows improvement. *(q)* Four days after the filling. Note the decrease in size and thickness of the scab. *(r)* Four days after the filling. Note the three areas showing opportunistic bacteria *(arrows)*. *(s)* Four days after the filling. Note that the color of the skin in the nose changed from bluish-red to red.

through masks and plastic helmets. In the case of monopatient chambers, the patient can also breathe the oxygen directly from the chamber atmosphere when it is pressurized with this gas.

Hyperbaric oxygen treatment consists of breathing 100% oxygen at a pressure of at least 2.5 times that of the atmospheric pressure. These conditions can only be reached inside the chamber, where the patients may undergo 10 to 40 sessions depending on how severe the condition is and also his or her response to the treatment. Patients should be at rest and breathing normally while inside the chamber, allowing large amounts of oxygen to be dissolved in the blood and reach areas with less oxygen.

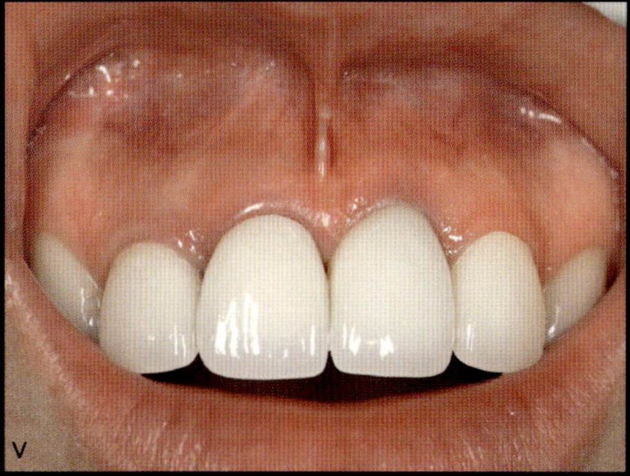

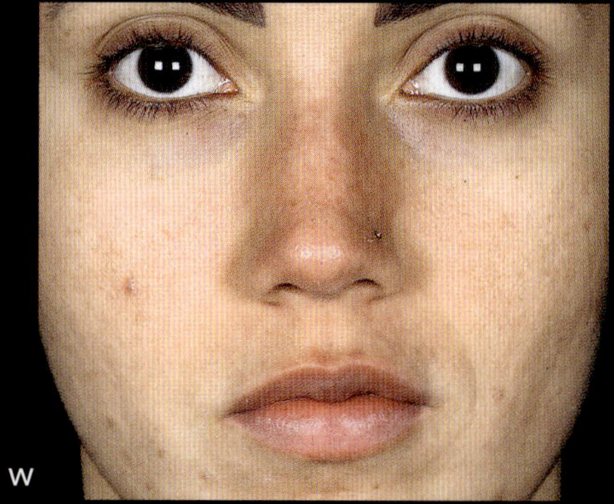

Fig 4-3 *(cont) (t)* Five days after the filling. Note that the three areas containing opportunistic bacteria reduced in size, even in the absence of antibiotic therapy. *(u)* Five days after the filling. Note that the necrosis area is reduced. *(v)* Fourteen days after the filling. Note the healthy-looking appearance of the tissues. *(w)* Fourteen days after the filling. Note the normal aspect of the epidermis.

5. Follow-up

The patient should be examined once a day until the tissue is back to normal (Figs 4-3n to 4-3q). The absence of signs and symptoms indicates tissue healing. All clinical findings and patient reports should be recorded during the daily consultation. Any necessary interventions should be accomplished based on the clinical findings.

The fourth day after the filling is fundamental for evaluation of the degree of necrosis. The skin over the area where the filler was injected might become darker. If this sign is observed, it means that the blood supply has not been re-established yet. Once this darkened scab is present, it cannot be removed because it will stimulate tissue proliferation over it. If the scab is removed later, it could result in a depression, that is, a concave scar. Because the patient in this clinical case did not have this darkened area, it was presumed that the blood supply was already being re-established.

On the fourth day, opportunistic bacteria were found on the surface of the skin (Figs 4-3r and 4-3s). An overgrowth of opportunistic bacteria is a sign that there is not enough blood reaching the tissues to fight the bacteria that infiltrate into dry skin. This is another event associated with necrosis. In the presence of a dark scab on the surface of the skin, it is important to use antibiotic creams to keep it protected from microorganisms, following the guidelines on the package insert. In more severe cases with a broad dark area on the surface of the skin and many areas of opportunistic infection, the administration of oral antibiotics, or injectable antibiotics in cases where the patient cannot receive oral therapy, is recommended in addition to topical antibiotic creams. Because the area of necrosis was progressively decreasing in this case and there were only a few infected areas, no antibiotic was used. If, on the fifth day, a decrease in the number of infectious foci is observed, this should be interpreted as a signal that the blood supply is back (Figs 4-3t to 4-3z).

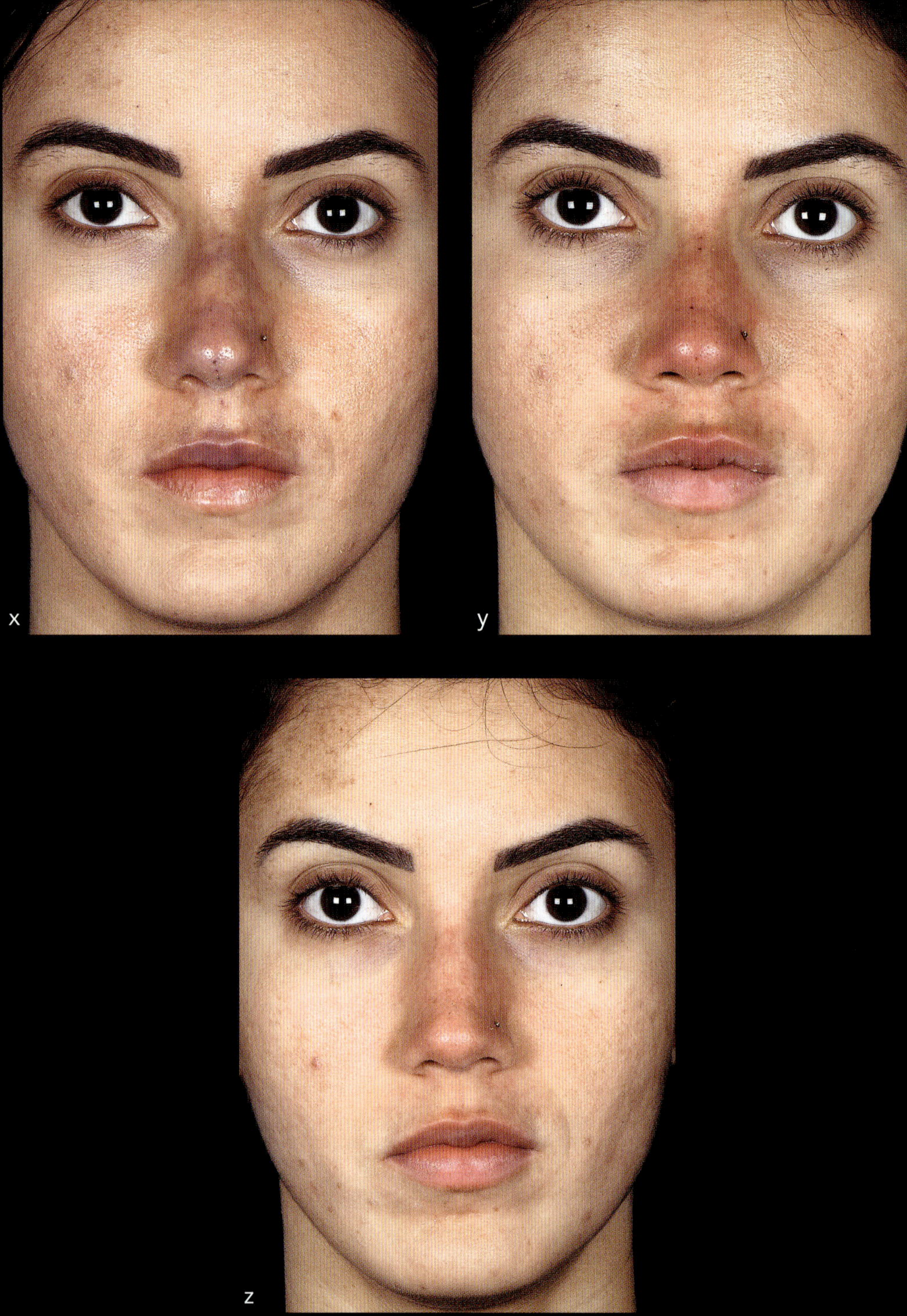

x y z

Fig 4-3 *(cont) (x to z)* Evolution of the case: 12 hours, 4 days, and 14 days after the filling, respectively.

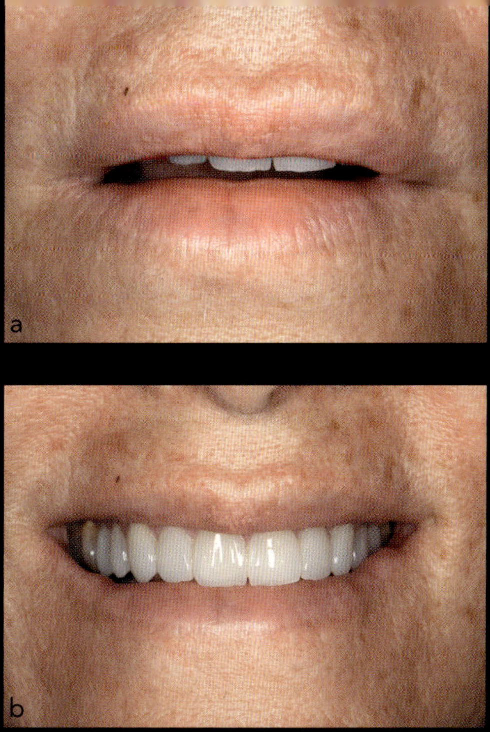

Fig 4-4 Two months after the filling. *(a)* Note the discreet nodules in the upper and lower lip vermilion. *(b)* When smiling, the nodules become even more evident.

Case Report: Lumps

A patient volunteered to be a patient in a course about filling using HA. Varioderm (Adoderm) was used to fill her lip vermilion.

Initially the patient reported that she was satisfied with the procedure result, but 2 months later she noticed the presence of small volumes in the vermilion of her upper and lower lips (Figs 4-4a and 4-4b). Because the nodules were formed 2 months later and they were stable in size, the hypothesis of infection was not considered. The other hypothesis was related to the fact that the HA was not biocompatible. Not all formulations of HA present an ideal biocompatibility, as it contains in its formula other substances that may lead to the formation of cystic capsules that isolate the HA from the tissues. These products are not reabsorbed over time. The ideal treatment for these lumps is simple:

1. Compress the lumps with your fingers and maintain the pressure (Fig 4-4c).
2. Use an 18G needle to lance several points in the lump (Fig 4-4d).
3. Squeeze the lump as much as possible to remove the contents inside (Figs 4-4e to 4-4g).

The application of hyaluronidase is not an option in these cases because it would have no effect on a product with low-purity HA.

All nodules were removed through perforation. The clinician should take note that this product in particular forms nodules that are not dissolved by hyaluronidase and do not disappear with time. They are encapsulated. If these nodules are under the lip vermilion, their removal is easy, but that is not true when they are under the skin in the face. Thus, Varioderm should not be used.

In case of doubt in relation to the diagnosis, the material collected can be sent for laboratory analysis in the culture medium and for a cytologic examination (Figs 4-4h to 4-4j). The samples examined in the laboratory were negative for the presence of infection. This result showed that the nodules were not caused by bacteria introduced during the injection.

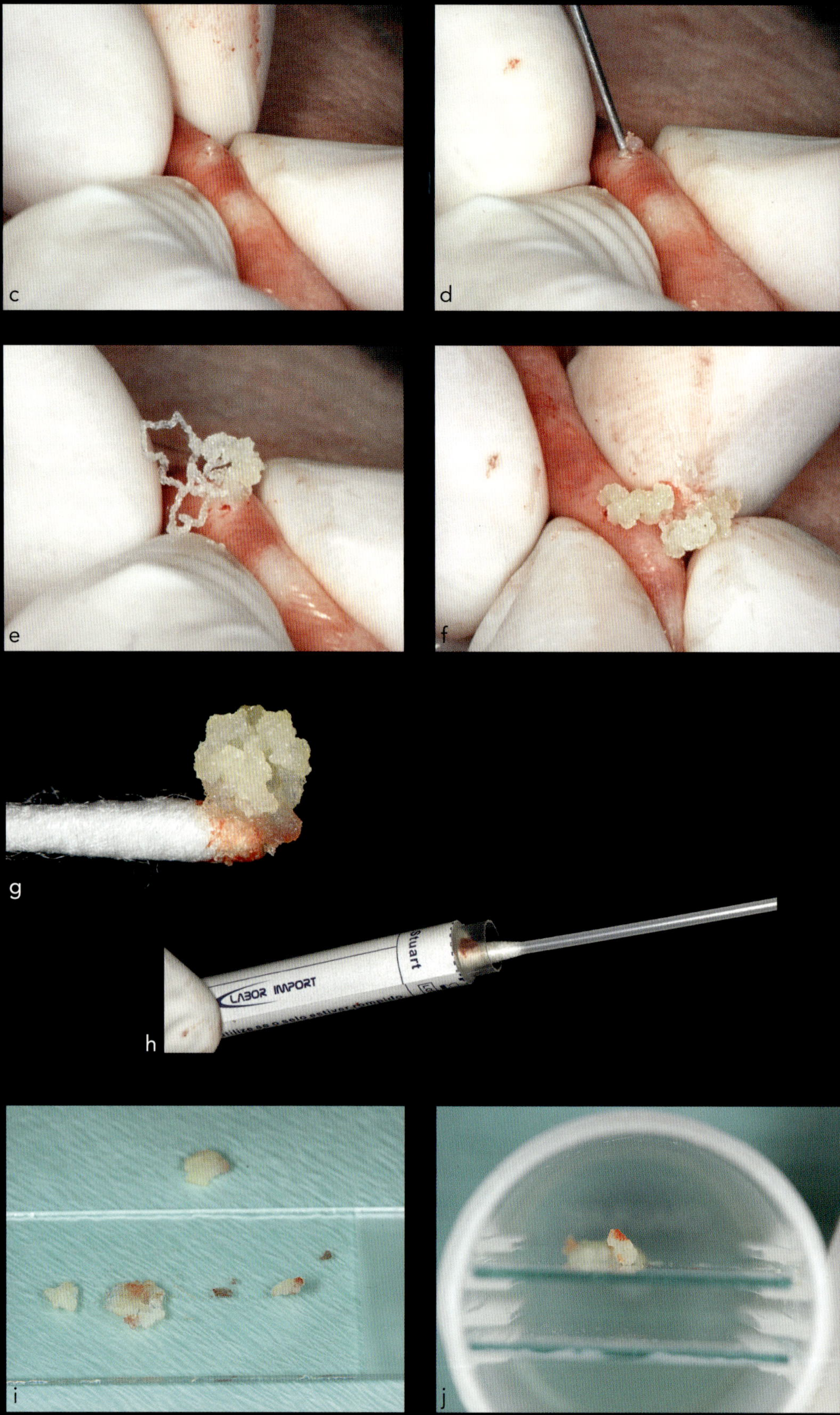

Fig 4-4 *(cont) (c)* Photograph showing two nodules of Varioderm. Continuous pressure should be maintained on these nodules to push their contents to the surface. *(d)* An 18G needle is used to puncture the nodule, as it might have additional pockets. *(e)* After being lanced, the Varioderm is removed from inside the nodule. *(f)* Note the change in color (from clear to yellowish) and consistency (from gel to paste). *(g)* Photograph showing the sample collected with a swab. *(h)* The sample being inoculated in a Stuart medium for further culture. *(i)* Contents removed from the nodules placed in a glass slide for microscopic testing. *(j)* Glass slides inside a sterile vial ready to be transported to the laboratory.

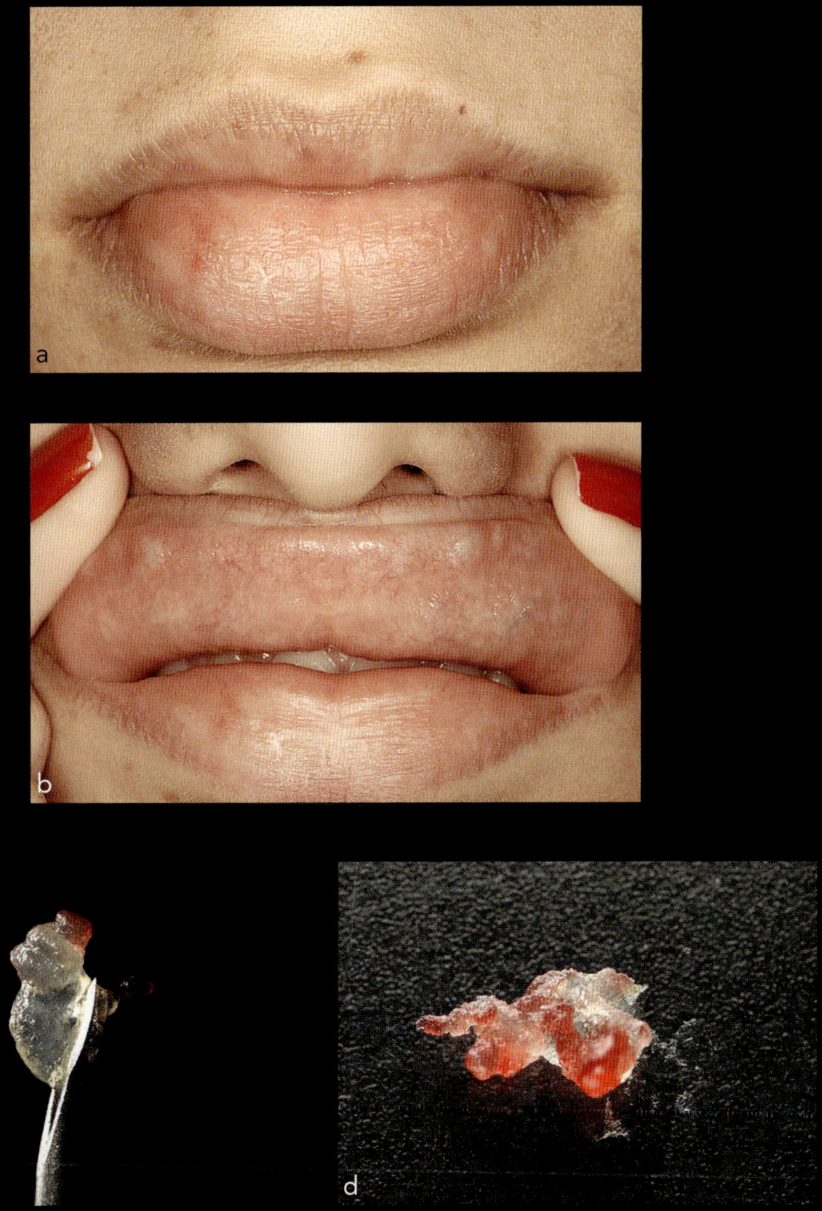

Fig 4-5 *(a)* Lips showing a normal aspect at rest. *(b)* When lifted, the lips show the presence of nodules. *(c)* The nodules were removed via compression, perforation, and further compression. *(d)* Varioderm nodule removed after 3 years.

Figure 4-5 shows the case of another patient whose lips were filled with Varioderm. According to the patient, nodules became visible 3 months after the injection, and 3 years later they were stable in terms of number, volume, and position (Figs 4-5a and 4-5b). A plastic surgeon injected hyaluronidase in the nodules, but the Varioderm did not react. If this product was a good-quality HA, it would have been reabsorbed by the body within 1 year. Instead the nodules had to be compressed and perforated to remove the contents (Figs 4-5c and 4-5d).

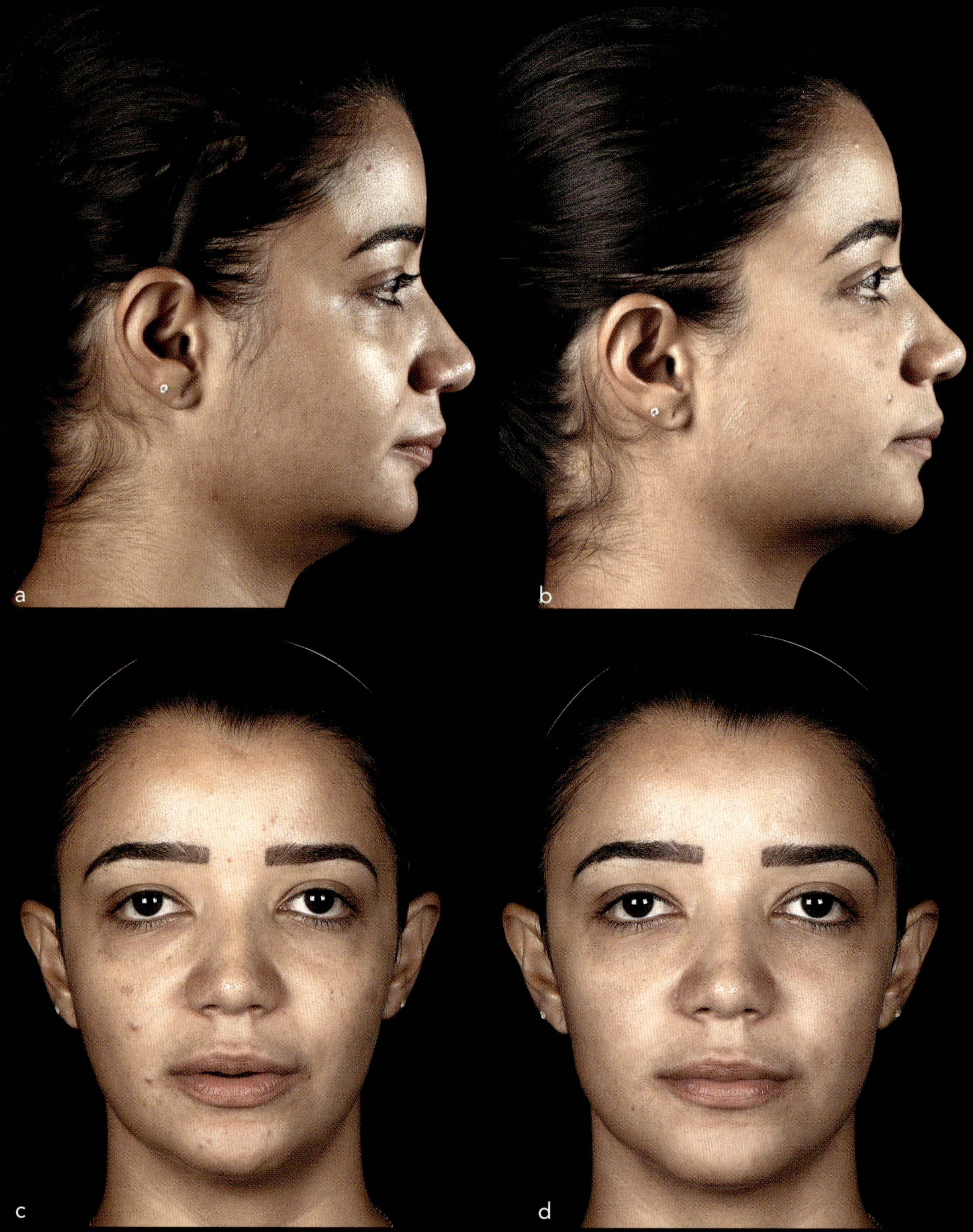

Fig 4-6 *(a)* Excessive volume in the tear trough 30 days after HA injection. *(b)* Seven days after the injection of hyaluronidase, the excessive volume disappeared. *(c and d)* Frontal views of the patient before and 7 days after hyaluronidase injection, respectively.

Case Report: Dissolution of Excessive Volume

A patient was treated with HA injection by another clinician. Thirty days after the injection, an excessive volume was still observed, which made the patient uncomfortable in terms of esthetics. In this case, the treatment chosen was the injection of hyaluronidase. The amount used was half that of the previously injected filler but to the same depth (Fig 4-6).

References

1. Johl SS, Burgett RA. Dermal filler agents: A practical review. Curr Opin Ophthalmol 2006;17:471–479.
2. Eppley BL, Dadvand B. Injectable soft-tissue fillers: Clinical overview. Plast Reconstr Surg 2006;118:98e–106e.
3. Urdiales-Gálvez lvez F, Delgado NE, Figueiredo V, et al. Preventing the complications associated with the use of dermal fillers in facial aesthetic procedures: An expert group consensus report. Aesthetic Plast Surg 2017;41:667–677.
4. Signorini M, Liew S, Sundaram H, et al. Global aesthetics consensus: Avoidance and management of complications from hyaluronic acid fillers—Evidence- and opinion-based review and consensus recommendations. Plast Reconstr Surg 2016;137:961e.
5. Lazzeri D, Agostini T, Figus M, Nardi M, Pantaloni M, Lazzeri S. Blindness following cosmetic injections of the face. Plast Reconstr Surg 2012;129:995–1012.
6. Glaich AS, Cohen JL, Goldberg LH. Injection necrosis of the glabella: Protocol for prevention and treatment after use of dermal fillers. Dermatol Surg 2006;32:276–281.
7. Bailey SH, Cohen JL, Kenkel JM. Etiology, prevention, and treatment of dermal filler complications. Aesthet Surg J 2011;31:110–121.
8. Sclafani AP, Fagien S. Treatment of injectable soft tissue filler complications. Dermatol Surg 2009;35(suppl 2): 1672–1680.
9. De Boulle K, Glogau R, Kono T, et al. A review of the metabolism of 1,4-butanediol diglycidyl ether–crosslinked hyaluronic acid dermal fillers. Dermatol Surg 2013;39:1758–1766.
10. DeLorenzi C. Complications of injectable fillers, part 2: Vascular complications. Aesthet Surg J 2014;34:584–600.
11. Kim DW, Yoon ES, Ji YH, et al. Vascular complications of hyaluronic acid fillers and the role of hyaluronidase in management. J Plast Reconstr Aesthet Surg 2011;64:1590–1595.
12. Kang MS, Park ES, Shin HS, et al. Skin necrosis of the nasal ala after injection of dermal fillers. Dermatol Surg 2011;37:375–380.
13. Cohen BE, Bashey S, Wysong A. The use of hyaluronidase in cosmetic dermatology: A review of the literature. J Clin Investig Dermatol 2015;3(2):7.
14. Schanz S, Schippert W, Ulmer A, Rassner G, Fierlbeck G. Arterial embolization caused by injection of hyaluronic acid (Restylane). Br J Dermatol 2002;146:928–929.
15. Park SW, Woo SJ, Park KH, et al. Iatrogenic retinal artery occlusion caused by cosmetic facial filler injections. Am J Ophthalmol 2012;154:653–662.e1.
16. Peter S, Mennel S. Retinal branch artery occlusion following injection of hyaluronic acid (Restylane). Clin Exp Ophthalmol 2006;34:363–364.
17. Hirsch RJ, Cohen JL, Carruthers JD. Successful management of an unusual presentation of impending necrosis following a hyaluronic acid injection embolus and a proposed algorithm for management with hyaluronidase. Dermatol Surg 2007;33:357–360.
18. Kang MS, Park ES, Shin HS, et al. Skin necrosis of the nasal ala after injection of dermal fillers. Dermatol Surg 2011;37:375–380.
19. Castro CM, Grilli H, Grois J. Intra-arterial hyaluronidase in the treatment of certain forms of lower limb ulcerations. Angiology 1963;14:277–284.
20. Narins RS, Coleman WP 3rd, Glogau RG. Recommendations and treatment options for nodules and other filler complications. Dermatol Surg 2009;35(suppl 2):1667–1671.
21. Requena L, Requena C, Christensen L, et al. Adverse reactions to injectable soft tissue fillers. J Am Acad Dermatol 2011;64:1–34.
22. Ozturk CN, Li Y, Tung R, et al. Complications following injection of soft-tissue fillers. Aesthet Surg J 2013;33: 862–877.
23. Pecharki D, Petersen FC, Scheie AA. Role of hyaluronidase in *Streptococcus intermedius* biofilm. Microbiology 2008;154(Pt 3):932–938.
24. Dayan SH, Arkins JP, Brindise R. Soft tissue fillers and biofilms. Facial Plast Surg 2011;27:23–28.
25. Rzany B, Becker-Wegerich P, Bachmann F, Erdmann R, Wollina U. Hyaluronidase in the correction of hyaluronic acid-based fillers: A review and a recommendation for use. J Cosmet Dermatol 2009;8:317–323.
26. Hyaluronidase. http://www.drugs.com/cdi/hyaluronidase.html. Accessed 30 January 2019.
27. Hyaluronidase enzyme. http://www.clinicalondon.co.uk/hyaluronidase-enzyme/. Accessed 30 January 2019.
28. Hyaluronidase protocol. https://aestheticsjournal.com/feature/hyaluronidase-protocol. Accessed 30 January 2019.
29. Csoka TB, Frost GI, Stern R. Hyaluronidases in tissue invasion. Invasion Metastasis 1997;17:297–311.
30. Makris G, Wright JD, Ingham E, Holland KT. The hyaluronate lyase of *Staphylococcus aureus*—A virulence factor? Microbiology 2004;150.
31. Wohlrab J, Finke R, Franke WG, Wohlrab A. Clinical trial for safety evaluation of hyaluronidase as diffusion enhancing adjuvant for infiltration analgesia of skin with lidocaine. Dermatol Surg 2012;38:91–96.
32. Rzany B, Becker-Wegerich P, Bachmann F, Erdmann R, Wollina U. Hyaluronidase in the correction of hyaluronic acid-based fillers: A review and a recommendation for use. J Cosmet Dermatol 2009;8:317–323.
33. Wohlrab J, Wohlrab D, Wohlrab L, Wohlrab C, Wohlrab A. Use of hyaluronidase for pharmacokinetic increase in bioavailability of intracutaneouslyapplied substances. Skin Pharmacol Physiol 2014;27:276–282.
34. Buhren BA, Schrumpf H, Hoff N P, Bölke, Hilton S, Gerber PA. Hyaluronidase: From clinical applications to molecular and cellular mechanisms. Eur J Med Res 2016;21:5.
35. Lambros V. Models of facial aging and implications for treatment. Clin Plast Surg 2008;35:319–327.
36. Lambros V. Observations on periorbital and midface aging. Plast Reconstr Surg 2007;120:1367–1376.
37. Dermal Fillers. https://emedicine.medscape.com/article/1125066-overview. Accessed 30 January 2019.

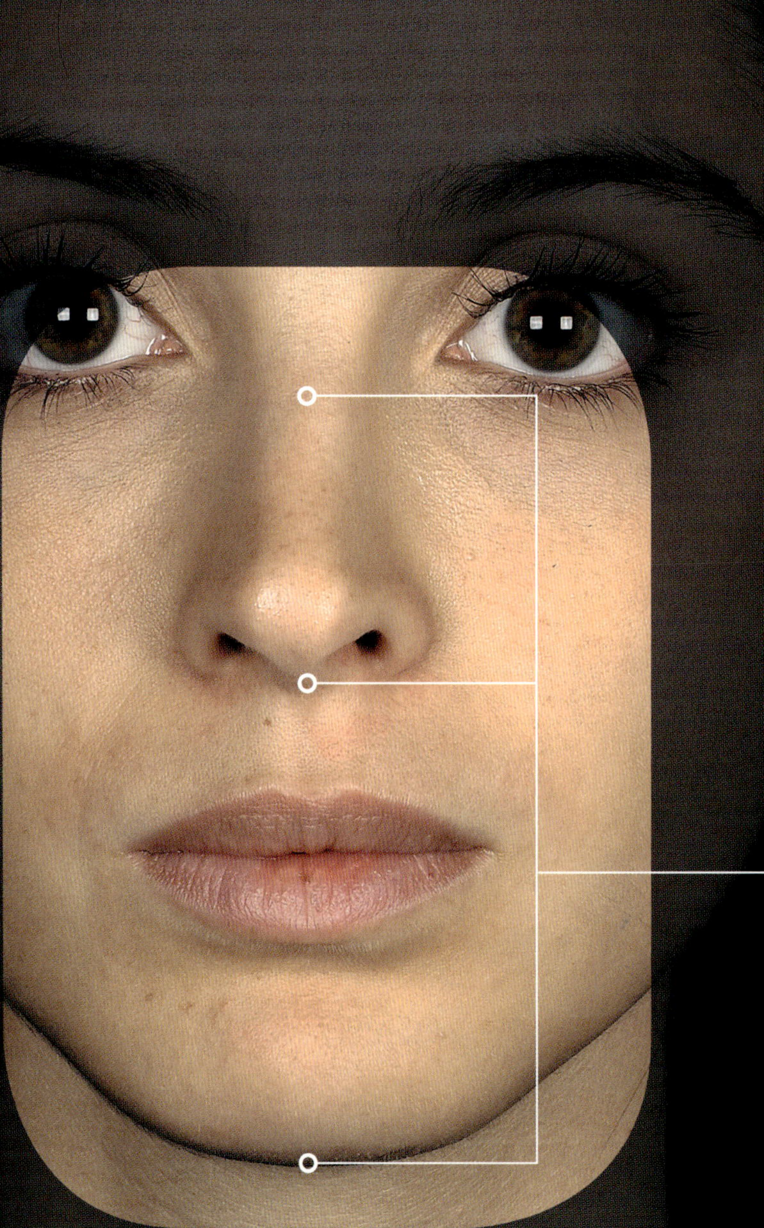

CHAPTER

05

Facial Analysis for Dermal Filler Injections

Prior to performing any filling procedures, the clinician must perform a thorough facial analysis of the patient. Figures 5-1 to 5-4 illustrate the workflow from initial consultation to presentation of the diagnosis.

The clinician should know the average facial dimensions of anatomical structures in order to be able to classify them as dominant, median, or slightly dominant. In general, a dominant anatomical structure suggests that all other structures are also dominant. A dominant anatomical structure gives the false idea that the structure next to it looks less dominant. In addition, the correct proportion between the dimensions of these structures should be understood so that the diagnosis and/or treatment can be performed to achieve harmony, which is very important in terms of esthetics. These parameters are obtained through the collection of data during the initial consultation (see Fig 5-2).

Consultation

The consultation begins with a sit-down conversation between the clinician and the patient, who should maintain a social distance. The clinician should ask the patient for permission to silently examine his or her face to prevent the patient's opinion from influencing this initial evaluation. All aspects that could be corrected with dermal fillers should be recorded, especially the most disharmonious feature of the face. This feature is very important because it is the first one to be socially noticed by other people (and is likely the main complaint of the patient). Write down all other issues in order of relevance.

During the second part of the consultation, the clinician should carefully listen to the patient's complaints. The following questions can be asked: In terms of esthetics, what bothers you the most? Do you get any criticism regarding your appearance? Do you avoid being photographed from a certain angle? What area of your face do you use makeup to correct or conceal?

The third part of the consultation involves taking facial measurements (see Fig 5-3a). The measurements can be taken using a caliper available for sale in a hardware store. The following measurements should be recorded: interpupillary, intercanthal, bizygomatic, and bigonial distances; gonial angle; width of the nose and the mouth; and length of the nose, upper lip, and lower lip. A measurement worksheet can be found via the QR code at right.

At the end of the consultation, a total of seven digital photographs necessary for the facial analysis are taken: a facial view from above and frontal and profile views of the face with lips closed, parted, and smiling. The photographic protocol can be found via the QR code at right. Once these photographs are taken, the patient is dismissed so that the clinician can evaluate the case and prepare a presentation (see Fig 5-3b). The assistant is responsible for preparing the photographs in a PowerPoint or Keynote presentation so the clinician can work on the analysis. The positions, dimensions, proportions, and angles of the facial anatomy should all be evaluated. If necessary, lines can be drawn using digital rulers. This analysis will influence the treatment plan and will be part of the presentation made to the patient.

Presenting the Esthetic Diagnosis and Treatment

A large screen (preferably at least 40 inches) should be used for the presentation. A screen smaller than 40 inches is not recommended because the photographs will look small; consequently, the patient will find it hard to observe the facial anatomy, and the details will not be so evident. The ideal setup is for the clinician to stand while the patient is comfortably seated (see Fig 5-4). For added convenience, the base of the monitor should be at the level of the patient's jaw, so the patient does not need to crane his or her neck to view the presentation.

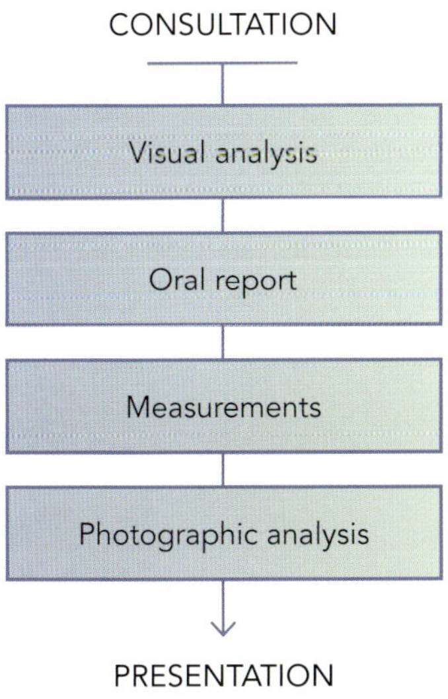

Fig 5-1 The workflow between the first consultation and the presentation of the diagnosis. This diagram is described in the following pages.

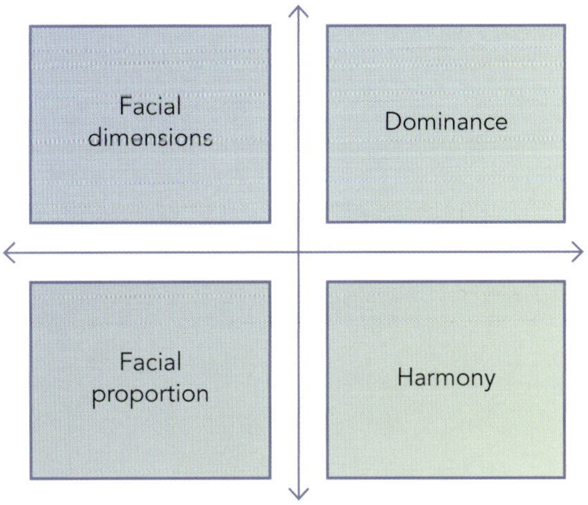

Fig 5-2 Anatomical structures are classified according to facial dimensions, facial proportion, dominance, and harmony.

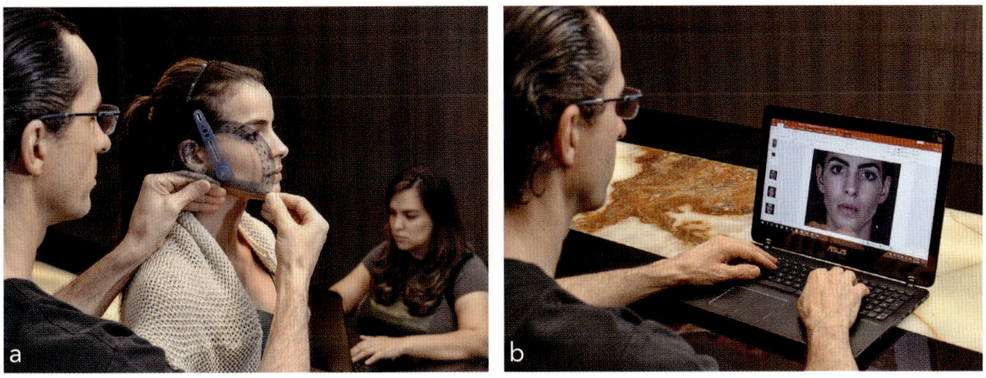

Fig 5-3 Important steps during the consultation. After performing a thorough visual analysis and recording the patient's responses during the oral report, various measurements are taken of the patient's face *(a)*. At the end of the consultation, digital photographs are taken of the patient's face. Once the patient has left the office, the clinician evaluates the photographs *(b)*.

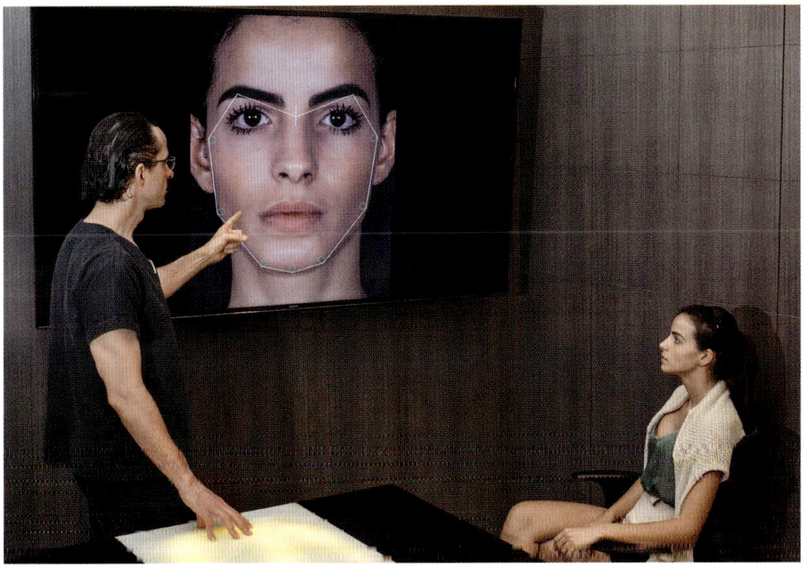

Fig 5-4 A possible setup for the treatment presentation.

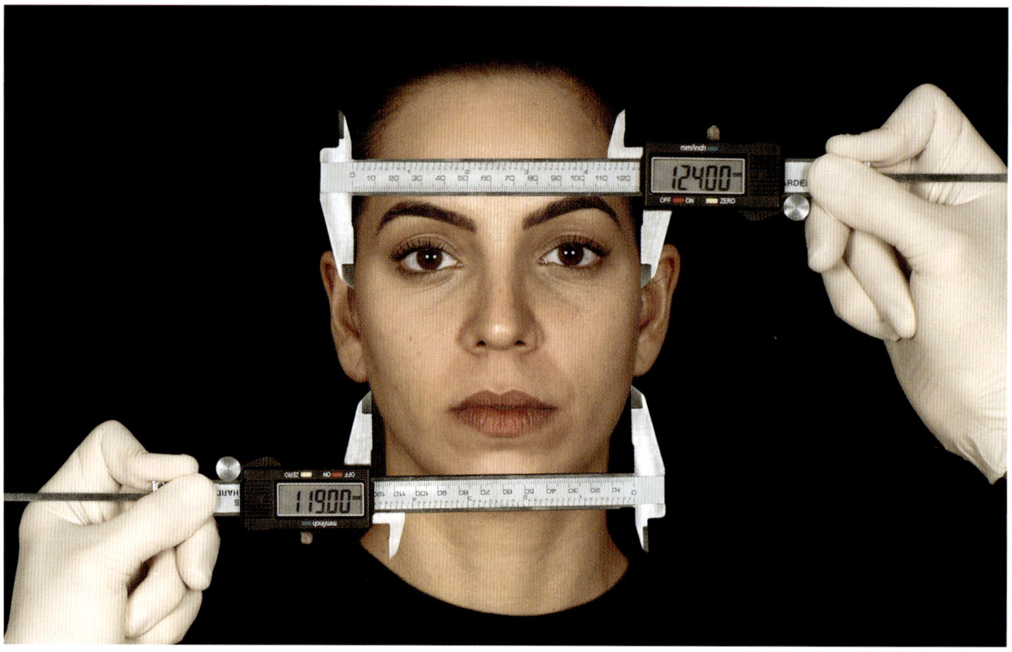

Fig 5-5 Example of facial measurements using a caliper.

A treatment plan presentation lasts 30 minutes on average. During this time, the clinician should summarize the conclusions drawn from the first consultation. These include the following:

1. Inform the patient about the most important point of the treatment.
2. Explain what will be done in regard to the patient's main complaints.
3. Show the measurement sheet and emphasize the correct measurements before talking about the deficiencies.
4. Show the photographs with tracings and any observations made.

During this presentation, the treatment plan is refined and adjusted according to the wishes and consent of the patient. At the end, the treatment plan should be documented and signed.

Facial Measurements

An individual's face is part of his or her identity, and its uniqueness helps to make all of us visually different from one another. Differences occur due to the diversity of shapes, colors, positions, gender, and also facial measurements. It is important that all clinicians interested in esthetic treatment know the average facial measurements while understanding that these measurements are not absolute. They differ according to different faces and ethnicities, and this is why studying facial proportions is so valuable. As a result, it can be said that a harmonious face is a proportional face, not a face that has accurate measurements. For instance, in a face where the nose is long and dominant and the chin is poorly defined in the horizontal direction, it is obvious that the nose, in this particular case, will look even more dominant. The professional can use a filler to advance the chin in a horizontal direction, decreasing the dominance of the nose and improving the esthetic profile of the patient.

In order to decide whether to use fillers in a particular region and determine the amount to be injected, the clinician must know the facial dimensions and proportions in the vertical and horizontal directions, frontal view, and profile. Facial measurements can be taken manually with a caliper or digitally with computer software (Fig 5-5). Knowing the exact place to be measured is also critical. Therefore, it is important to know the cephalometric points.

Table 5-1 Important cephalometric points for filler injections

POINT	ABBREVIATION	DESCRIPTION
Median points		
Trichion	Tr	Midline of hairline
Ophryon	Oph	Point in the center of the frontal diameter; the deepest part of the frontalis
Glabella	G'	In the center of the middle frontal protuberance; the most protuberant midpoint on the frontal bone
Nasion	N	Over the frontonasal suture (craniometry); the deepest point at the nasal root
Apex nasi	AN	Most anterior point on the soft tissue nose
Subnasale	Sn	Point where the nasal septum and the upper lip meet
B point	B'	The deepest part of the mentolabial fold
Stomion	St	The most inferior point in the upper lip
Gnathion	Gn'	The most anterior point on the chin
Mental eminence	ME	The most anterior curve of the tegument tissue of the chin (cephalometry)
Menton	Me'	The lowest point on the chin as seen on a frontal view or profile
Lateral points		
Frontotemporal	Ft	The temporal crest at the level of the eyebrow tail; located at the most anterior point of the temporal line on the frontal bone
Zygion	Zy	The most lateral points of the zygomatic arch
Gonion	Go	The most posterior and inferior point of the mandible in the anteroposterior direction; located at the bisecting angle formed by tangents to the lower and posterior borders of the mandible
Menton lateral	Mel'	Point of union between the chin and lateral jaw

Cephalometric points

While craniometric points (bone) are important, in the case of a facial analysis for dermal filler injections, the cephalometric points (facial) should be the priority. Cephalometric points help build a facial identity and are most important when a facial analysis is being performed for dermal filler injections.[1] The most important cephalometric points for dermal filler analysis are listed in Table 5-1 and illustrated in Fig 5-6. Fillers applied in the facial cephalometric points can enhance them with better definition and also create appropriate proportions between points.[2–4]

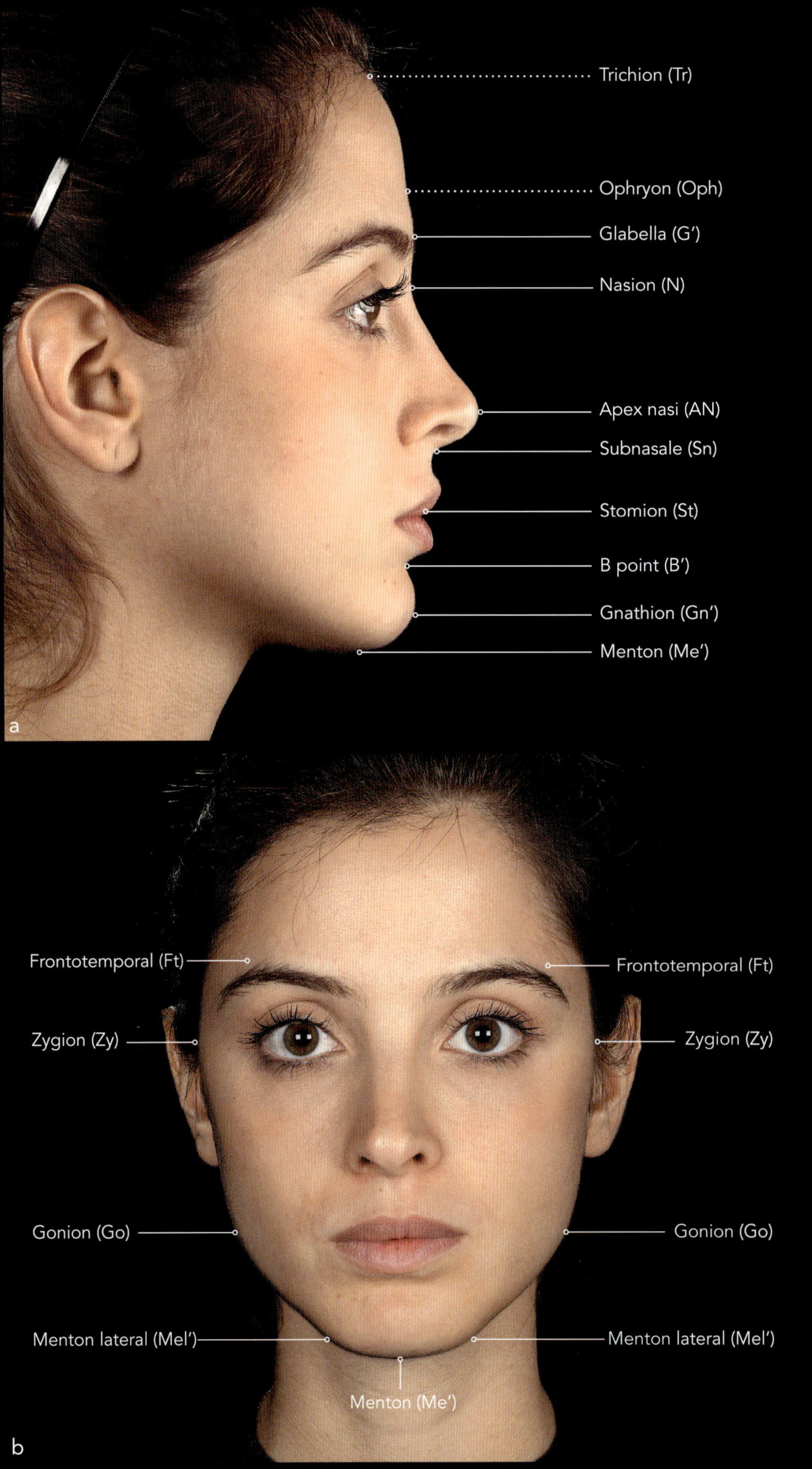

Fig 5-6 *(a)* Lateral view of cephalometric points that can receive fillers *(solid lines)* and that cannot receive fillers but can be used as landmarks *(dotted lines)*.[2–4] *(b)* Frontal views of cephalometric points that can be filled with dermal fillers to provide better facial definition and appropriate proportions between points.

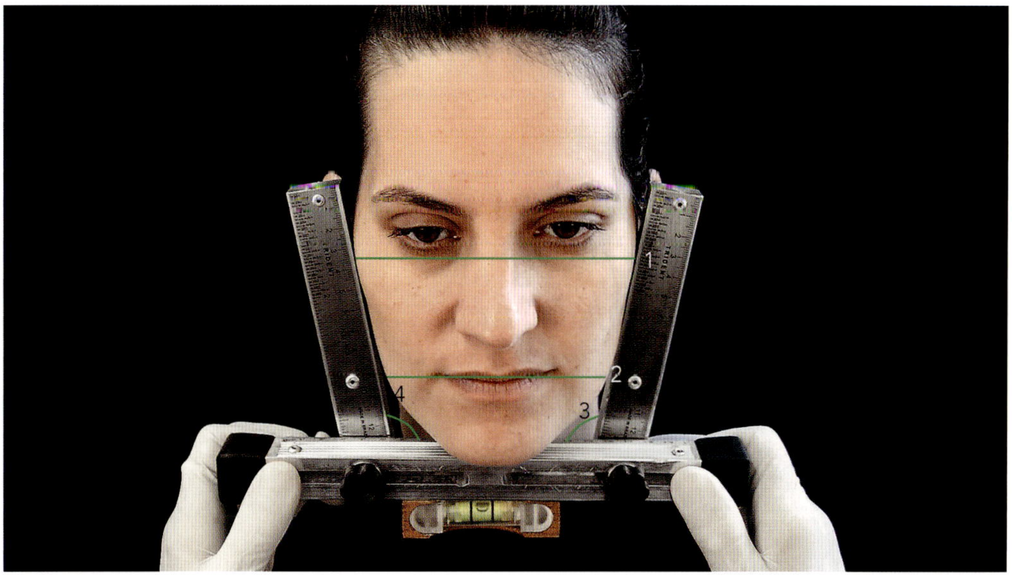

Fig 5-7 Use of a V-shape measurer to measure the following: 1, bizygomatic distance; 2, bigonial distance; 3, angle of the zygion and gonion line to the horizontal plane on the left side; 4, angle of the zygion and gonion line to the horizontal plane on the right side.

Facial cardinal points

The V-shape facial measurer is a device consisting of a horizontal aluminum base and a fixed metallic ruler to measure the width of the lower third of the face (ie, the bigonial distance). There are two vertical rods that also have metal strips attached to them. These slides are attached to the aluminum base by means of two pivot bolts. At the bottom, there is an instrument showing the level. The horizontal base must be parallel and level in equilibrium. The angle of the patient's face is determined by the intersection of the lines that are tangent to the most lateral facial points of the bizygomatic and bigonial distances (Fig 5-7).

The main functions of the V-shape measurer are the following:

1. To measure the bigonial distance

Use the metal ruler located at the base to measure this distance.

OBJECTIVE: To research and diagnose the masseter hypertrophy and to classify the facial shape as square, tapered, or ovoid.

2. Measure the bizygomatic distance

Mark on both sides of the vertical rods the height at which they touch the zygion. Use a marker for this step. After that, couple a common ruler positioned horizontally on the two marks and measure with the ruler to determine the bizygomatic distance.

OBJECTIVE: To research and diagnose masseter hypertrophy and asymmetries and to determine the need to use fillers at the zygomatic arch and bone.

3. Measure the angle between the zygion and gonion

Place a protractor in the horizontal aluminum base and check the angulation of the vertical rods.

OBJECTIVE: To research and diagnose the masseter hypertrophy and determine the need to use fillers at the zygomatic arch and bone.

4. Check for asymmetries between the two sides of the face in frontal view

Make a comparison of the angles between the zygion and the gonion, on the right and left side.

OBJECTIVE: Check for significant differences between the angles by comparing the measurements on both sides and decide on possible treatments such as botulinum toxin, facial fillers, and suspension sutures and also confirm asymmetries caused by unilateral chewing.

5. Check the shape of the jaw

Turn around the device until the vertical rulers are positioned horizontally, and position the device horizontally until the zero number of the aluminum base rulers touch the patient's chin.

OBJECTIVE: To investigate and confirm the diagnosis of masseter hypertrophy and to evaluate the need to cause traction at the lower lateral fat of the jaw (jowl fat) and the need to use fillers at the gonion and at the prejowl area.

6. Diagnose possible facial harmonization procedures

Check the measurements obtained to diagnose whether a facial harmonization procedure, such as botulinum toxin in the masseter muscle or use of facial fillers in the zygion and gonion, is necessary.

OBJECTIVE: To provide determinant mathematical parameters for the performance of facial harmonization procedures.

7. Diagnose the numerical difference between the bizygomatic and bigonial distances

Use the measurements obtained to verify the ratio between these two distances.

OBJECTIVE: To research and diagnose the masseter hypertrophy, determine the need to use fillers at the zygomatic arch and bone, and help with the diagnosis of facial type.

8. Measure the vertical distance between the gonion and the zygion

Use a marker to mark bilaterally on the vertical rods the height at which the rods touch the gonion and the zygion. After that, attach a common ruler positioned vertically on the two marks and read the measurement.

OBJECTIVE: To research and help with the classification of facial type.

9. Create mathematical parameters to classify faces as mesocephalic, brachycephalic, or dolichocephalic

Search the literature for information that may contribute to the elaboration of these parameters. Also, make measurements on faces that typically have all three facial patterns.

OBJECTIVE: To research and contribute to the classification of facial type.

10. Evaluate the need to move by traction the lower lateral fat of the mandible (inferior jowl fat)

Tilt the device until the vertical bars are positioned horizontally, positioning the device in the horizontal plane until the number zero of the aluminum base rulers touches the patient's chin. The rulers should touch the most posterior part of the jaw. To harmonize a face in this circumstance, one can use suspension sutures to traction the lateral fat of the face (jowl fat). In cases like this, the gonion could receive fillers to make the posterior part of the mandible the widest part.

OBJECTIVE: To aid the diagnosis with the use of suspension wires for facial harmonization.

Frontal Facial Diagram

One of the ways we recognize an object is through the points that constitute its anatomy. Every geometric figure is formed by a group of points. Straight lines are originated from points displaced in a determined plane, without a curve. A *line segment* is defined as a segment connecting two points. The more noticeable these points and straight lines, the more defined a face and, therefore, the more esthetic. Rounded and less defined faces are less esthetic and more childlike. However, a face can become more defined and esthetic with the use of fillers when they are applied to value these strategic points, resulting in points that are more evident and that show an adequate proportion.

The union of cephalometric points results in a facial diagram suggested by the author to help with the facial analysis (Fig 5-8). According to the author, connecting these cephalometric points

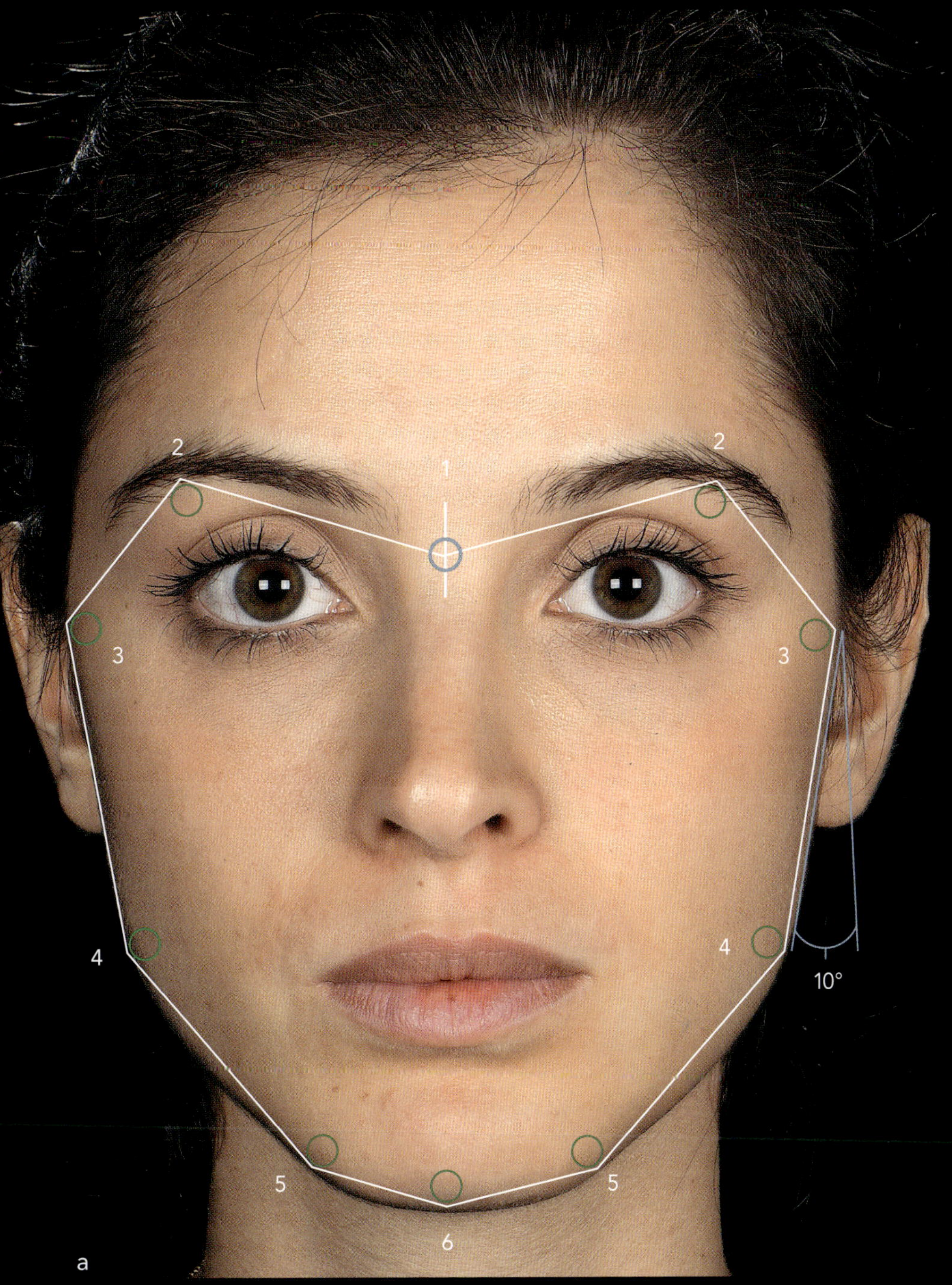

Fig 5-8 *(a)* The union of cephalometric points to create a facial diagram: 1, nasion; 2, eyebrow arching point; 3, zygion; 4, gonion; 5, menton lateral; 6, menton. The points were placed inside the facial contour to indicate where the filler should be injected. In this case, the mandible body asymmetry is not significant. A small asymmetry at the horizontal level of the eyebrow is observed, where the right side is lower than the left side. The angle formed by the difference between the bizygomatic and bigonial distances is 10 degrees.

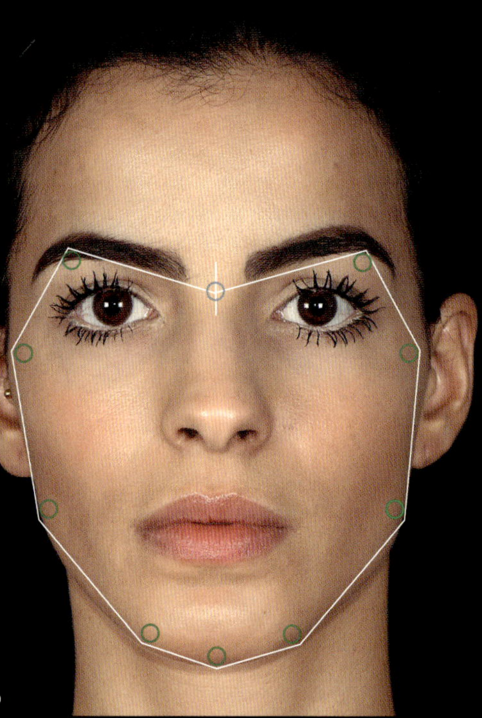

b

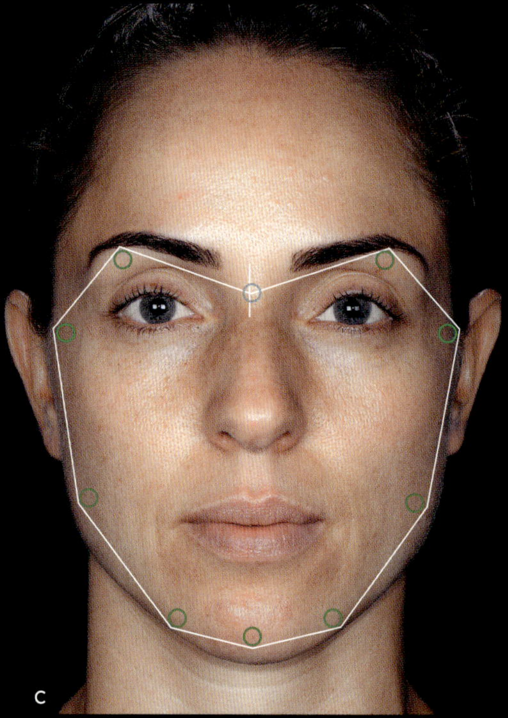

c

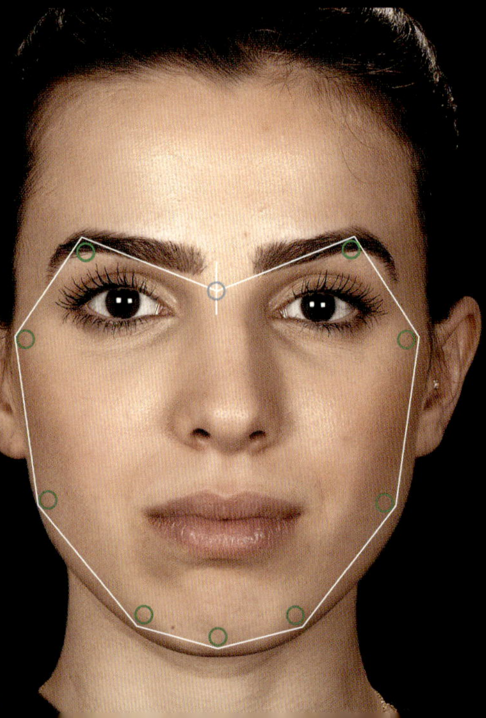

d

Fig 5-8 *(cont) (b)* Facial diagram in a different individual. In this case, there is a small asymmetry in the gonion, where the left gonion is more prominent. Note that although there is a slight asymmetry in the level of the eyebrows, the arching is ideal. *(c)* Facial diagram in a different individual. Note that the eyebrows are perfectly symmetric, the face is long, and the patient shows a masseter hypertrophy. *(d)* Facial diagram in a different individual. Because the face is wide, the eyebrow could be more arched to make the face look longer.

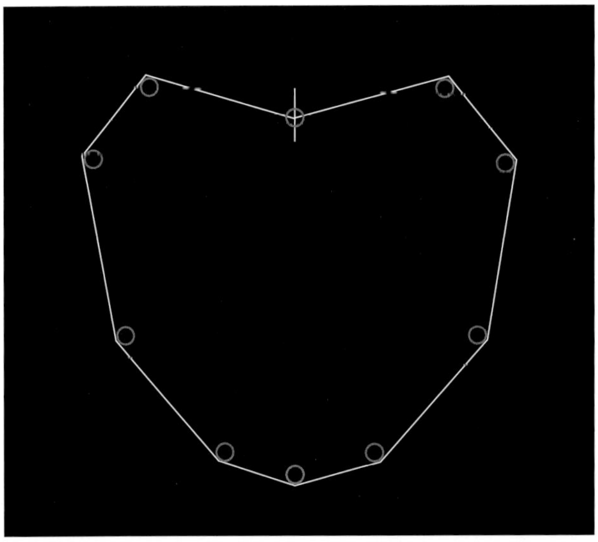

Fig 5-9 Figure available via QR code. The *green circle* is the point where the filler could be injected, and the *vertical line* is the midline. Measure the distance between the inner canthus of the eye and position the midline in the center of the measurement.

with straight lines forms a geometric figure with the approximate shape of a heart. This figure can be used as a diagram placed over the patient's face to do the following:

- Help the operator decide whether to inject a filler in a certain area
- Define the location of points to be filled
- Evaluate the proportion among the points
- Verify facial asymmetries
- Classify a face as mesocephalic, dolichocephalic, or brachycephalic
- Search for masseter hypertrophy

How to use it:

1. Copy the image available via QR code (Fig 5-9).
2. Paste the diagram over the photograph of the patient to be evaluated.
3. If using a PC, hold the Shift key while adjusting the figure. If using a Mac, use the function "constrain proportions." This will maintain the photographic proportions.

The cardinal points in the face might be filled so that they become more noticeable, improving the face contouring. This might influence the inclination of the lines between the points (Fig 5-10). Single or multiple filler injections can be performed depending on the goal of the treatment. After the injections, the skin tends to be more stretched, smoothing out wrinkles and furrows.

EYEBROW ARCHING POINT

Location: Following the path of the eyebrow, between the middle and outer third.

The use of fillers in this case might:

1. Change the face shape into a more dolichofacial pattern.
2. Help lift the brow and project it horizontally.
3. Diminish the dominance of the eyeball.

ZYGION

Location: Laterally and over the zygomatic arch.

The use of fillers in this case might:

1. Make the face more triangular.
2. Accentuate the depression between the zygomatic bone and the gonial angle.
3. Accentuate the temporal fossa.

GONION

Location: Gonial angle.

The use of fillers in this case might:

1. Change the face to a more square shape.
2. Accentuate the depression between the zygomatic bone and the gonial angle.
3. Help define the contour and mandibular ramus.

MENTON LATERAL

Location: Between the chin and mandibular body.

The use of fillers in this case might:

1. Change the chin to a more square shape.
2. Help define the contour of the mandibular body.

MENTON

Location: Base of the chin along the midline.

The use of fillers in this case might:

1. Result in a longer face.
2. Equalize the proportion of the lower third of the face.

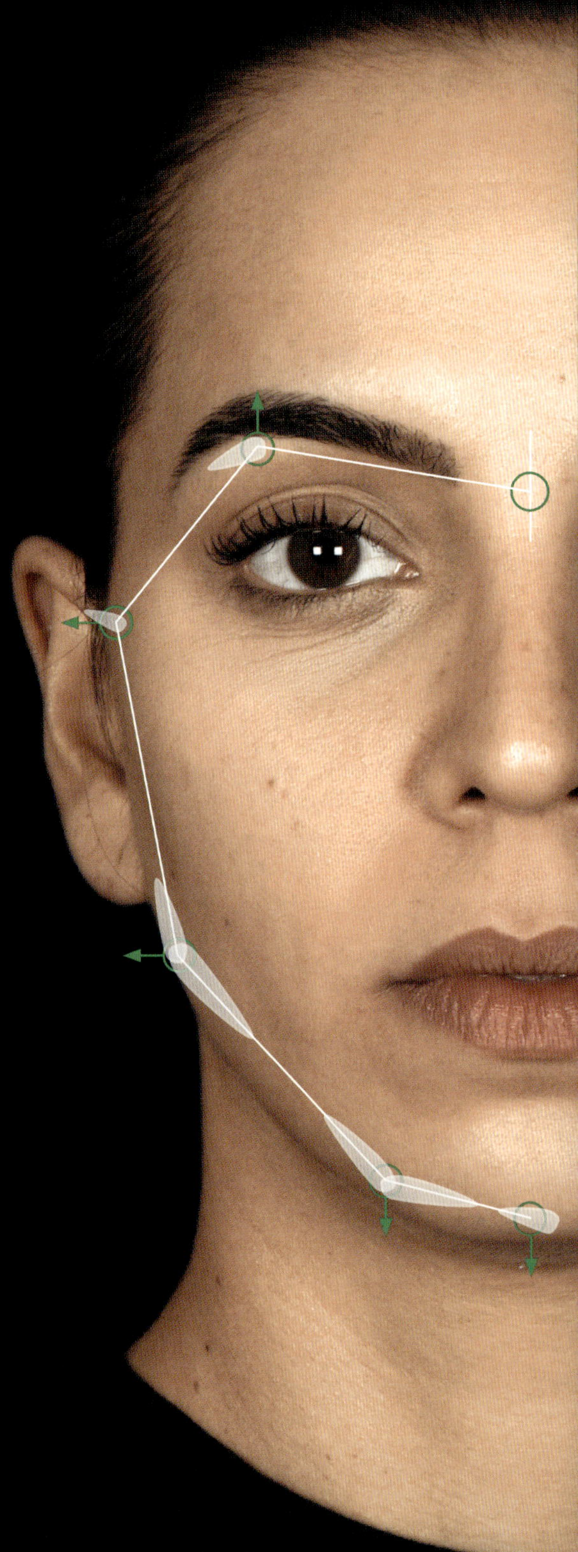

Fig 5-10 Dermal filler injection into the cardinal points can change the contouring of the face.

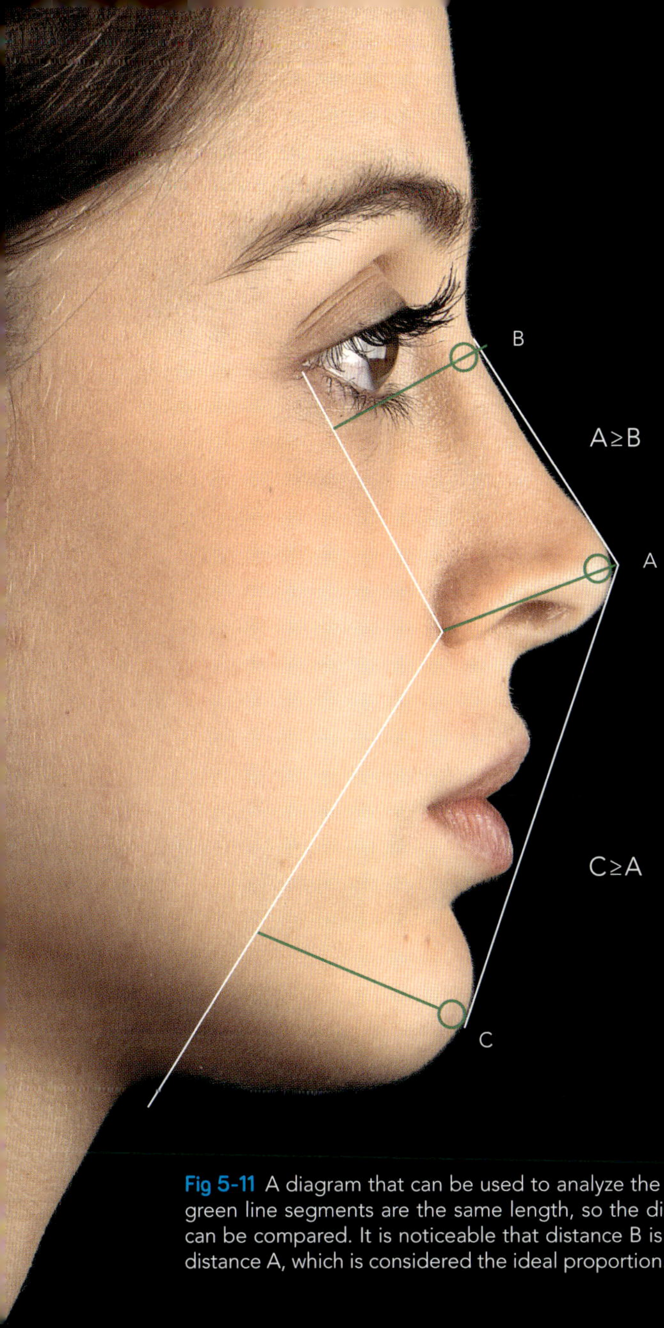

NASAL ROOT

Location: It lies between the end of the glabella and beginning of the nose at the nasion point.

The use of fillers in this case might:

1. Increase the projection of the nasal bridge.
2. Reduce a dominant nasal tip.
3. Regulate a dominant eye globe.
4. Smooth out the curvature in aquiline noses.

This is a dangerous procedure (see chapter 7).

NASAL TIP

Location: Tip of the nose.

The use of fillers in this case might:

1. Increase the projection of the nasal tip.
2. Reduce a dominant nasal bridge and chin.
3. Accentuate a convex profile.
4. Smooth out the curvature in aquiline noses.
5. Decrease the apparent width of the nose.

This is a dangerous procedure (see chapter 7).

SOFT TISSUE POGONION

Location: The most anterior point of the chin.

The use of fillers in this case might:

1. Decrease the profile convexity.
2. Highlight the limit between the head/neck and the mandibular body.
3. Reduce a dominant nose.

Fig 5-11 A diagram that can be used to analyze the external and internal profiles. In the diagram, all three green line segments are the same length, so the distances between the white lines at points A, B, and C can be compared. It is noticeable that distance B is smaller than distance A, and distance C is larger than distance A, which is considered the ideal proportion.

Profile Proportions and Diagram

In general, the profile is evaluated according to three external landmarks: the nasal root, the nasal tip, and the soft tissue pogonion. The analysis should include these landmarks, but it should be supplemented with the balance of the "internal profile" formed by three other landmarks: the outer canthus, the beginning of the ala nasi, and the mentocervical angle. The external profile can be adjusted with fillers. Figure 5-11 shows a diagram that can be used to analyze these profiles.

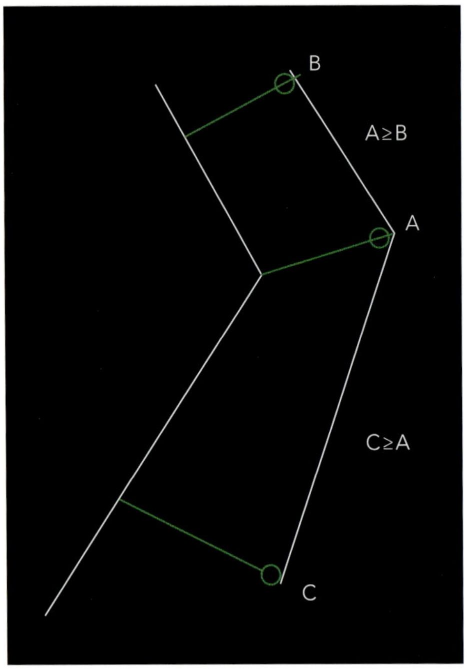

Fig 5-12 Diagram available via QR code. See below for instructions.

How to use it:

1. Copy the image available via QR code (Fig 5-12).
2. Paste the diagram over the photograph of the patient to be evaluated.
3. Adjust the figure to the patient's profile, clicking and dragging the corners of the white lines. Based on the position of the final intersection of these lines, the green circles should be positioned.
4. Repeat the step above for the nasal tip line. Delete other green lines.
5. Copy line A and paste the duplicates in the positions B and C, always maintaining the same length for the three lines.
6. Read the results: Line A should be greater (ideal) or equal to line B. Distance C should be equal or greater (ideal) than distance A.

Figure 5-13 shows various examples of interpretation of the results.

True vertical line

The true vertical line is often used to evaluate the facial profile. The true vertical line is created by drawing a vertical line that passes by the subnasale point. From this line, a digital ruler can be used to measure the distances from facial points to the line (Fig 5-14).[5-10] The line position can be slightly changed by injecting a filler at the subnasale angle. Ideally, the line should not touch the glabella; otherwise, the profile might look straight and boring.

E-line

A line that touches the nasal tip and the chin can be used to evaluate the treatment plan with fillers (Fig 5-15). For the measurement to be considered acceptable, the lower lip should be 0 to 4 mm short of this line, while the upper lip is 2 to 6 mm short of it. A profile considered desirable is one where the distance up to the E-line is as small as possible within the limits mentioned above.[11,12]

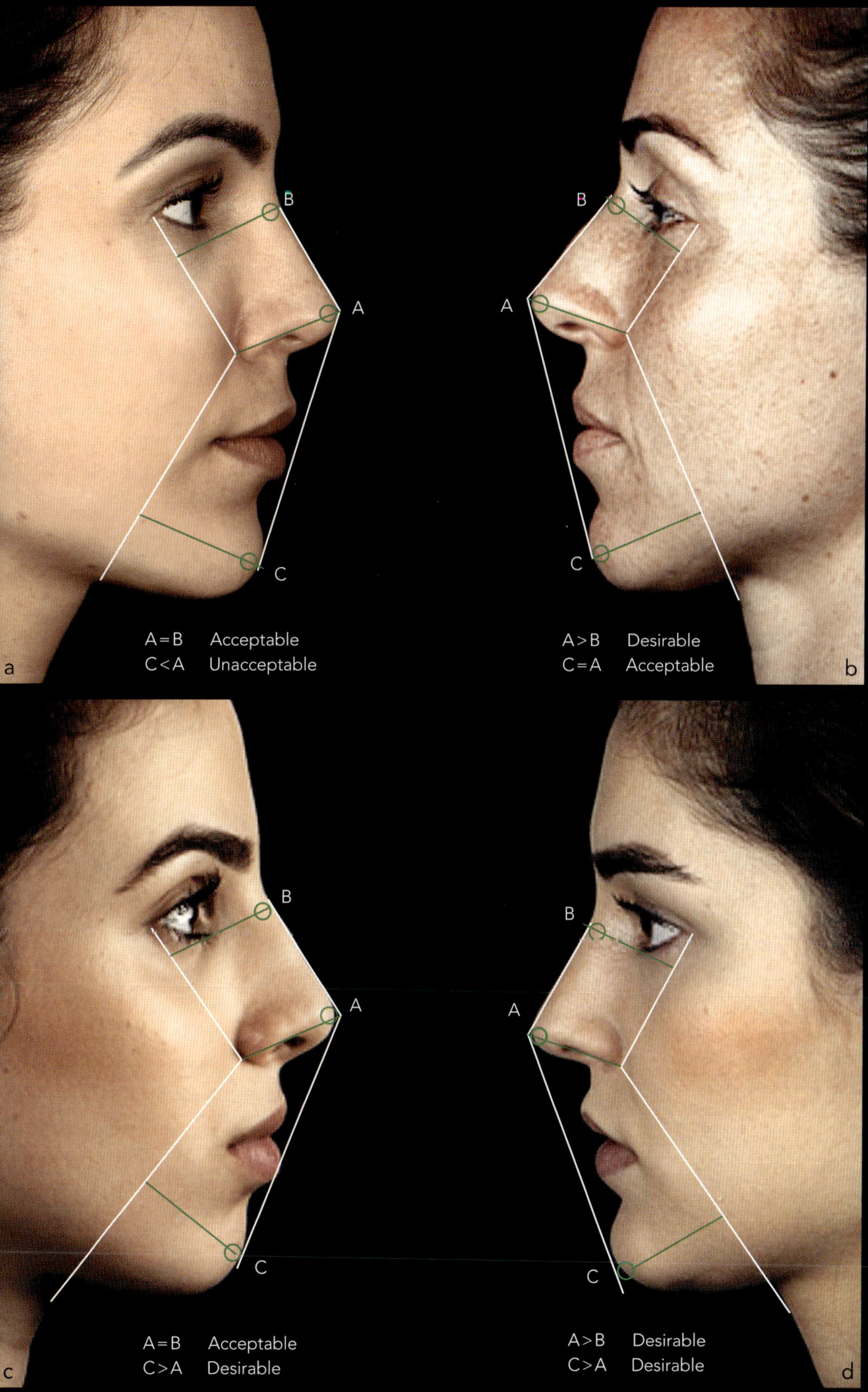

Fig 5-13 Interpretation of the results in four examples. The ideal proportions are A > B and C > A. *(a)* Distance A is equal to distance B, which is considered acceptable but not desirable. A possible solution would be to use fillers at the nasal tip. On the other hand, distance C is shorter than distance A, which is unacceptable. In this case, a possible solution would be to use fillers at the chin. *(b)* Distance A is greater than distance B, which is considered desirable. Distance C is equal to distance A, which is acceptable, but a small amount of filler injected in the chin would define C as being visibly larger than A. *(c)* Distance A is equal to distance B, which is acceptable. In order to make it desirable, a filler could be injected at the nasal tip. Distance C is greater than distance A, which is desirable. *(d)* Distance A is greater than distance B, which is desirable. And distance C is greater than distance A, which is also considered desirable.

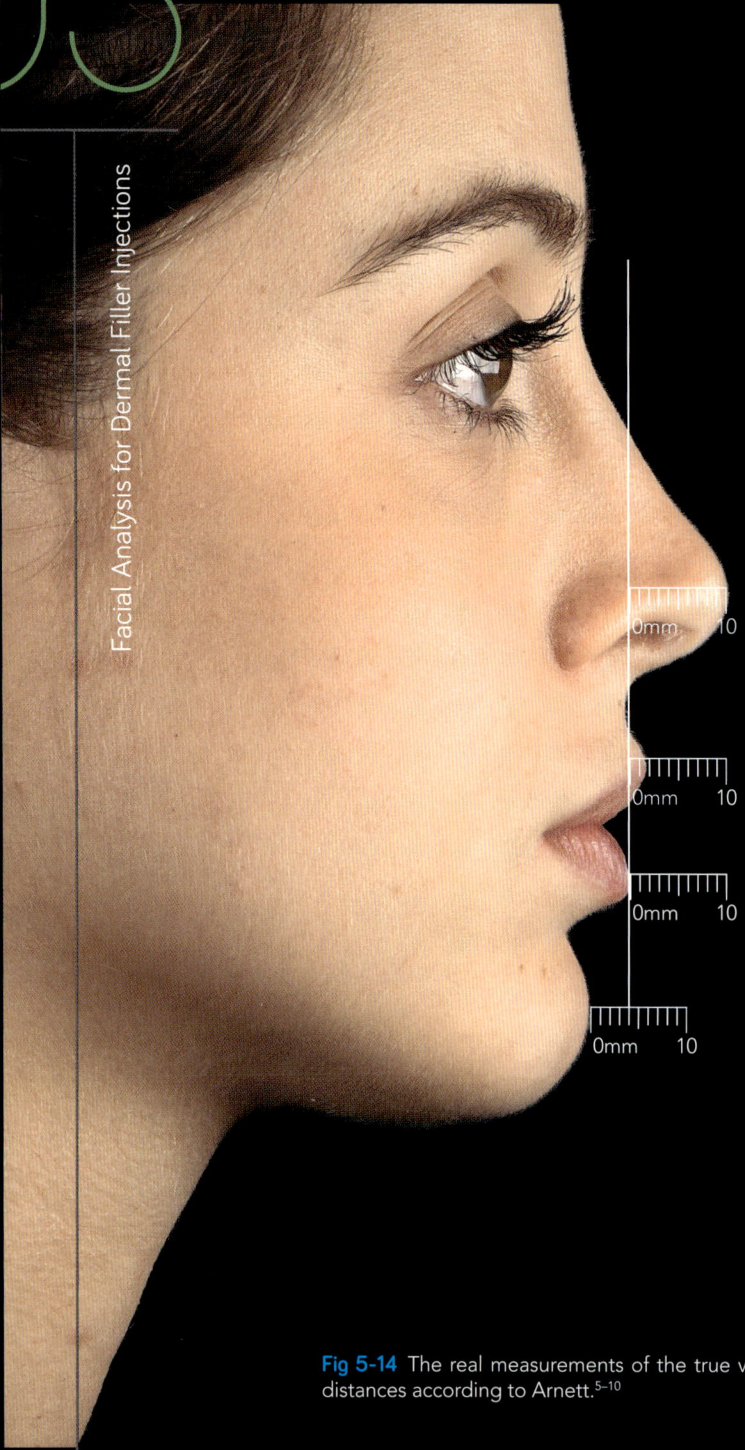

NOSE

Distance: It should be 8 to 10 mm past the line. The filler could be injected at the nasal tip and supratip in order to:

1. Horizontally project the nose.
2. Increase the profile convexity.
3. Reduce the chin dominance.

UPPER LIP

Distance: It should be 2 to 5 mm past the line. The filler could be injected to evert the upper lip in order to:

1. Horizontally project the upper lip.
2. Improve the definition of the white roll.
3. Smooth out lip rhytids.

LOWER LIP

Distance: It should be 0 to 3 mm past the line. The filler could be injected to evert the lower lip in order to:

1. Horizontally project the lip.
2. Improve the definition of the skin/vermilion.
3. Smooth out lip rhytids.

SOFT TISSUE POGONION

Distance: It should be 0 to 4 mm short of the line. The filler could be injected to advance the chin in order to:

1. Horizontally project the chin.
2. Decrease the nose dominance.
3. Improve the contour of the head/neck and mandibular body.
4. Decrease the profile convexity.

Fig 5-14 The real measurements of the true vertical line in this patient. See QR code for the average distances according to Arnett.[5–10]

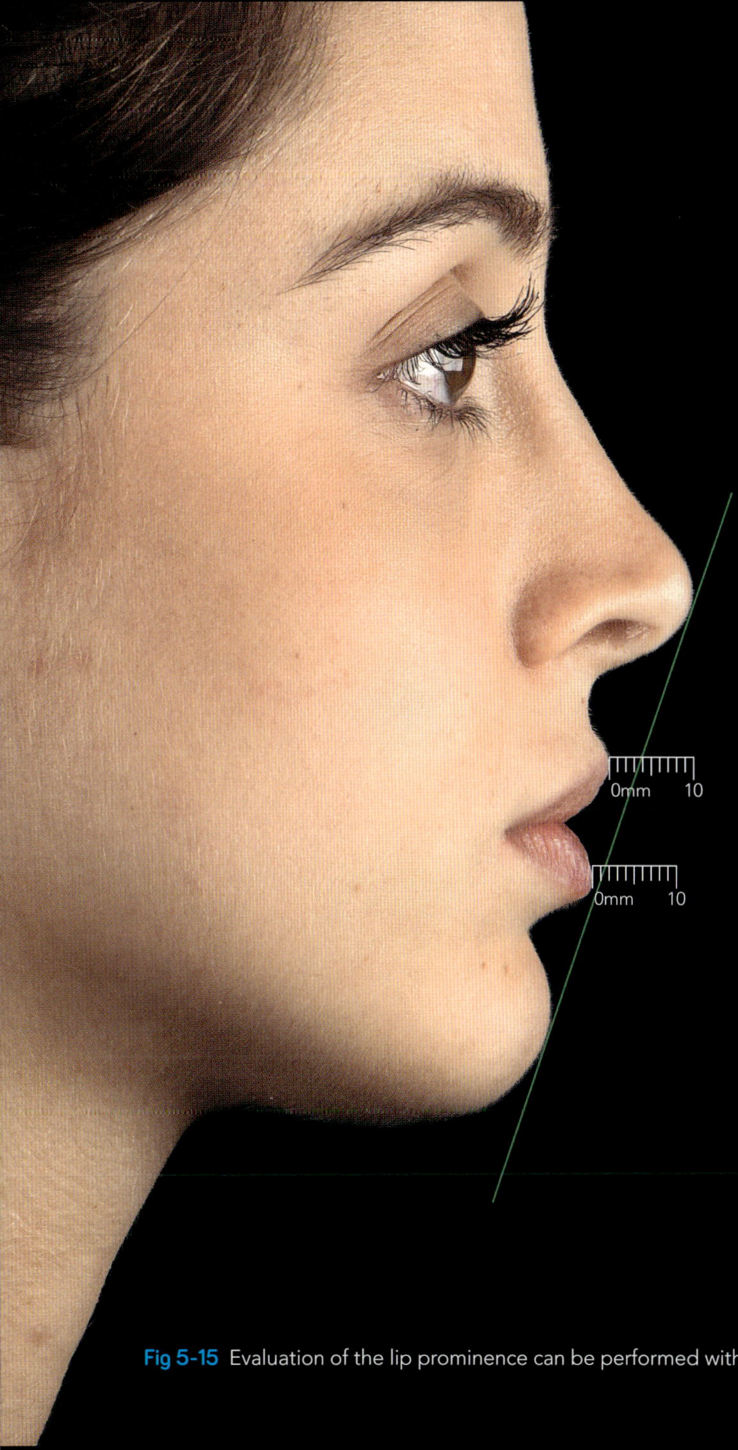

E-LINE

According to Ricketts analysis, the E-line or esthetic line runs from the tip of the nose to the soft tissue pogonion.

This measurement is an indication of soft tissue balance between the lips and the facial profile.

It can be useful as an indicator of functional abnormalities of the lip.

The lips are analyzed depending on their distance from this line.

In the average Caucasian, the lower lip is 2 mm short of this line, while the upper lip is 4 mm short of this line. Variations are normal for patients of different ethnic backgrounds, but there are still some common aspects that could be applied to all patients.

Fig 5-15 Evaluation of the lip prominence can be performed with the E-line.

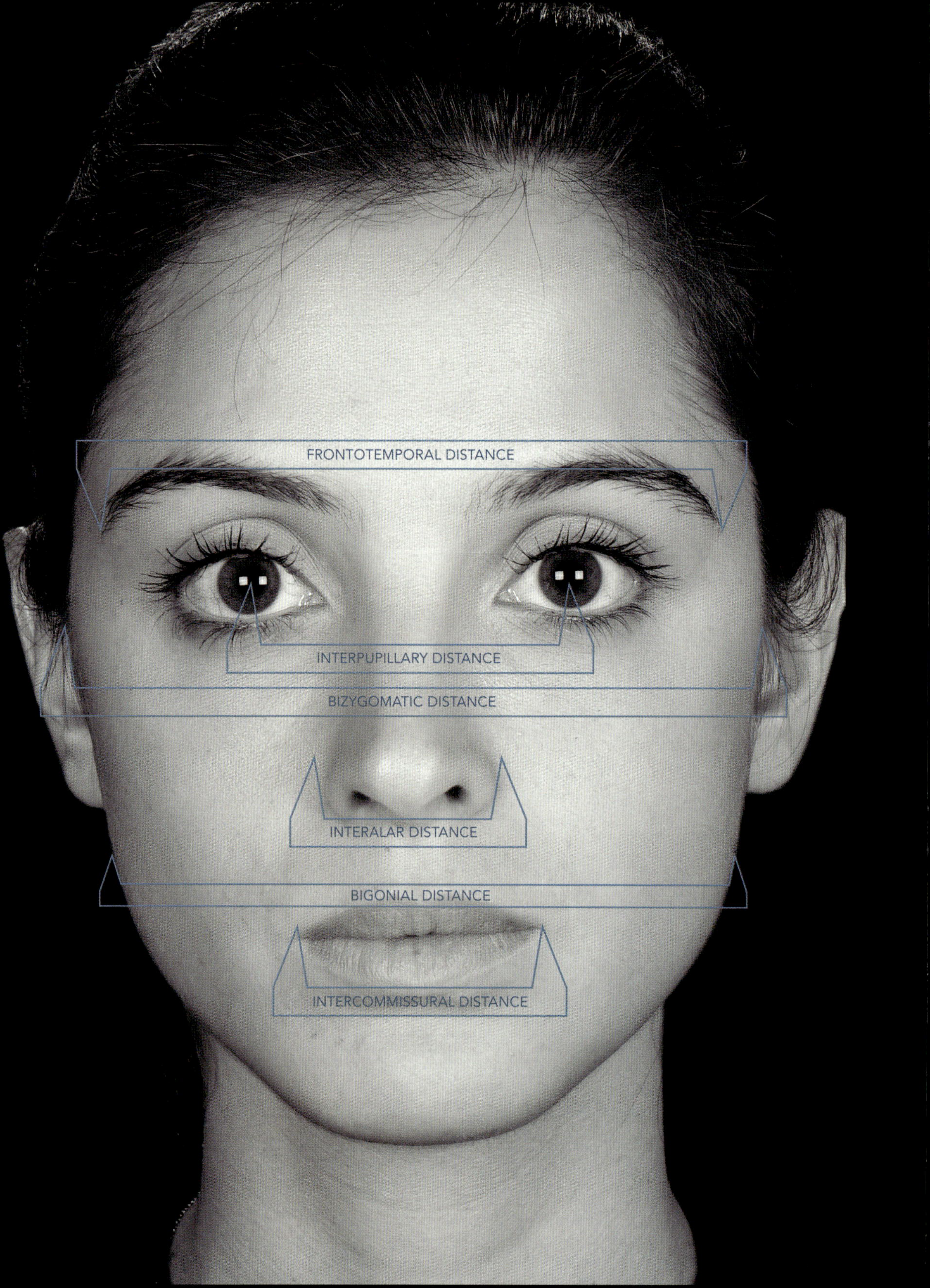

Fig 5-16 Ideal position of the caliper for horizontal facial measurements.

Average Horizontal Dimensions in Frontal View

Several horizontal dimensions are important when considering and planning filler treatments (Fig 5-16).

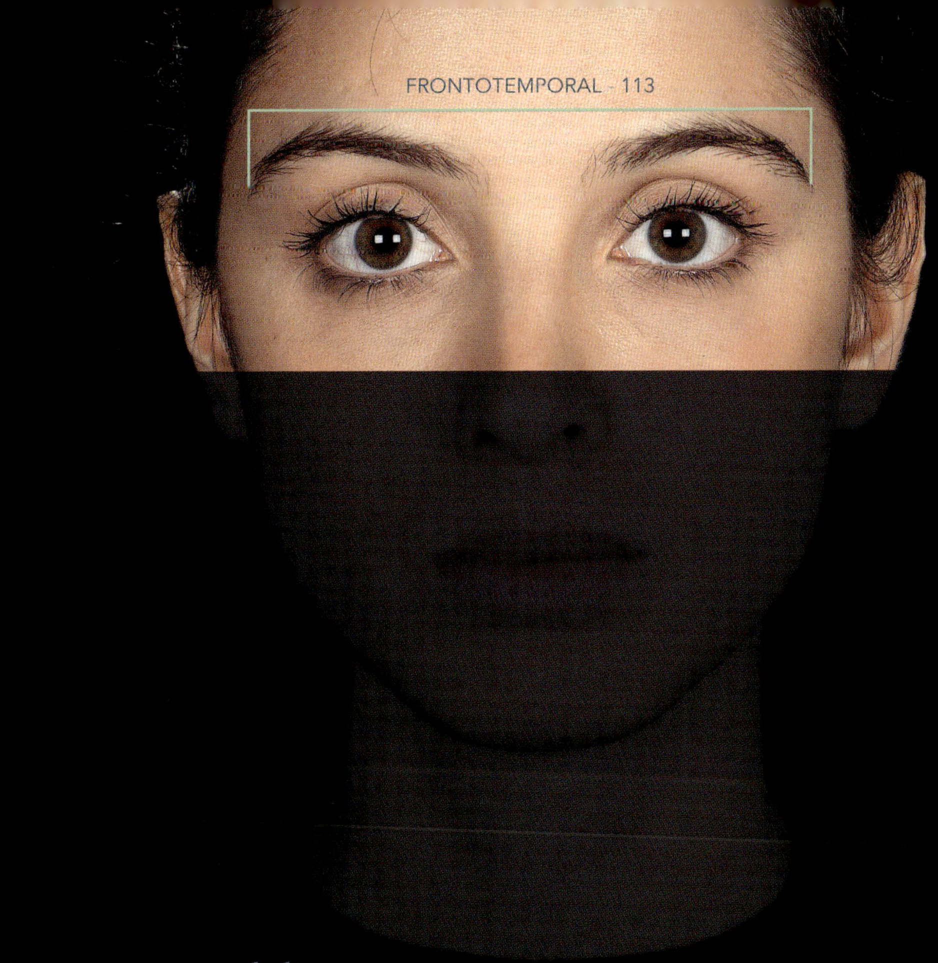

Frontotemporal distance (bitemporal width)

n a frontal view, the lateral contour of the face, given by a line drawn from the frontotemporal point to the mandible gonion, originates the external contour of the face, which is a result of the proportional relationship between the width of the upper, median, and lower parts of the forehead. The bitemporal width, measured from the most lateral point of the face (frontotemporal, Ft), represents 80% to 85% of the bizygomatic distance and should be the widest distance found in the face.[13]

Importance of the measurement

- Gives the observer the perception of age: In older patients, this distance is decreased due to the flattening of the bony orbit.
- Influences the ocular dominance: The greater the distance, the less dominant the eyes will be.

Example of applicability

Around the age of 35 years, individuals tend to show a bone loss in the lateral upper part of the bony orbit. Flattening of this area will make the face look older. On the other hand, a filler injected in this area would rejuvenate it.

How to measure

Consider the orbital bone at the level of the eyebrow tail.

Rule

The ideal difference between the frontotemporal distance and the bizygomatic distance should be approximately 16%.

Use of fillers at the frontotemporal area

- Frontal view: It causes a slight increase in volume that contributes to brow arching. The area becomes brighter. It can also stretch the skin so that the eyelid ptosis can be slightly reduced.
- Lateral view: It increases the space between the eyelid and the brow.

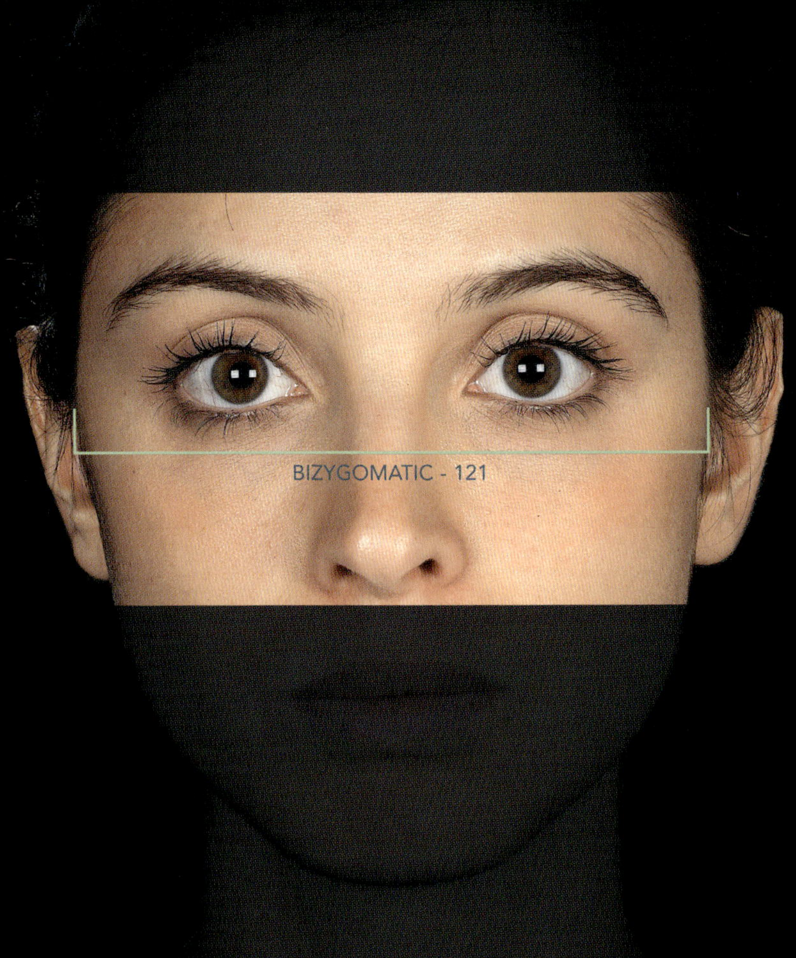

Bizygomatic distance

The bizygomatic distance is the distance between the two zygion (Zy) points. It should be the widest part of the face. This distance is 119.2 ± 4.9 mm in women and 127.5 ± 5.9 mm in men.[4]

Importance of the measurement

- Helps with the perception of a more defined face.
- Suggests that the individual is not overweight.
- A visible zygomatic volume suggests a more adult face.

Examples of applicability

- In cases of masseter hypertrophy, botulinum toxin can be injected at the masseter muscle. The injection will decrease the bigonial distance. The bizygomatic distance can also be increased with linear filler injections over the zygomatic area in the superficial fat to confirm that the bizygomatic distance is greater than the bigonial distance. This procedure is a good tool when deciding whether to use a filler at the zygomatic area. The bigonial distance, measured from the soft tissue overlying the most lateral point on the angle of each mandible (soft gonion, Go), in general represents 70% to 75% of the bizygomatic distance.[13]
- An excessive interpupillary distance can be improved by using fillers at the zygomatic area.
- Fillers injected at the zygomatic area could be used to decrease the perception of a round face.
- Fillers injected at the zygomatic area can slightly smooth out wrinkles in the side of the face.

How to measure

In frontal view, consider the widest point in the face at the level of the zygomatic bones.

Rules

- Bizygomatic distance – 11% = bigonial distance: According to the literature, the bigonial distance is 70% to 75% of the bizygomatic distance.[8,9,13] However, the average found in the models studied by the author was different. For further details, see the section on facial proportions.
- The length/height and width proportion is 1.3:1 in women and 1.35:1 in men.[8,9] That is, the bizygomatic distance is 70% of the height of the face.

Use of fillers at the zygomatic area

- Frontal view: A lateral bump is formed in relation to the temporal and cheek regions.
- Lateral view: It helps to create a depression between the zygomatic and jugal area similar to the one observed after a bichectomy.
- The area where the filler was injected becomes brighter.

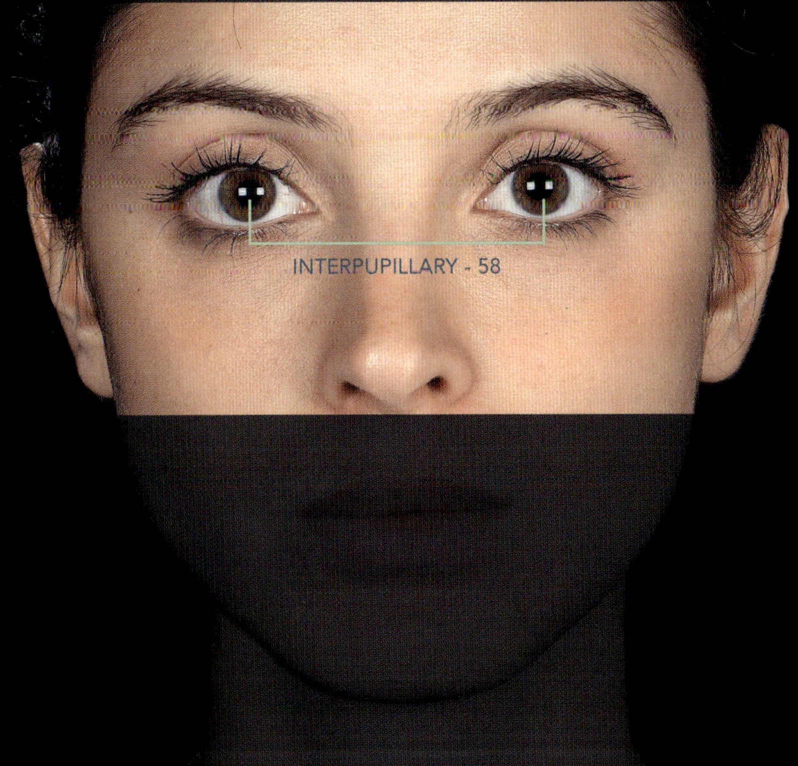

Interpupillary distance

The interpupillary distance is the distance measured between the two pupils. The average interpupillary distance is 60 mm.

Importance of the measurement

- Helps with the perception of the face width.
- Because it becomes stable after the age of 6 to 8 years, this measurement becomes a reference for other measurements that can change over time.[14,15]

Example of applicability

An interpupillary distance greater than 60 mm is above the average and requires that the mouth, lower jaw, bony rim of the orbit, malar area, and teeth are dominant in terms of width.[16] In order to be dominant, their measurements should be proportionally greater than the average width. This helps identify the points that need to be treated with fillers.

How to measure

Consider the center of each pupil to correctly position the caliper.

Rules

- The interpupillary distance divided by 6.6 equals the width of the maxillary central incisor.
- The width of the maxillary central incisor times 16 is the facial width. This parameter was established in a study performed by Cesario and Latta[15] in a North American population.

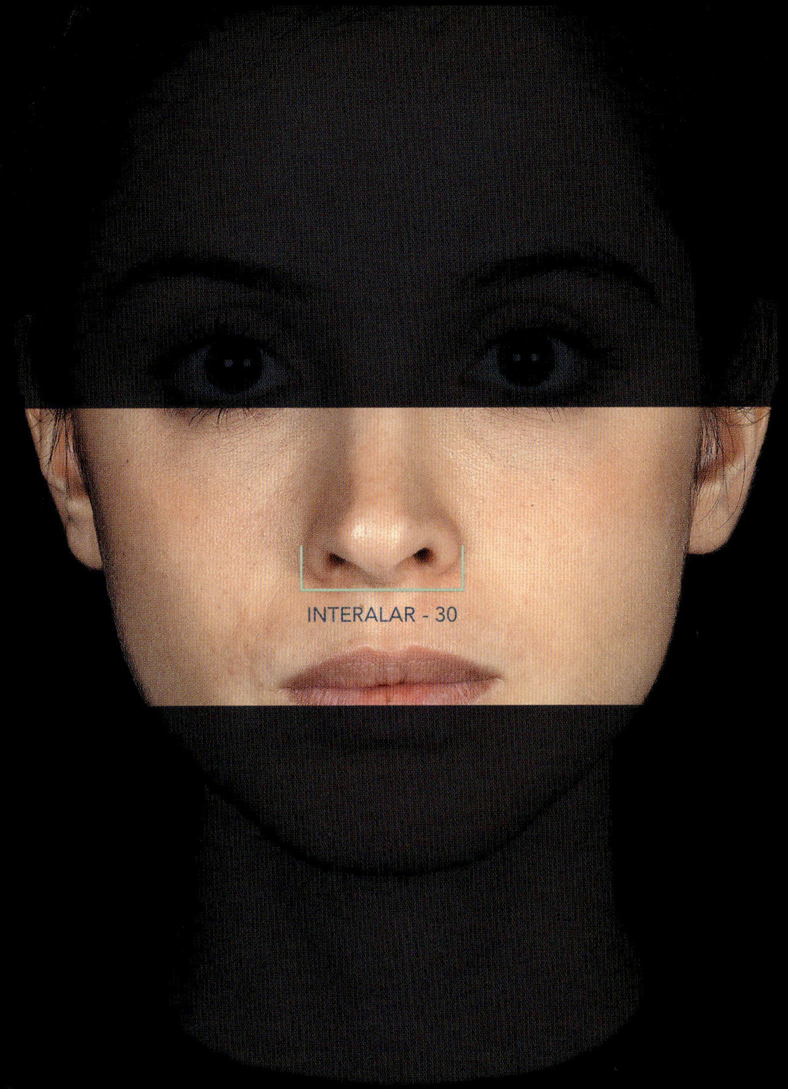

Interalar distance

The interalar distance is the distance between the two alae nasi. The ala nasi is the lateral prolongation of the lobe, and it consists primarily of cartilage. The average measurement between the two nasal wings is the nose thickness, which based on the classic anthropometry standards corresponds to one-fifth the width of the face in frontal view.[16] The average interalar distance found by Galantucci et al[2] was 31.6 mm in Caucasian women. The average nose width according to Fradeani[17] is 34 to 36 mm.

Importance of the measurement

The nasal width influences the perception of the mouth width.

Examples of applicability

- A dominant wide nose suggests that the mouth should also be dominant, which can be made by injecting fillers at the lips.
- A very narrow nose suggests that in case a labial filling is needed, only a small amount of the filler should be used.
- An excessively wide nose can be reshaped by injecting fillers at and above the nasal tip (supratip area). However, this type of procedure is very dangerous (see chapter 7).

How to measure

With the patient at rest, place the caliper in a way that it gently touches the side of the alae nasi.

Rules

- In most cases, the nasal width is greater than its length (from the base of the nose to the tip). When the nose is longer than it is wide, it will look too long.
- In a frontal view, a line tangent to the ala nasi at rest should touch the medial palpebral fissure or the semilunar fold in the corner of the eye. If it touches the sclera, it means that the nose is too wide for this face. If the patient does not want to undergo a rhinoplasty to narrow the nose, the use of fillers at the nasal tip or lip vermilion can smooth out the excessive width.

Use of fillers in the supratip area

- Can decrease the apparent nasal width.
- Can give the impression of an upturned nose.
- Can produce a supratip break, depending on the desired sculpture.

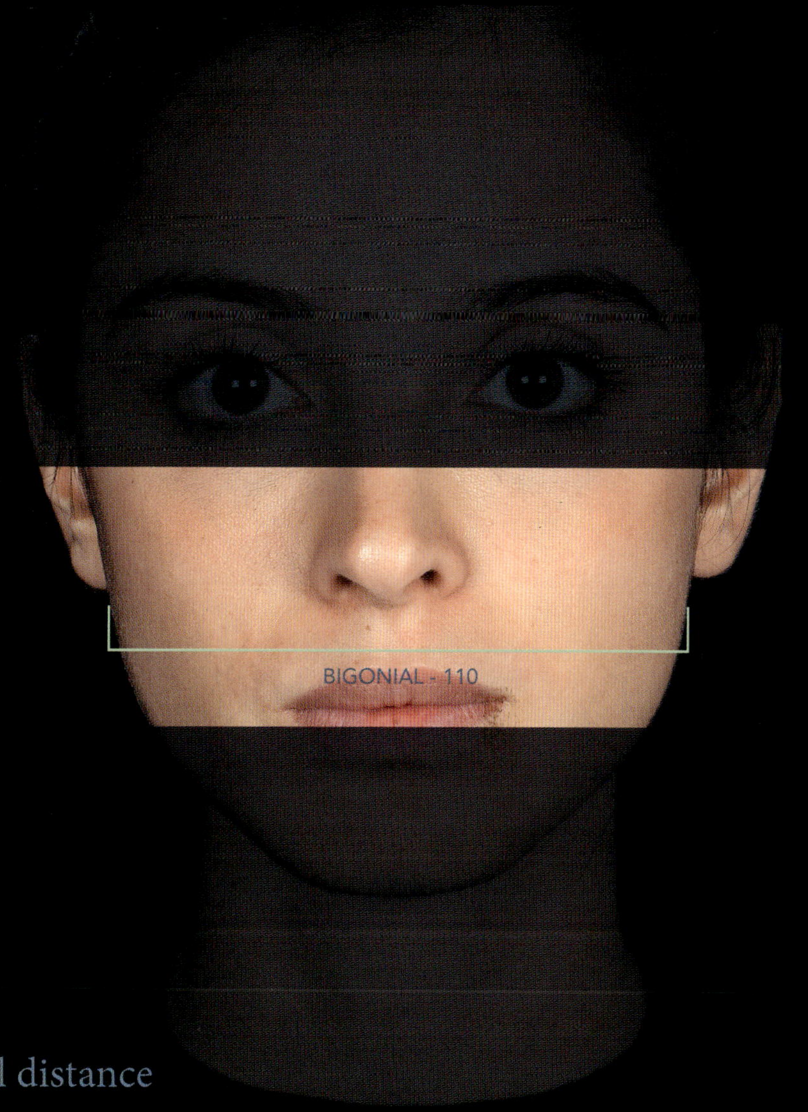

Bigonial distance

The bigonial distance is the distance between the right and left gonion (Go-Go). The average bigonial distance is 89.3 ± 5.7 mm in women and 97.7 ± 6.3 mm in men.[4]

Importance of the measurement

- Helps with the perception of a defined face because it contributes to the definition of a limit between the head and neck.
- Helps to give the impression that the individual is thin.
- A marked gonial angle suggests a more adult face.
- Because seniors have a poorly defined jawline, this helps differentiate the young from the elderly.

Examples of applicability

- In cases of a poorly defined jawline, a filler can help redefine this contour.
- An excessive bizygomatic distance can be improved with fillers injected at the gonial angle.
- In round faces, fillers injected at the gonial and zygomatic angles lead to a concavity between these two areas, showing a result similar to a buccal fat pad reduction.
- A visibly defined gonial angle gives the observer the perception of strength.
- Smooth out wrinkles in the side of the face

How to measure

In a lateral view, mark a point in the gonial angle using a makeup pencil. Then from a frontal view, position the caliper and measure the distance between these two points.

Rules

- Bigonial distance = bizygomatic distance – 11%: When this difference is less than 4%, it might suggest a masseter hypertrophy. If the masseter is hyperkinetic, it can show an increased volume, causing an increase in the bigonial distance and resulting in a smaller difference between the bizygomatic and bigonial distances.
- A bizygomatic distance larger than the bigonial distance might indicate a masseter hypertrophy.
- A very narrow gonial angle might indicate a mandibular deficiency, suggesting the injection of a filler and potentially also a chin advancement or the use of fillers at the chin.

Use of fillers at the gonial angle

- Frontal view: It creates a lateral bump in relation to the jugal area.
- Lateral view: It creates an angle between the mandibular ramus and body.

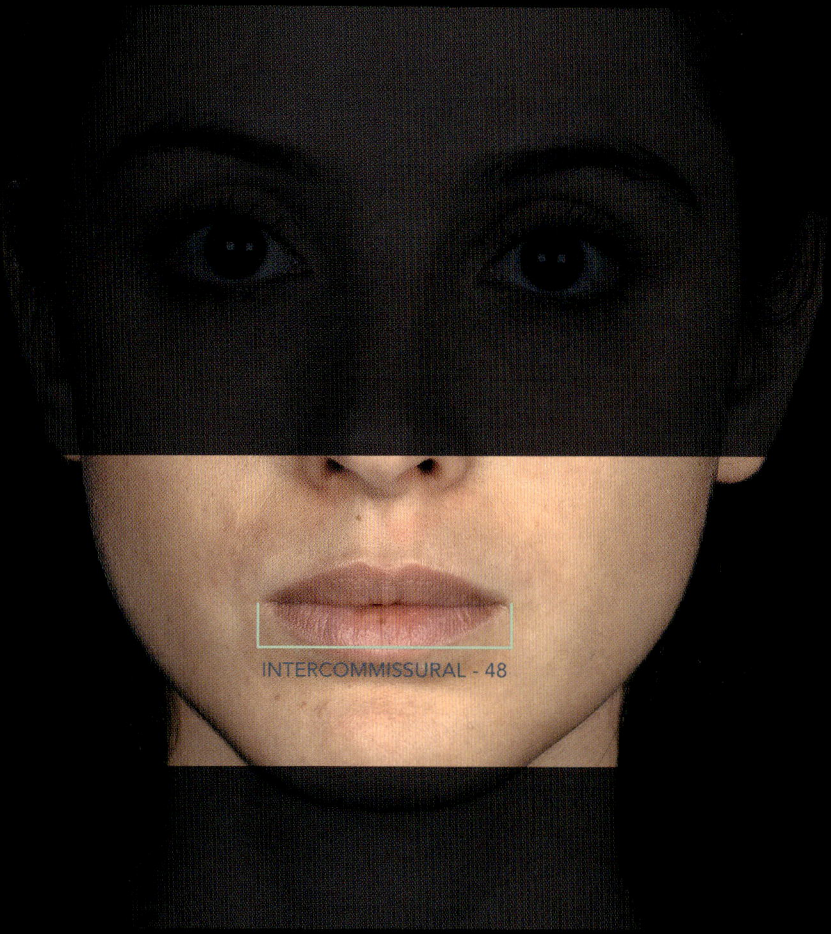

Intercommissural distance

The oral intercommissural distance is the mouth width. The average oral intercommissural distance is 45.70 ± 2.77 mm in Caucasian women.[2] In men, this average is 50 mm.

Importance of the measurement

- Helps with the perception of sensuality.
- Increases the sensuality.
- Balances the dominance of the nasojugal region.

Examples of applicability

An increase in the mouth width can:

- Decrease the dominance of a very dominant nose.
- Provide harmony for a wide lower third of the face.
- Smooth out labial wrinkles.

How to measure

Consider the widest point in the mouth at the level of the oral commissures.

Rules

- In a frontal view and with the face at rest, a vertical line tangent to the medial part of the iris of the eye should touch the oral commissure. If the commissure is short of the line, the mouth is considered narrow, suggesting that fillers should be used to increase its length. On the other hand, if the commissure is beyond this line, in case a filler injection is needed, the width of the mouth should not be increased.
- A mouth wider than 50 mm is considered a dominant mouth in terms of width, suggesting that the bigonial and bizygomatic distances should also be dominant. This can be achieved by using fillers in this region.
- According to Suguino,[14] the ideal mouth width (at rest) is equal to the distance between the irises.

Use of fillers at the lips

- Frontal view: By using a filler from the lip vermilion to the commissure, the mouth width is increased by up to 2 mm on each side. To use a filler at the lip vermilion without increasing the width of the mouth, leave 3 mm in length of vermilion in the commissures free of fillers.
- Lateral view: The horizontal position of one or both lips can be advanced to adjust the patient's profile to the true vertical line.

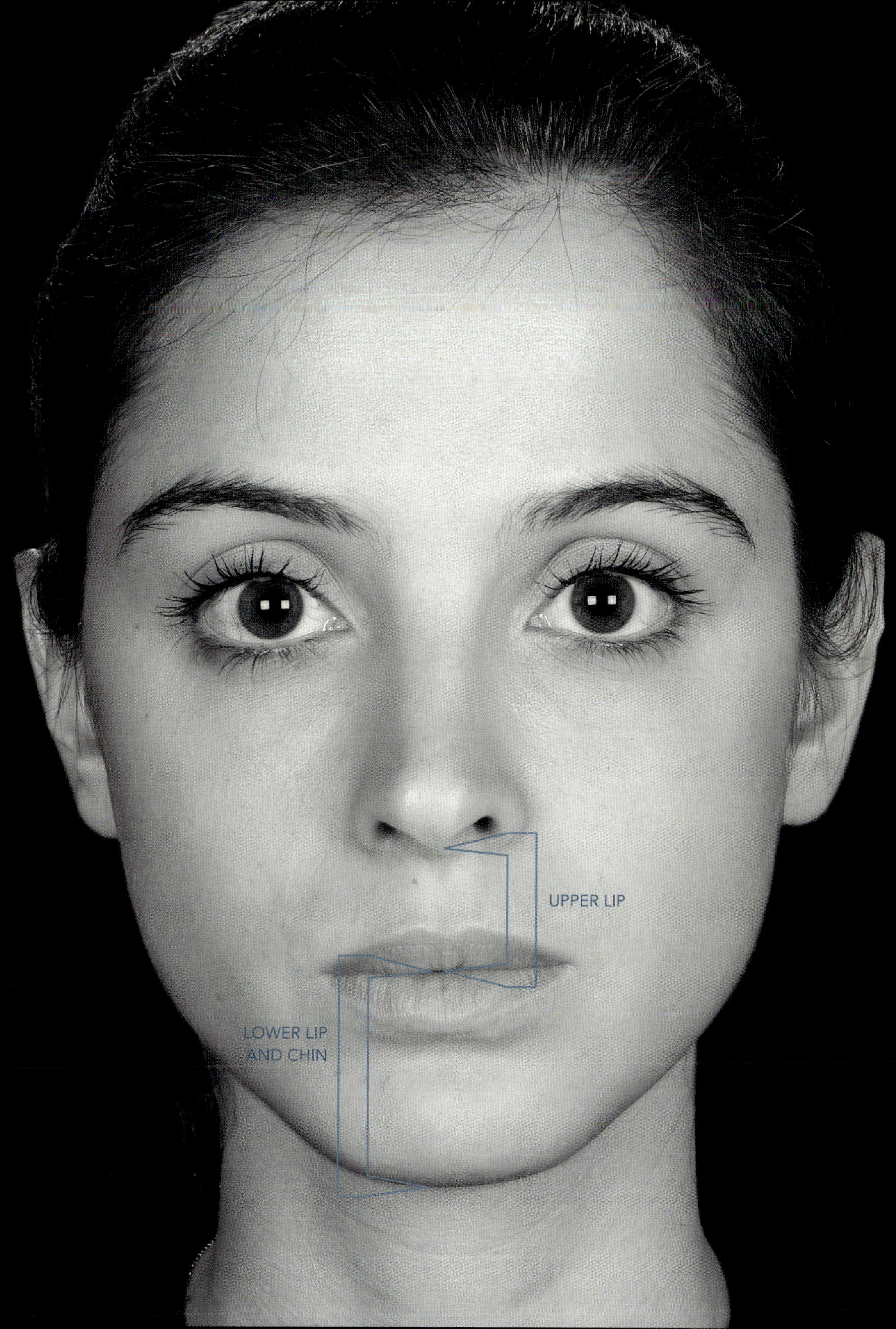

Fig 5-17 Ideal position of the caliper for vertical facial measurements, corresponding to the distance from the subnasale point to the stomion and from the stomion to the menton.

Average Vertical Dimensions in Frontal View

Multiple vertical dimensions are important when considering and planning filler treatments (Fig 5-17).

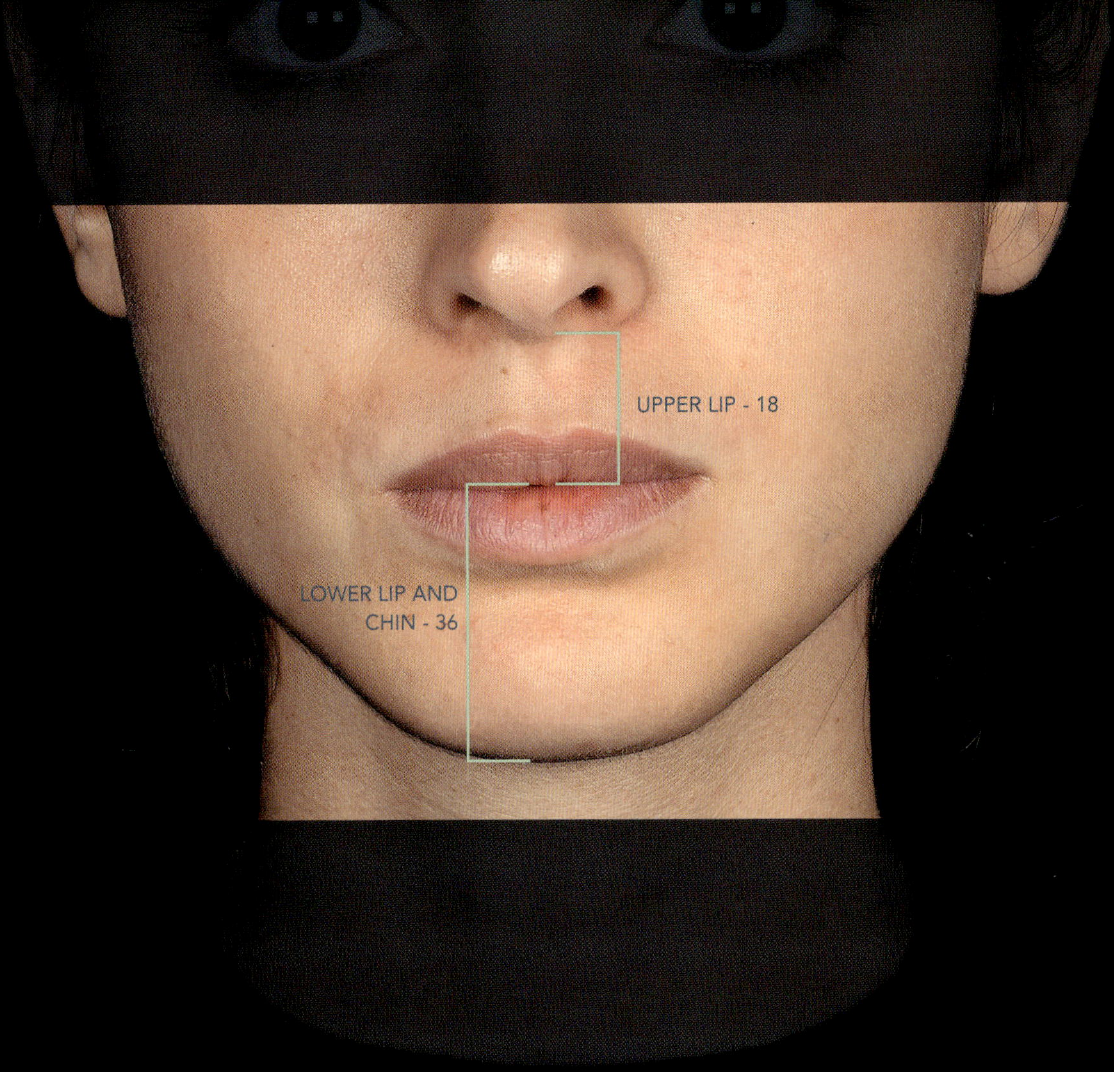

Upper and lower lips

The upper lip corresponds to the region located between the subnasale and the stomion, which should occupy one-third of the subnasale-chin distance.[18,19] Its normal length, measured from the subnasale to the most inferior point at the lip, is 19 to 22 mm.[8,9] The average length in young women in 19.5 mm, while the length in young men is 22 to 24 mm. The lower lip to chin is approximately twice this length. According to Landgraf et al,[19] the lower lip and the chin correspond to two-thirds of the subnasale point–menton distance. The regular length from the most superior point of the upper lip to the soft tissue menton (Li-Pg') is 38 to 44 mm.[8,9]

Importance of the measurement

The proportion between these two measurements results in harmony of the lower third of the face.

Examples of applicability

- In patients with a short face (brachycephalic) and/or shortening of the lower third of the face, the increase in these measurements might make the face look longer, improving its esthetics. This can be achieved by using a filler in the nasolabial sulcus or increasing the volume of the lips and using fillers at the base of the chin.
- It might favor the passive labial sealing in patients lacking it.
- The use of fillers in the mandibular base in patients with a double chin makes it difficult to visualize this unesthetic aspect.

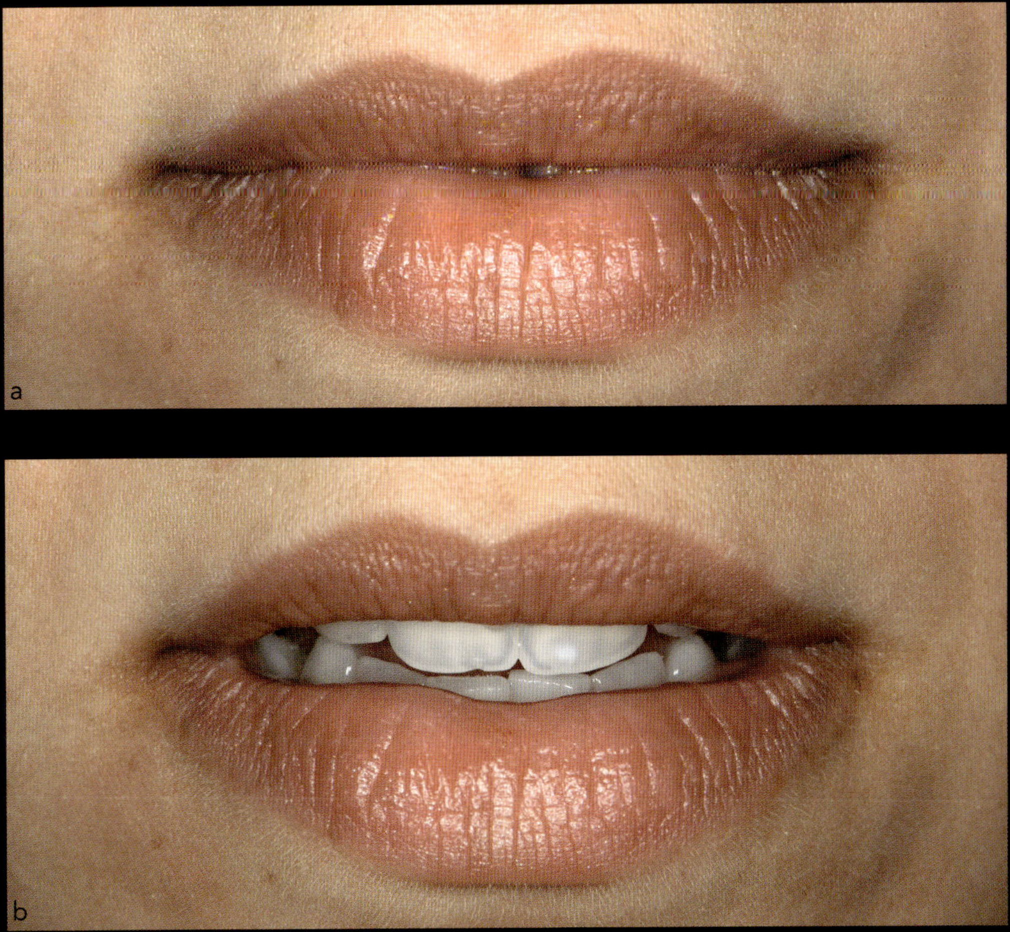

Fig 5-18 *(a)* Detail of the proportion of volumes between the vermilion of the lips. *(b)* Detail of the ideal amount of tooth display for young women.

How to measure

- Upper lip: From the subnasale point to the stomion.
- Lower lip and chin: From the upper border of the lower lip to the base of the chin at the facial midline.

Rules

- The sum of the vertical length of the upper lip, skin, and vermilion should be approximately 50% of the length of the lower lip, according to Arnett and Bergman.[8,9]
- The vertical length of the upper lip vermilion should be 50% of the vertical length of the lower lip vermilion. This difference between the lips should be at least 25%, according to Epker et al[20] (Fig 5-18a).
- According to Vig and Bruno,[21] the amount of maxillary central incisor display with the lips at rest is 3.4 mm in young women (Fig 5-18b) and 1.9 mm in young men.

Use of fillers at the lips

In a frontal view, the use of fillers will increase the volume of the vermilion, which can increase the lip width if the filler is also injected in the commissures.

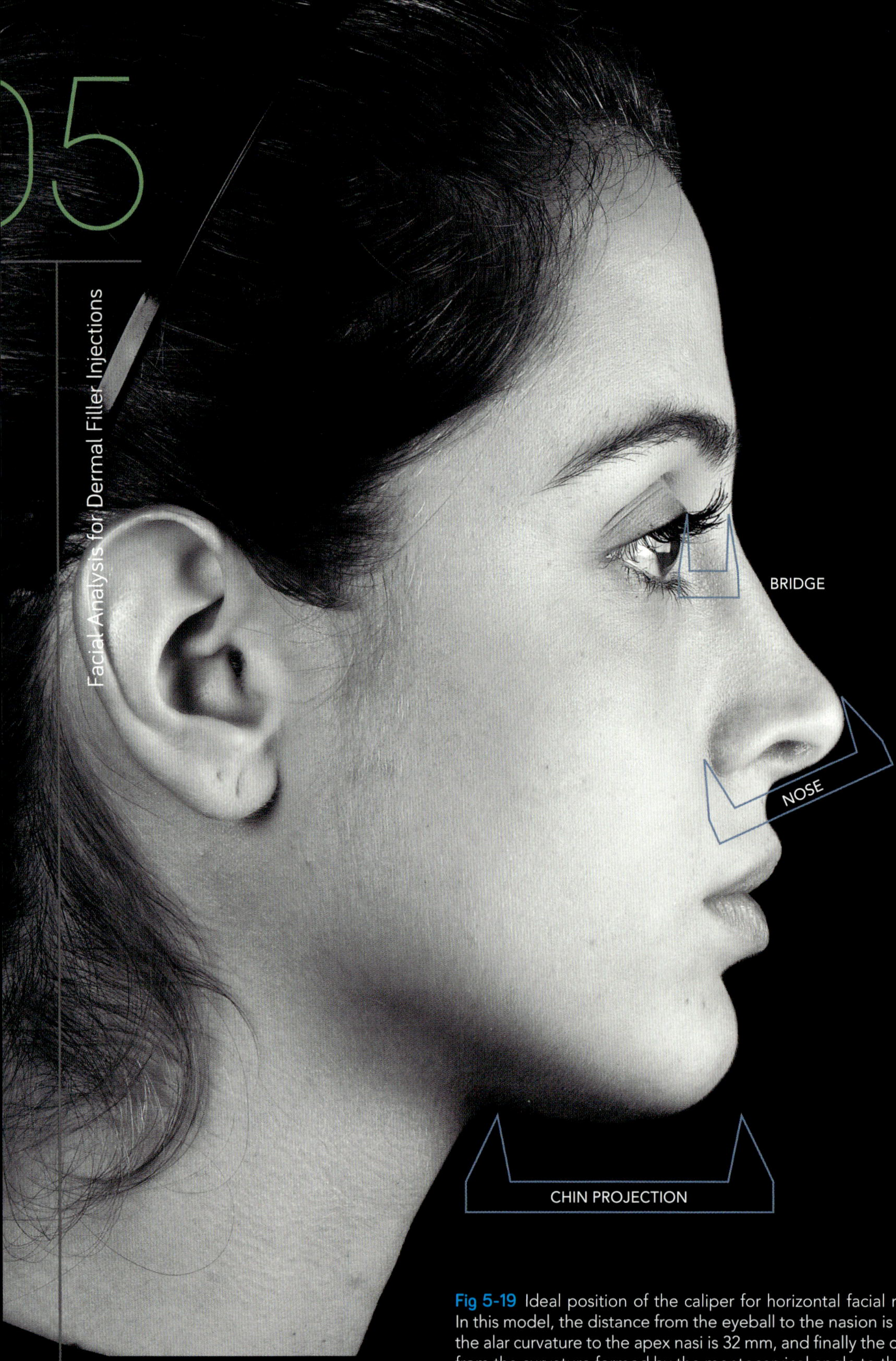

Fig 5-19 Ideal position of the caliper for horizontal facial measurements in profile. In this model, the distance from the eyeball to the nasion is 8 mm, the distance from the alar curvature to the apex nasi is 32 mm, and finally the chin projection measured from the curvature formed by the mentocervical angle to the menton is 45 mm.

Average Horizontal Dimensions in Profile

Figure 5-19 illustrates the horizontal dimensions in profile that are important when planning filler treatments.

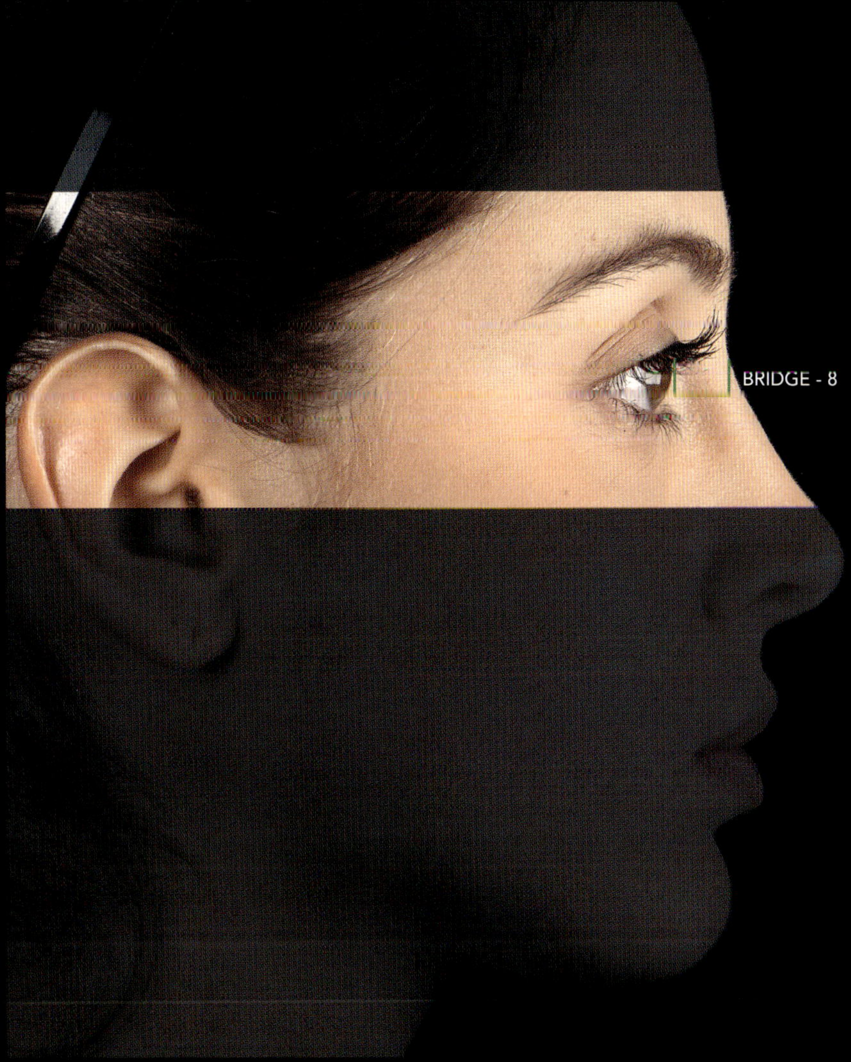

Ocular/nasal bridge distance

The ocular/nasal bridge distance is the distance between the eyeball and the nasion.

Importance of the measurement

- Regulates the dominance of the forehead.
- Regulates the dominance of the nose.

Examples of applicability

- In patients whose eyes look excessively projected in the horizontal plane, the use of fillers can help to decrease this projection.
- It can be used to decrease the appearance of a nose tip, chin, and/or forehead excessively projected in the horizontal plane.
- In patients with an aquiline nose, the use of fillers decreases the excessive curvature.
- It can help decrease glabellar wrinkles.
- It smoothes out the aspect of a stern face.

How to measure

Position the caliper with the patient in profile, next to but not touching the eyeball. Consider the most anterior part of the eye globe and the deepest part of the nasion.

Rules

- The nasion (N) is the deepest point of the frontonasal angle (4 to 6 mm below the glabella). The ideal position of the nasion follows the same horizontal level of the eyelash of the upper eyelid (where the eyelash meets the upper eyelid), so this is the point for fillers.
- To evaluate how deep the nasion is, trace two vertical lines—one tangent to the glabella and one tangent to the nasion.
- With this analysis, it is easy to observe whether the increase in this area is necessary so that the dominance of the nose in relation to the forehead can be worked by improving the proportions.

Use of fillers at the nasion

Lift the skin at the level of the nasion, decreasing the curvature at this point. Never use a filler to the point that the curve becomes a straight line. The use of fillers in this area is very dangerous (see chapter 7).

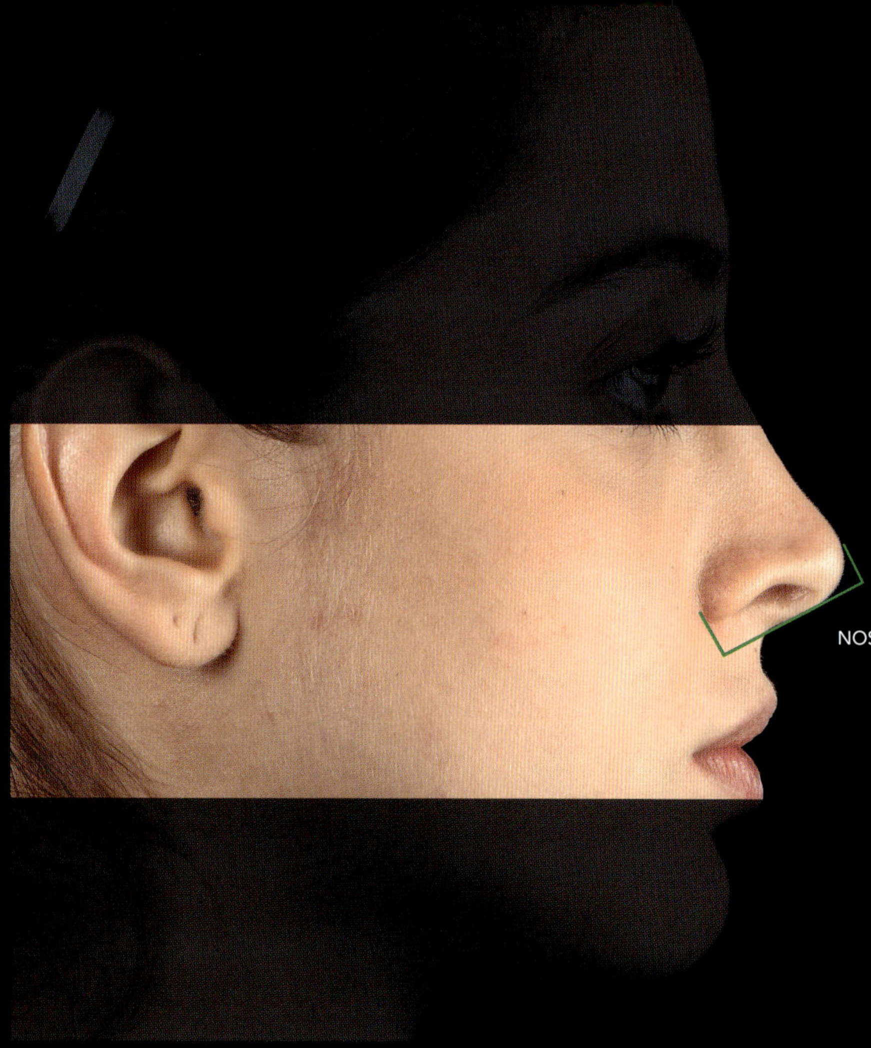

Length of the ala nasi

The length of the ala nasi is the distance from the alar curvature (AC) to the most prominent point of the nasal tip (pronasale, PRN) at the median axis of the apex nasi. The AC point according to Guyuron[22] varies a lot depending on the racial group, making it difficult to establish an average.

Importance of the measurement

- It helps with the perception of a more defined face.
- It influences the convexity of the profile.
- It balances the nose width.

Examples of applicability

- Patients with an excessively wide nose who do not want to undergo a rhinoplasty can have their nose length increased to hide the width.
- The use of fillers in the nasal tip can smooth out the excessive nasal bridge.
- It can be used to give the nose an upturned look.
- In patients with an aquiline nose, the use of fillers decreases the excessive curvature

How to measure

From the most posterior part of the ala nasi to the nasal tip.

Rules

- The *nasal index* is the ratio between the nasal breadth and the length times 100 (ie, breadth/length × 100). This index classifies the nose in three types: leptorrhine when the index is less than 60%, mesorrhine when the index is between 60% and 80%, and platyrrhine when the index is over 80%.[16]
- When noses are longer than they are wide, they seem to be excessively long.

Use of fillers in the supratip area

- Decreases the apparent nose width.
- Gives the impression of an upturned nose, which might result in a supratip break, depending on the desired sculpture.

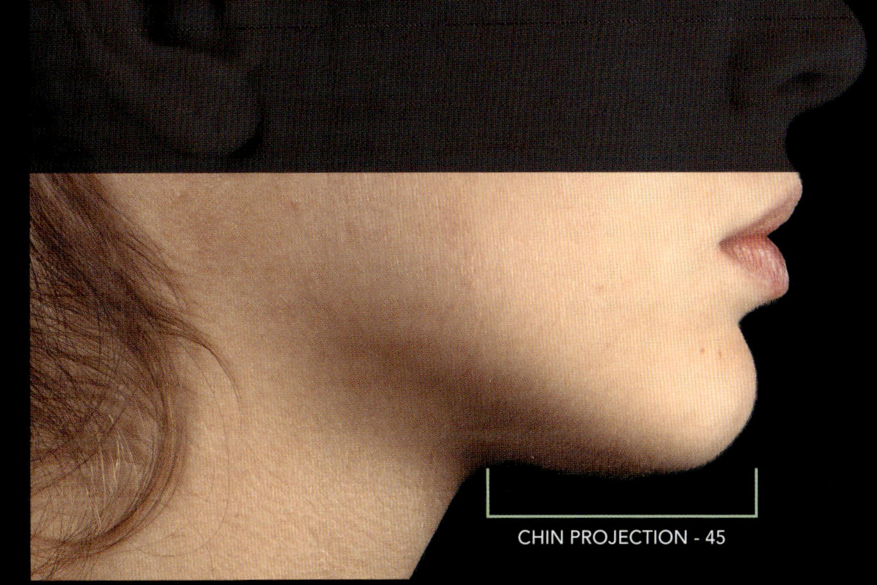

Chin projection

The chin projection is the distance from the neck to the tip of the chin.

Importance of the measurement

- Helps with the perception of a more defined face, because it better accentuates the mandible.
- A longer projection suggests that the patient is not overweight.
- A larger projection suggests that the patient is young.
- A smaller projection in young patients might indicate a horizontal deficiency of the chin.

Examples of applicability

- In horizontal deficiencies of the chin, it can fill the soft tissue pogonion to hide the deficiency.
- In cases of a very small distance, the correction should be surgical with the chin advancement and/or liposuction.

How to measure

Consider the point of union between the submental region and the neck. Then measure from this line to the soft tissue pogonion.

Rule

The ideal size of the submental region is like four fingers in a horizontal position placed parallel to the frontal plane.

Use of fillers at the chin

The use of fillers results in the formation of a volume that advances the chin in a horizontal plane.

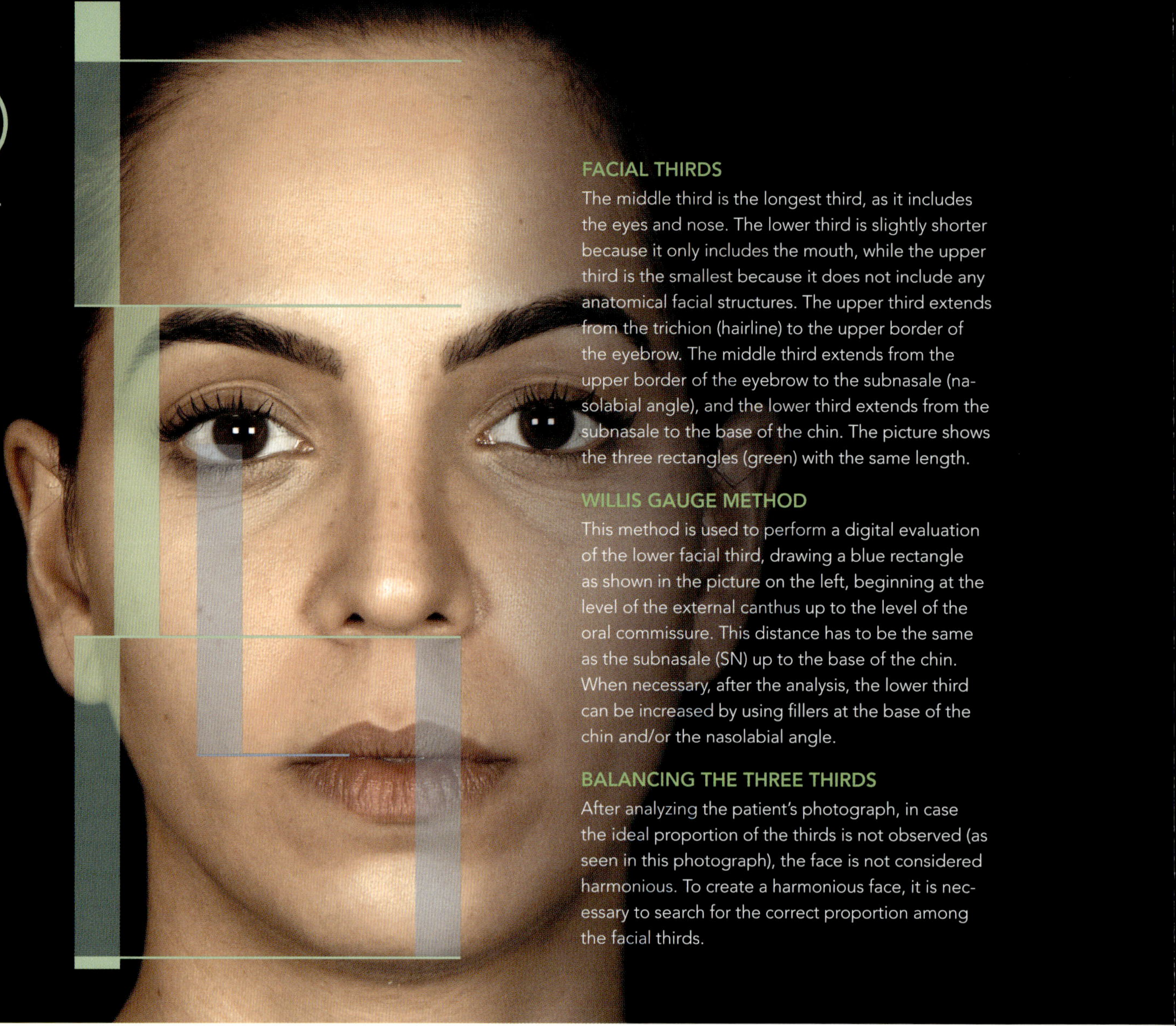

Fig 5-20 Facial thirds.

Important Facial Proportions for Filling Procedures

Facial thirds

To understand facial proportions, it is necessary to understand the concept of the facial thirds. The face is divided in upper, middle, and lower thirds (Fig 5-20). In a balanced face, the thirds are within a range of 55 to 65 mm vertically.

The upper third is located between the trichion (hairline) and the eyebrow line.[10] Because it is affected by the hair and it is highly variable, it is considered the least important third by Arnett and Bergman.[8,9]. The middle third, on the other hand, extends from the eyebrow line to the subnasion point (SN).[10] The eyes, orbits, nose, cheeks, and ears are systematically analyzed. In order for an optimal proportion to occur, the width of the nasal base should be approximately the same as the intercanthal distance.[14] Asymmetry of the eye globes suggests the existence of poor development of the mandible on the affected side, which might be caused by the presence of crossbite or mixed or oral breathing.[10]

As for the lower third, which extends from the SN to the menton (M), it is examined for symmetry, vertical relationships, and morphology. In general, the chin is more prominent than the rest of the face.[8,9] If the lower third is increased or even decreased, this lack of harmony might suggest the presence of a malocclusion.[10]

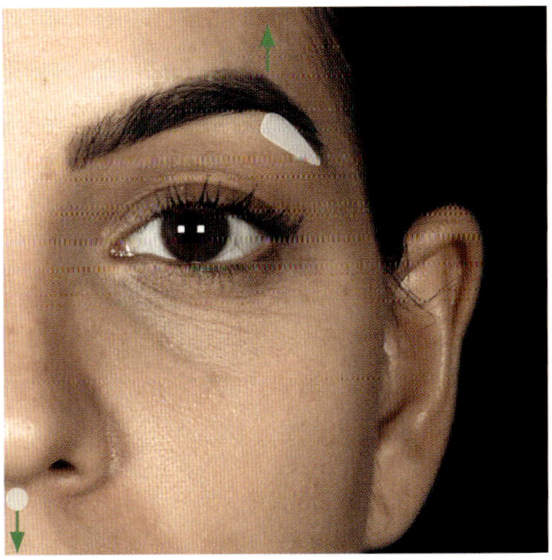

Fig 5-21 Increasing the middle third with fillers. Fillers at the side of the orbit will raise the horizontal level of the eyebrow, and fillers at the nasolabial angle will lower the horizontal level of the columella.

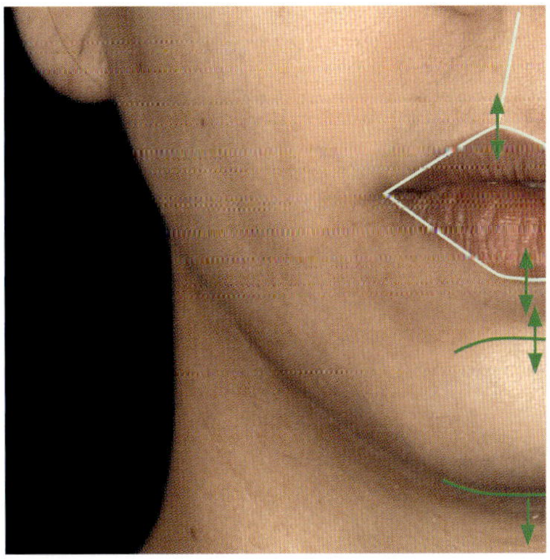

Fig 5-22 Increasing the lower third with fillers. Fillers can be used at the lip vermilion to increase thickness, at the philtrum to make the upper lip longer, at the mentolabial sulcus to make the lower lip longer, and at the base of the chin to make the chin longer.

Therefore, in addition to the facial dimensions, the clinician should understand that proportional measurements create harmony in the face. If after an analysis of the facial proportions, the clinician concludes that the proportion among the measurements is not the ideal, a treatment plan should be offered to the patient that might involve orthodontic treatment or surgery or, in simple cases, the use of fillers to increase the measurements that are shorter, thereby resulting in a more proportional face. For example, if the bizygomatic distance is less than the ideal when compared with the bigonial distance, the bizygomatic distance can be increased with the injection of hyaluronic acid.

Increasing the middle third and the lower third will make the patient look younger. In general, this can be explained by the fact that the face will become more defined and the skin will show fewer wrinkles. Also, older people tend to show a shorter face because of loss of occlusal vertical dimension. So by increasing the length of the face, it will look younger.

Increasing the middle third

When using fillers at the side of the orbit, the horizontal level of the eyebrow is increased (Fig 5-21). Other consequences include:

- Increased eyebrow arching
- Longer face (dolichofacial type)
- Balanced dominance of the eyes
- Smoothing of the dominant upper third

When using fillers at the nasolabial angle, the horizontal level of the columella is lowered. Other consequences include:

- Opening of the nasolabial angle
- Smoothing of retracted columella

Increasing the lower third

When using fillers at the lip vermilion, the lip thickness is increased, making the lips look fuller and more sensual (Fig 5-22). Wrinkles at the lip skin are also smoothed.

When using fillers at the mentolabial sulcus, the lower lip becomes longer and the mentolabial angle more opened.

When using fillers at the base of the chin, the chin becomes longer. In addition, the frontal view of a double chin is reduced, and the patient's facial pattern becomes more dolichofacial.

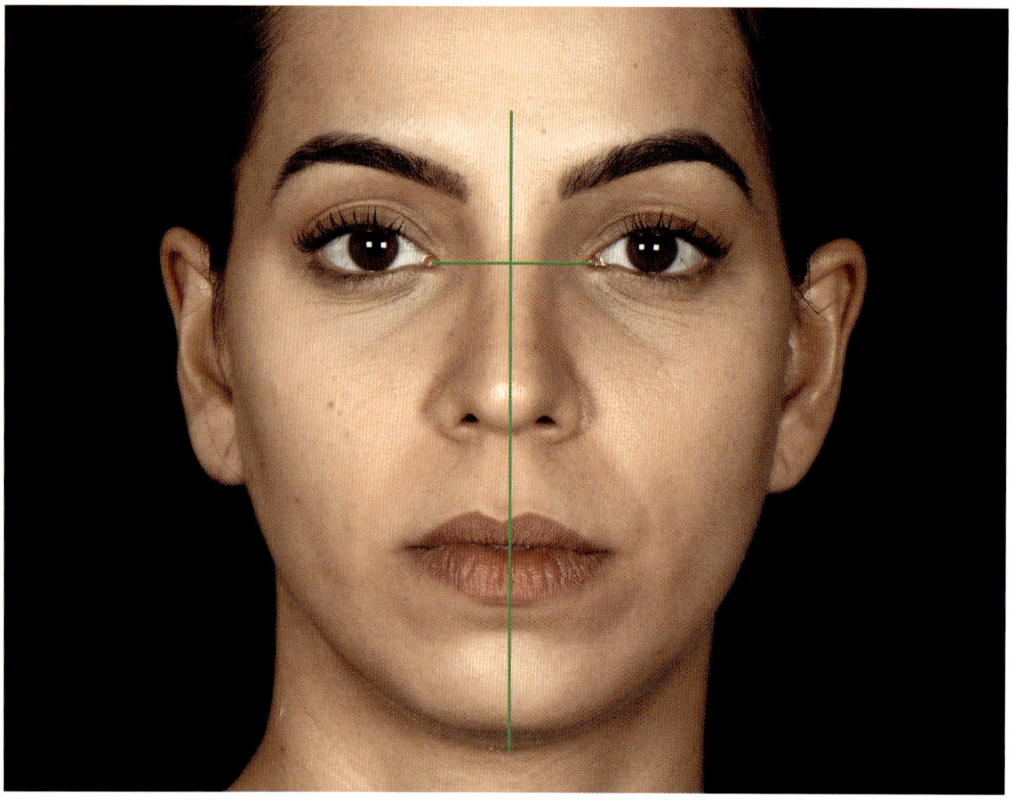

Fig 5-23 Facial midline. Note the asymmetry of the Cupid's bow in the upper lip.

Facial midline

Position

The facial midline is the equidistant point between the internal corners of the eyes (Fig 5-23). The nose, mouth, and chin should not be considered. The midline helps to diagnose the differences in the width and position of the anatomical structures of the face.

Rule

Both sides of the nose, mouth, and chin should have the same width and horizontal level.

Applicability

- When one side of the mouth is wider than the other, the filler will only be injected at the commissure in the narrower side.
- Fillers are used in patients with a chin, gonial, malar, or zygomatic angle narrower and/or higher on one side than the other.

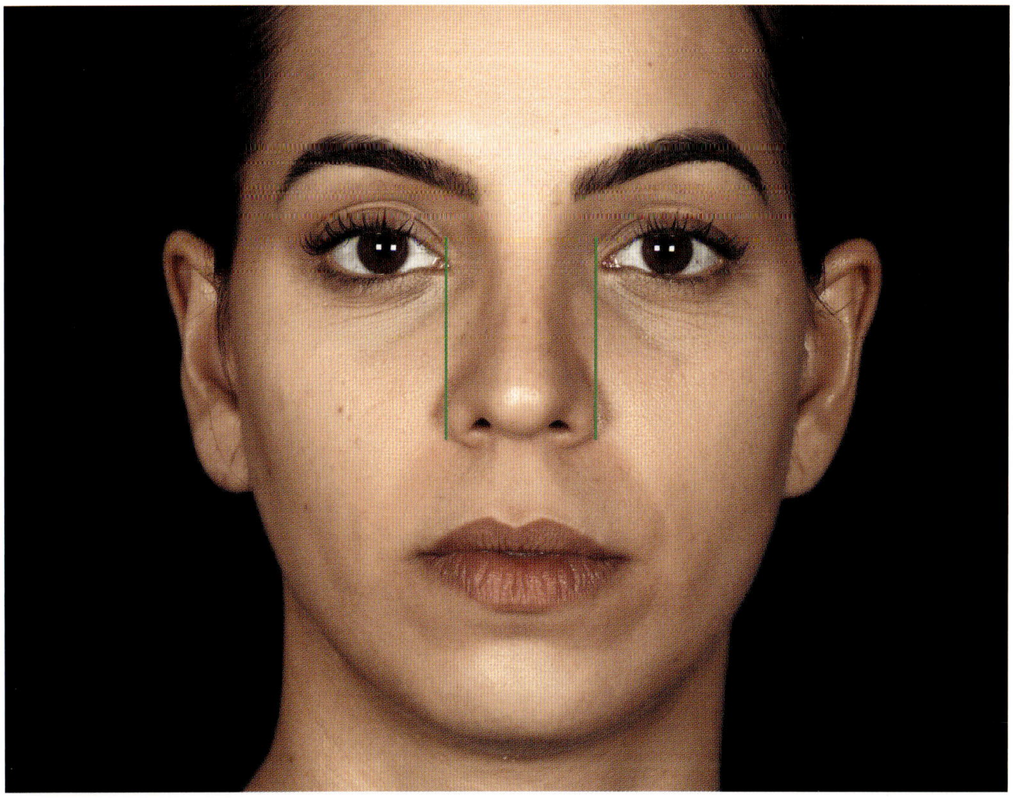

Fig 5-24 Alar line. This line should go through the semilunar fold.

Alar line

Position

The alar line is tangent to the ala nasi (Fig 5-24). It diagnoses the nasal width and symmetry.

Rule

The nose has the width of the intercanthal distance (distance between the eyes). If the alar line goes through the skin, the patient has a narrow nose. If it goes through the semilunar fold, the patient has an average nose. And if it goes through the sclera, the patient has a wide nose.

Applicability

A wide nose suggests that the filler should be injected at the nasal tip and supratip to increase its length. It also indicates the need to increase the labial dominance, because when it is wide, the mouth looks narrower. An additional approach consists of using fillers at the columella to open the nasolabial angle.

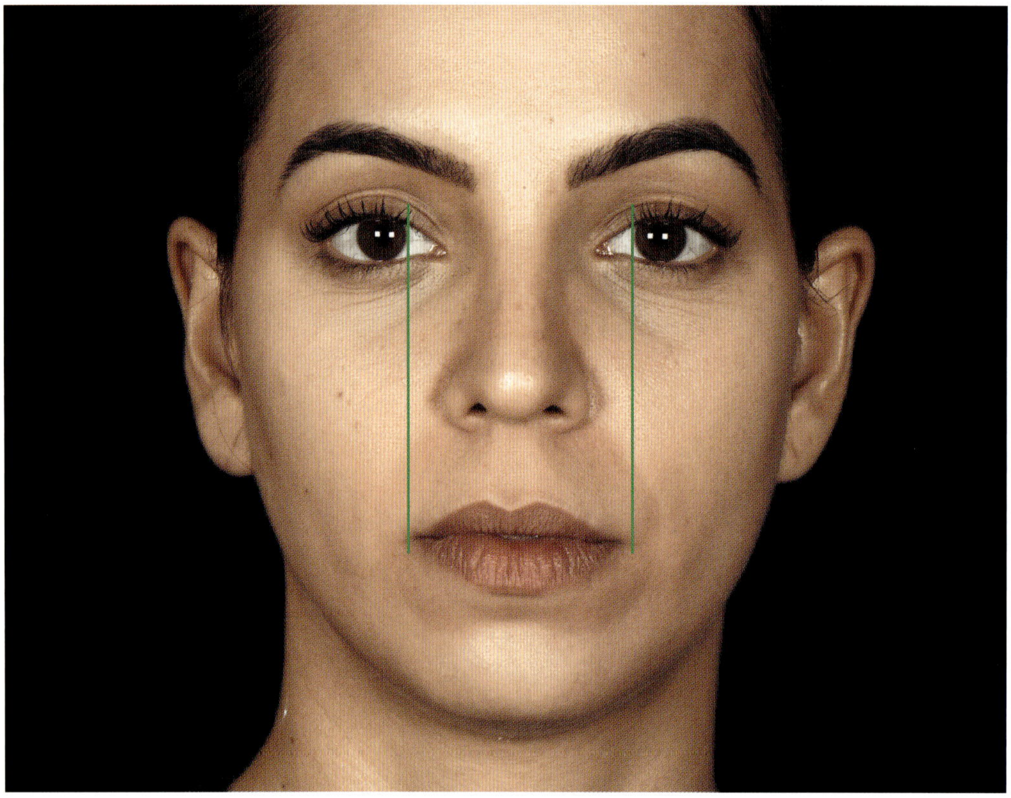

Fig 5-25 Medial iris line. This line should touch the oral commissure.

Medial iris line

Position

The line is drawn along the vertical plane, tangential to the iris (Fig 5-25). It diagnoses oral asymmetries and classifies the mouth in terms of dominant width.

Rule

If the oral commissure is short of the line, the mouth is narrow. If it touches the line, the mouth is proportional to the face. And if it extends beyond the line, the mouth is wide.

Applicability

The mouth width can be increased by using fillers up to the commissure.

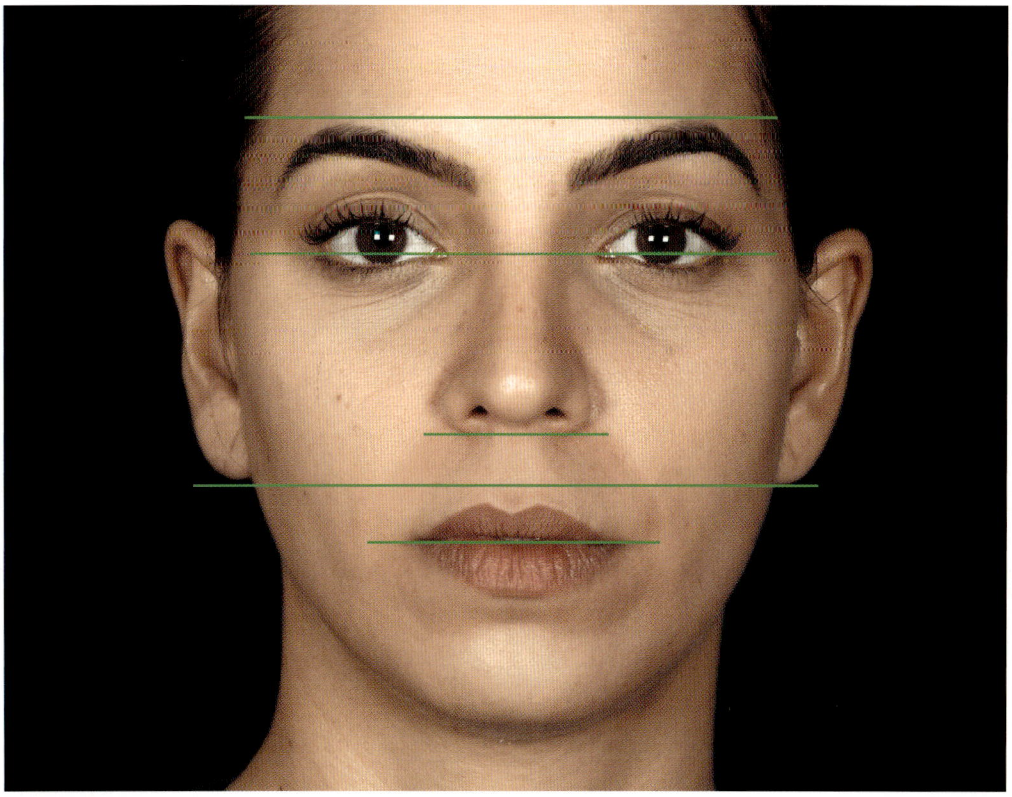

Fig 5-26 Level lines. These lines help to diagnose facial asymmetry.

Level lines

Position

They are horizontally tangent to the external canthus, alae nasi, oral commissures, eyebrows, and ear lobes (Fig 5-26). They diagnose horizontal facial asymmetries.

Rule

The more symmetric the face, the better the facial harmony.

Applicability

Show the patient his or her preexisting asymmetries, or take a photograph prior to treatment to document the change in symmetry with the use of fillers. Explain to the patient that these asymmetries cannot be corrected only by using a filler. Other treatments should be combined with the use of botulinum toxin.

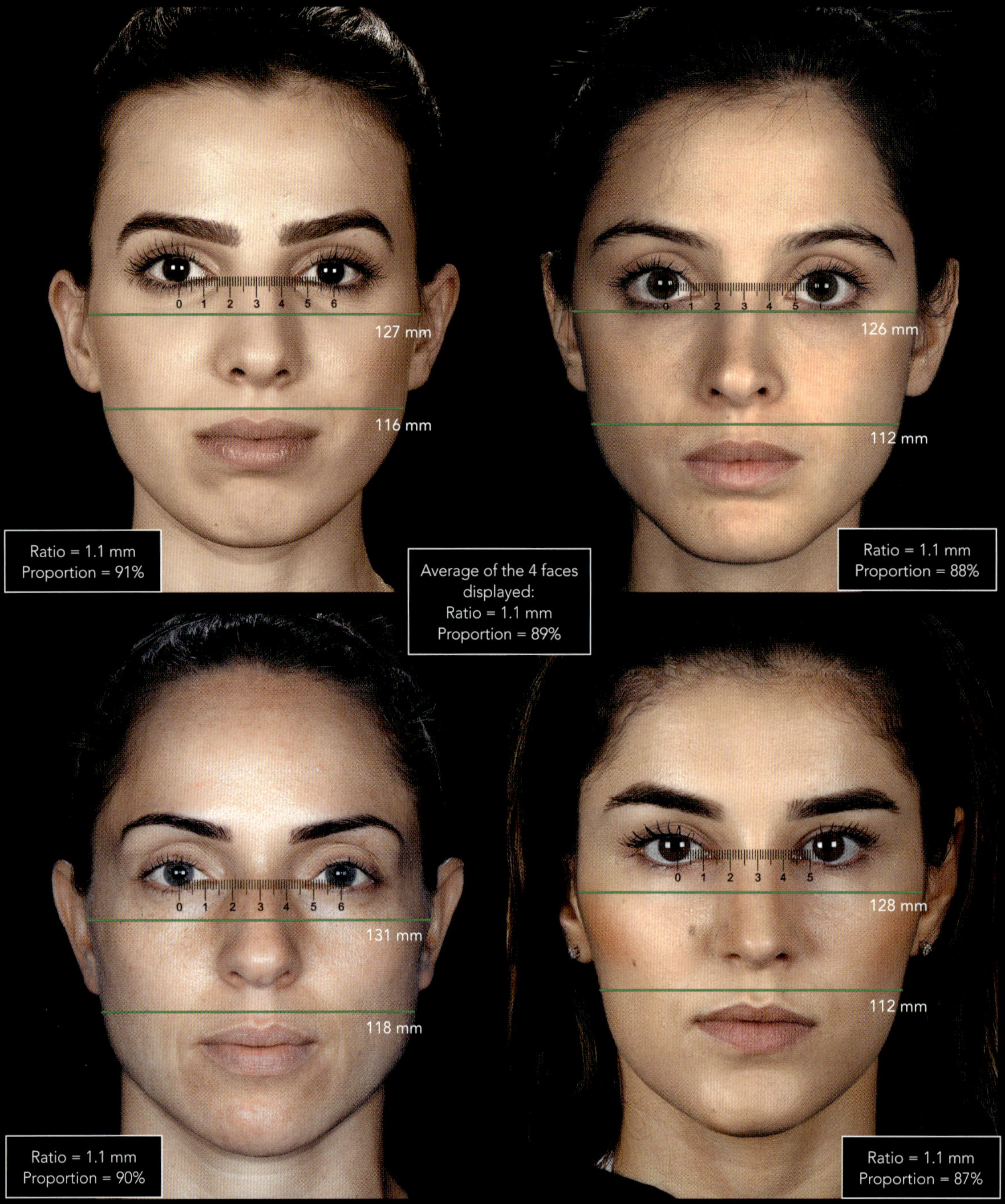

Fig 5-27 On average, the bigonial distance in these faces is 11% smaller than the bizygomatic distance, which is the ideal proportion. The top horizontal line shows the bizygomatic distance, and the bottom horizontal line shows the bigonial distance.

Important Facial Ratios for Filling Procedures

The ratio between the bizygomatic distance and the bigonial distance is important for establishing facial harmony (Fig 5-27). The ratio between facial height and width is also key (Fig 5-28).

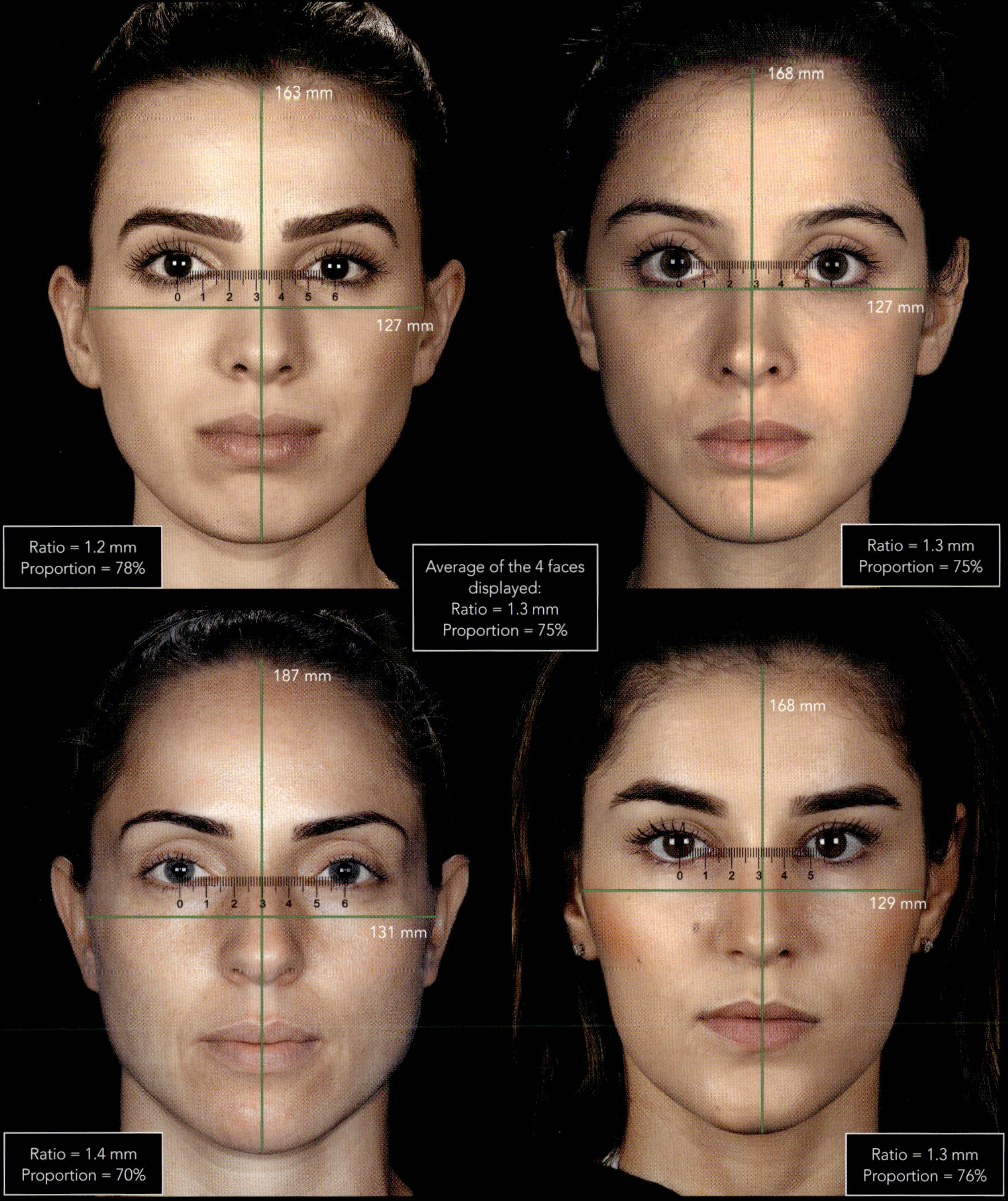

Fig 5-28 The average width of the four faces shown here is 25% narrower than the length. The width should be defined as the bizygomatic width and not the width between the ears (intertragus) because the hair might be covering the area as shown in *d*. Farkas et al[23] state that the ideal ratio of facial height to width is 1.3:1 for females and 1.35:1 for males. Therefore, the bizygomatic width should correspond to approximately 78% of the facial height.

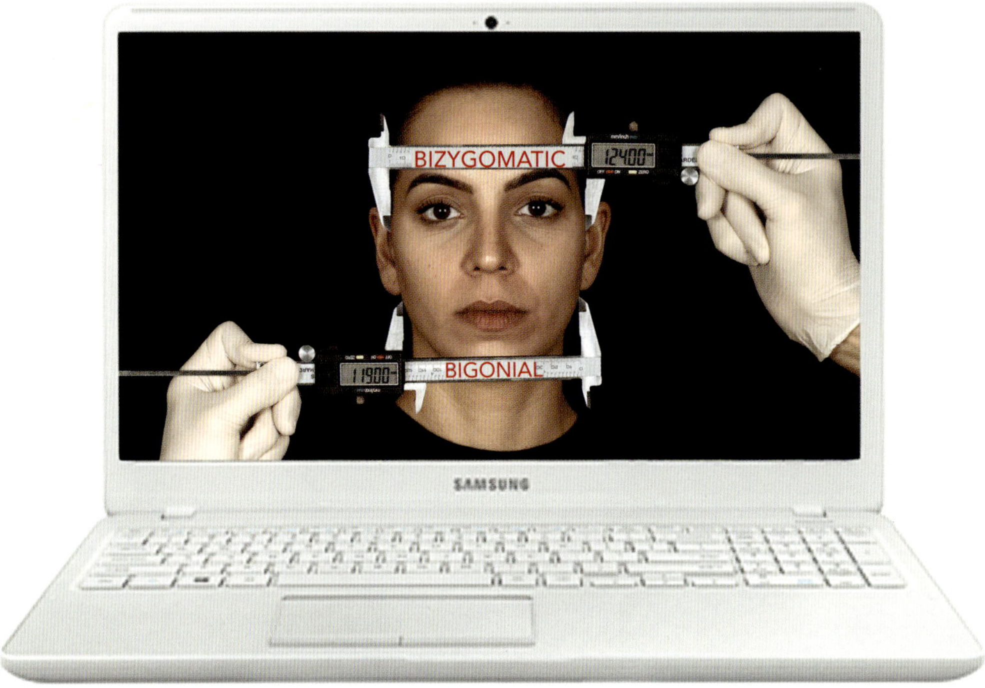

Fig 5-29 PowerPoint, Keynote, or any similar program can be used for the facial analysis.

Photographic Analysis

A full dedication to esthetic treatment is not possible without the use of photographs. After taking any relevant measurements directly on the patient's face, digital photographs should be taken so that the patient's face can be analyzed digitally. The clinician or assistant can take the photographs, but only the clinician is able to perform the facial analysis when the patient is not present to avoid distractions. Because a photograph is a static image, several measurements, proportions, and angles can be analyzed in the same position and with the help of tools, such as digital rulers, straight lines, and angles, which could not be done directly on the patient's face (Fig 5-29). Before a facial analysis is performed, the professional should correctly position the photograph on the computer monitor and magnify the image as large as possible before correcting its lateral inclination. This is intuitively done. Only then should the lines be drawn and other tools be used for analysis.

References

1. Borbolla RR, Faltin Junior K, Costa C, Ortolani CLF, Kamitsuji IKN, Rodrigues CPF. Normatização e padronização da localização e abreviação dos pontos cefalométricos utilizados nas análises cefalométricas em norma lateral de Ricketts e Schwarz-Faltin. Rev Inst Ciênc Saúde 2008;26:328–233.
2. Galantucci LM, Deli R, Laino A, et al. Three-dimensional anthropometric database of attractive Caucasian women: Standards and comparisons. J Craniofac Surg 2016;27:1884–1895.
3. Mosle MAA, Baba MS, Malek S, Almaktari RA. Ceph-X: Development and evaluation of 2D cephalometric system. BMC Bioinformatics 2016;17(suppl 19):499.
4. Volkmann O, Cotrim-Ferreira FA, Villi ER, Ferreira-Tormin AC, Junior HS, Vellini-Ferreira F. Correlations of linear measures in the palate, the cranium and the face: An anthropometric study. J Bras Ortodon Ortop Facial 2003;8:307–314.
5. Marianetti TM, Gasparini G, Midulla G, et al. Numbers of beauty: An innovative aesthetic analysis for orthognathic surgery treatment planning. Biomed Res Int 2016:6156919. https://www.hindawi.com/journals/bmri/2016/6156919/. Accessed 14 February 2019.

6. Alam MK, Noor NFM, Basri R, Yew TF, Wen TH. Multiracial facial golden ratio and evaluation of facial appearance. PLoS One 2015;10(11):e0142914.
7. Arnett GW, Jelic JS, Kim J, et al. Soft tissue cephalometric analysis: Diagnosis and treatment planning of dentofacial deformity. Am J Orthod Dentofac Orthop 1999;116:239–253.
8. Arnett GW, Bergman RT. Facial keys to orthodontic diagnosis and treatment planning. Part I. Am J Orthod Dentofac Orthop 1993;103:299–312.
9. Arnett GW, Bergman RT. Facial keys to orthodontic diagnosis and treatment planning. Part II. Am J Orthod Dentofacial Orthop 1993;103:395–-411
10. Almeida RC, Almeida MHC. Assimetria facial no exame clínico da face. Ortodontia 1999;32:82–86.
11. Ricketts RM. Provocations and Perceptions in Craniofacial Orthopedics. Denver, CO: Rocky Mountain Orthodontics, 1989.
12. Ricketts RM. Cefalometria progressiva paradigma 2000. California: Instituto Americano para Educação Bioprogressiva, 1996:64–120.
13. Naini FB. Estética Facial—Conceitos e Diagnósticos Clínicos. Rio de Janeiro: Elsevier, 2014.
14. Suguino R, Ramos AL, Terada HH, Furquin LZ, Maeda L, Filho OGS. Análise facial. Rev Dental Press Ortod Ortop Facial 1996;1:86–107.
15. Cesario Jr VA, Latta Jr GH. Relations between the mesiodistal width of maxillary central incisor and interpupillary distance. J Prosthet Dent 1984;52:641–643.
16. Furtado IR. Morfologia nasal—Harmonia e proporção aplicada a rinoplastia. Rev Bras de Cir Plást 2016;31:599–608.
17. Fradeani M. Análise Estética: Uma Abordagem Sistemática para o Tratamento Protético, vol 1. São Paulo: Quintessence, 2006.
18. Costa LAL, Fernandes GO, Kanazawa LS, Miranda JG, Pretti H. Análise facial—Uma revisão de literatura facial analysis—A literature review. J Bras Ortodon Ortop Facial 2004;9:171–176.
19. Landgraf ME, Filho MV, Junqueira JLC, Valdrighi HC, Vedovello SAS. Análise facial, elemento chave no diagnóstico ortodôntico contemporâneo. Ortodontia 2002;29:147–160.
20. Epker BN, Stella JP, Fish L. Dental Facial Deformities: Integrated Orthodontic and Surgical Corretion, ed 2. St Louis: Mosby, 1995.
21. Vig RG, Bruno GC. The kinetics of anterior tooth display. J Prosthet Dent 1978;39:502–504.
22. Guyuron B. Precision rhinoplasty. Part I: The role of life-size photographs and soft-tissue cephalometric analysis. Plast Reconstr Surg 1988;81:489–499.
23. Farkas LG, Bryson W, Klotz J. Is photogrammetry of the face reliable? Plast Reconstr Surg 1980;66:346–355.
24. Ricketts RM. Divine proportion in facial esthetics. Clin Plast Surg 1982;9:401–405.

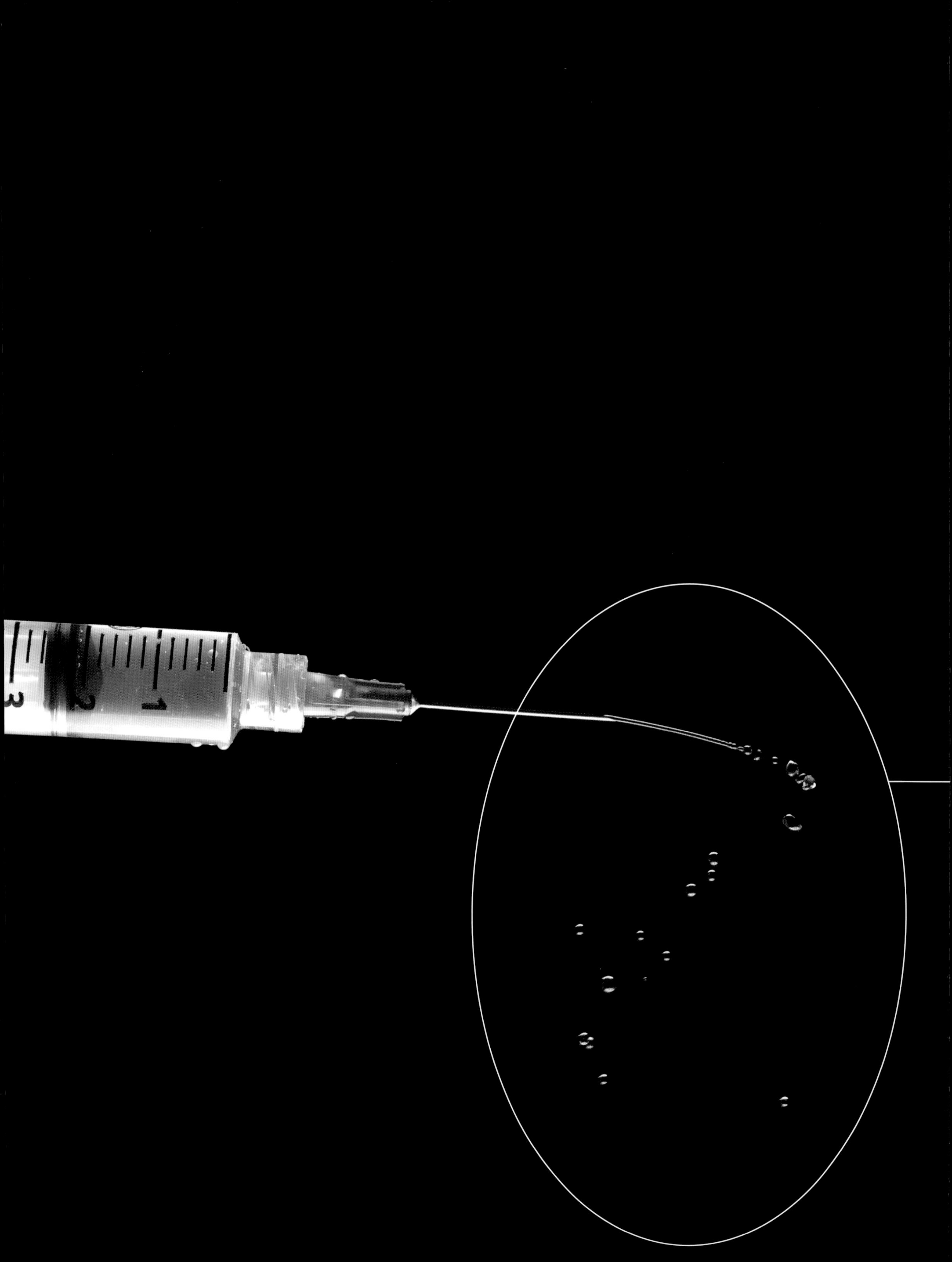

CHAPTER

06

Facial Anesthesia for Filling Procedures

Several medical and dental surgery procedures require local anesthesia because of unpleasant physiologic and emotional feelings associated with pain. When the patient is assured that the esthetic technique proposed is painless, the fear of pain is no longer an obstacle, thereby improving the acceptance of these procedures.

The effectiveness of local anesthesia depends on the clinician's awareness of the sensory innervation of the face (see Fig 6-1). Effective local anesthesia prevents the nociceptive impulse from reaching the patient's brain, and understanding the exact location of the innervation means that fewer injection points (and less anesthesia) can be used.

The use of an appropriate health questionnaire can determine if the patient has any contraindications to receiving local anesthesia.

Before performing anesthesia in a patient, several steps must be followed:

1. Clean the face for correct asepsis using 2% chlorhexidine. If the procedure is intraoral, an antiseptic mouthwash (0.2% chlorhexidine) can be used.
2. Apply a topical anesthetic cream to the face (eg, 4% lidocaine). Wait until it is absorbed by the skin. If the procedure is intraoral, apply the cream using a disposable applicator. Wait for the requested time as recommended by the manufacturer.
3. Once the cream is fully absorbed and the skin is dry, use a facial marker or makeup pencil to mark the area to be injected.

Box 6-1 provides hints for an optimized anesthetic procedure.

Box 6-1 Hints for an optimized anesthetic procedure

- Asepsis and topical anesthesia can be performed by a duly accredited oral health technician, saving time for the clinician.
- The area to be injected should *always* be marked before the anesthesia is performed so that the temporary volumization resulting from the anesthetic does not interfere with this procedure.
- The anesthesia point of nerves that emerge through the foramina must be determined so that all of their branches will be numbed using only one point. For the nerves that do not emerge from the foramina, the anesthesia can be performed only posterior to the area to be injected because most of the nerve branches run posterior to anterior toward the facial midline.
- Intraoral accesses are preferable to extraoral because they result in less pain and do not cause injury to the skin.
- Needles that have been used for intraoral anesthesia should not be used to puncture the facial skin. Instead, they should be discarded as they may contain biofilm.
- Before applying anesthetics in the face and/or neck, see Fig 6-1.

Innervation of the Face

Table 6-1 lists important nerves of the face to be blocked during the injection of fillers, and Fig 6-1 illustrates the innervation.

Table 6-1 **Nerves in the face to block before filler injection**

POINT IN FIG 6-1	NERVE	ORIGIN	ANATOMICAL REFERENCE	ACCESS	QUANTITY OF ANESTHETIC
1	Supratrochlear	Ophthalmic	Anterior to the orbit, inferior and medial to the forehead. It emerges to the face through the medial portion of the orbit.	Extraoral	0.05 mL
2	Infratrochlear	Ophthalmic	Lacrimal sac and lacrimal caruncle. It runs toward the face through the medial portion of the orbit under the supratrochlear nerve.	Extraoral	0.05 mL
3	Medial branch of the supraorbital nerve	Ophthalmic	Above the upper medial aspect of the orbital rim. It runs toward the face through the supraorbital foramen or fissure.	Extraoral	0.05 mL
4	Lateral branch of the supraorbital nerve	Ophthalmic	Above the upper lateral aspect of the orbit margin. It runs toward the face through the orbit below the supraorbital margin.	Extraoral	0.05 mL
5	Auriculotemporal	Mandibular	It traverses the upper part of the parotid gland and becomes superficial when crossing the posterior portion of the zygomatic arch.	Extraoral	0.2 mL
7	External nasal branch of the anterior ethmoidal nerve	Ophthalmic	Medial rim of the orbital roof in a descending direction. It becomes superficial at the nasal dorsum immediately below the osseocartilaginous junction.	Extraoral	3 drops
8	Infraorbital	Maxillary	Infraorbital groove and infraorbital canal emerging to the face through the infraorbital foramen.	Intraoral or extraoral	0.9 mL
9	Zygomaticofacial	Maxillary	Anteriorly in the pterygopalatine fossa, emerging toward the face through the zygomaticofacial foramen.	Extraoral	0.2 mL
10	Buccal	Mandibular	Medial surface of the mandibular ramus. It becomes superficial at the base of the coronoid process, following the descending path on the lateral aspect of the buccinator muscle.	Intraoral	0.9 mL
11	Mentonian	Mandibular	It runs in the mandibular canal and becomes superficial, emerging from the mental foramen, following an anterior path.	Intraoral	1.8 mL
12	Anterior superior alveolar nerve	Maxillary	It emerges from the infraorbital nerve approximately 6 to 10 mm before arising through the infraorbital canal. It descends through the anterior wall of the maxillary sinus.	Intraoral	0.9 mL
13	Nasopalatine	Maxillary	It descends toward the mucosa of the anterior hard palate, innervating this region and also the mucosa of the anterior nasal septum. In its final path, it crosses the incisive foramen.	Intraoral	0.9 mL
14	Mylohyoid	Mandibular	It branches from the inferior alveolar nerve just before it enters the mandibular canal. It then follows the mylohyoid groove and innervates the skin of the mental protuberance.	Intraoral	0.9 mL

The three nerves at the bottom of the table require extra anesthesia due to possible fiber crosslinking, which may lead to anesthetic failure.

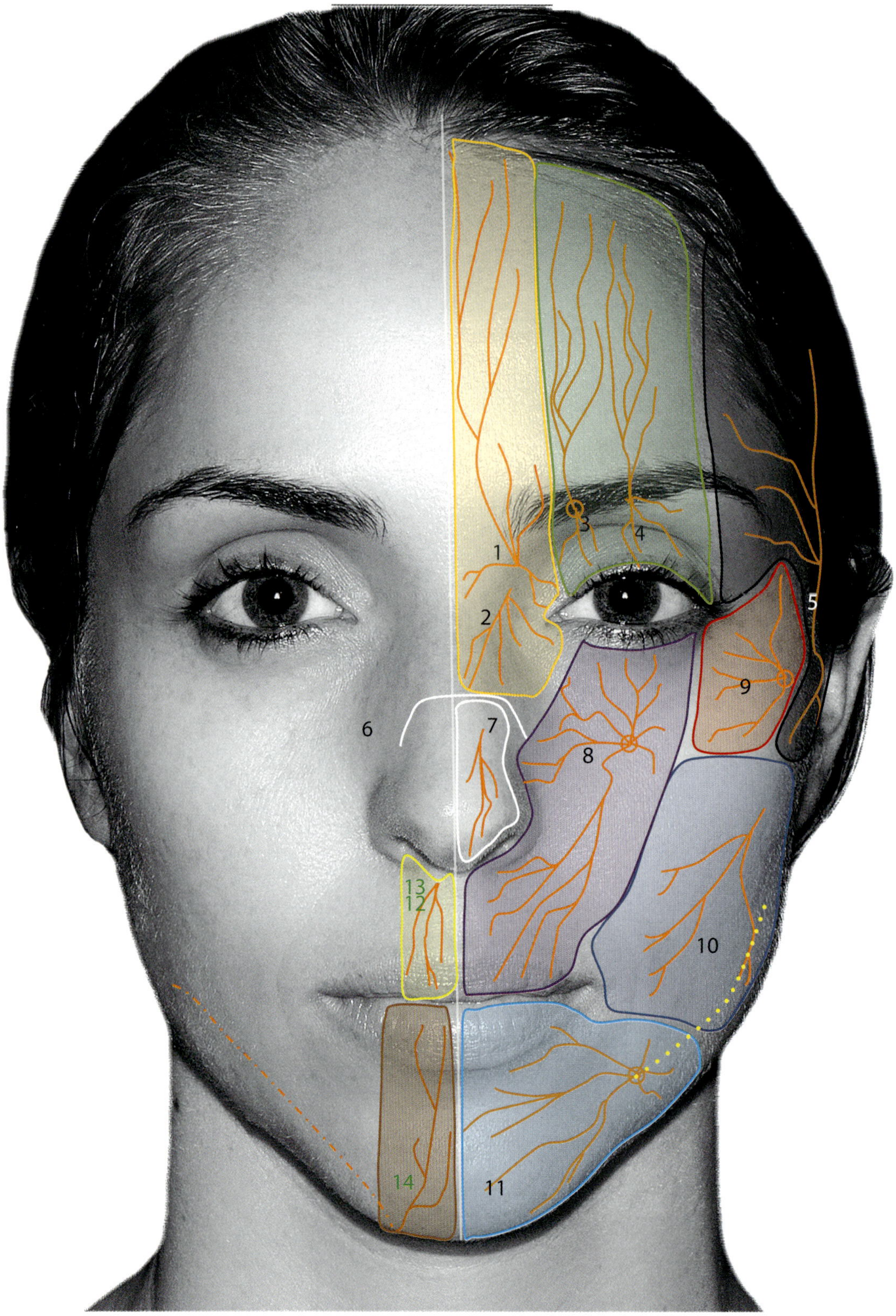

Fig 6-1 General view of sensory pathways of the face. It is important to anesthetize any areas to be injected with fillers. The small circular points show the points at which the sensory innervation emerges on the face through the foramina, becoming superficial. These points are described in Table 6-1. Point 6 is an anatomical reference only, the osseocartilaginous junction. The right hemiface shows the complementary points of anesthesia due to the intercrossing of nerves. The *dotted line* shows the course of the mylohyoid nerve, a branch of the inferior alveolar nerve that detaches immediately after its entry into the mandibular canal. The *orange dot* shows that the mental nerve is the final part of the inferior alveolar nerve, so the operator can anesthetize it posteriorly via the intraoral technique, at the most posterior part of the mandibular canal. This will avoid undesired volumes created by the presence of the anesthetic liquid in the jowls and prejowls, marionettes, and lateral part of the chin. If some of these are target areas for filling, the anesthetic volume could disturb the procedure.

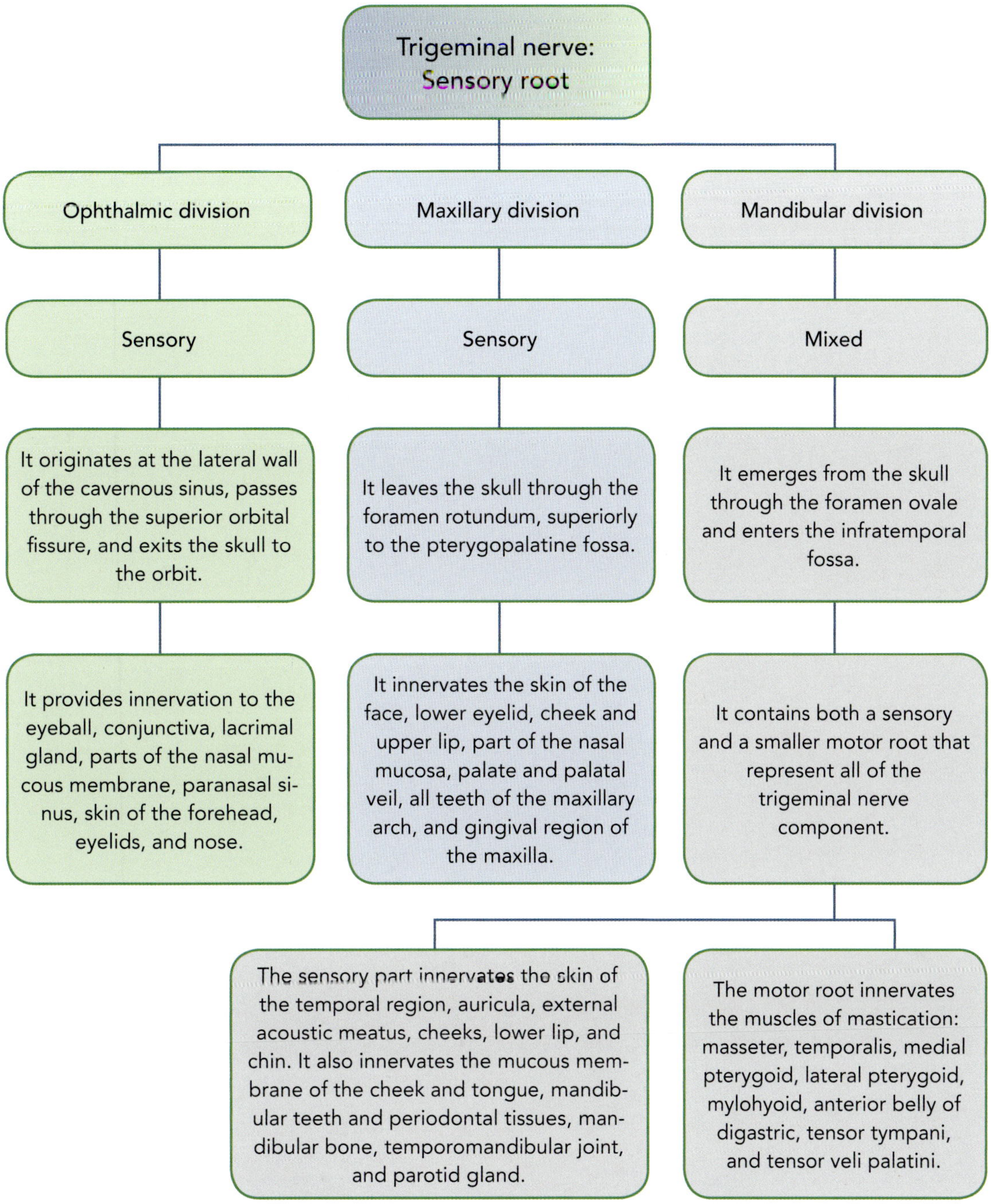

Fig 6-2 Three divisions of the sensory root of the trigeminal nerve.

The **facial nerve** provides the motor innervation to the muscles of facial expression through its many branches: temporal, zygomatic, buccal, marginal mandibular, and cervical.

The **trigeminal nerve**, the fifth cranial pair, is the largest of the cranial nerves. Its neurons are responsible for the exteroceptive sensations of pain, pressure, touch, and temperature. It consists of a motor and sensory root, but mainly it is sensory. The sensory root has three branches—ophthalmic, mandibular, and maxillary—that exit the Meckel cavity on the anterior surface of the petrous portion of the temporal bone, providing sensation for the skin of the face. The trigeminal nerve is also responsible for the motor innervation of the muscles of mastication through the mandibular trunk and its branches. Figure 6-2 and Table 6-2 show this division as well as the branches of important nerves present in the areas susceptible to filling procedures.

Table 6-2 Branches of the sensory root of the trigeminal nerve

BRANCH	ANATOMICAL REFERENCE	NERVES IT GIVES OFF	INNERVATION
Ophthalmic division			
Nasociliary	It travels along the medial border of the orbital roof, ending in the skin at the root of the nose.	Anterior ethmoidal nerve (internal nasal nerve)	Mucous membrane of the anterior part of the nasal septum and the lateral wall of the nasal cavity
		External nasal nerve	Skin of the lacrimal sac and caruncle
		Infratrochlear nerve	Ethmoidal and sphenoidal sinuses
		Posterior ethmoidal nerve	Skin over the tip and the ala of the nose
Frontal	It travels anteriorly in the orbit.	Supratrochlear nerve	Conjunctiva, skin over the lower and mesial aspects of the forehead
		Supraorbital nerve	Upper eyelid, from the scalp up to the parietal bone and lambdoid suture
Lacrimal	Lacrimal canal	Lacrimal nerve	Lateral part of the upper eyelid and a small area of the adjacent skin
Maxillary division			
Branches at the pterygopalatine fossa	It emerges from the foramen rotundum and crosses the pterygopalatine fossa.	Zygomatic nerve—zygomaticotemporal and zygomaticofacial	Skin on the side of the forehead and skin on the prominence of the cheek
		Pterygopalatine nerves	Orbit, nose, palate, and pharynx
		Posterior superior alveolar nerve	Buccal gingiva in the maxillary molar region and adjacent facial mucosal surfaces; mucous membranes of the maxillary sinus; alveoli; periodontal ligaments; pulpal tissues of the maxillary third, second, and first molars (in 28% of the patients, with the exception of the mesiobuccal root of the first molar)
Branches in the infraorbital canal	It surpasses the infraorbital canal.	Middle superior alveolar nerve	Two maxillary premolars and perhaps the mesiobuccal root of the first molar and periodontal tissues to the buccal soft tissues and bone
		Anterior superior alveolar nerve	Maxillary incisors, canine, and periodontal tissues to the buccal bone
Branches on the face	The infraorbital nerve emerges in the face through the infraorbital foramen and is then divided.	Inferior palpebral nerve	Skin of the lower eyelid
		External nasal nerve	Skin of the lateral aspect of the nose
		Superior labial nerves	Skin and mucous membrane of the upper lip
Mandibular division			
Branches from the undivided nerve	On leaving the foramen ovale, it gives off two branches during its 2- to 3-mm course.	Nervus spinosus	Dura mater and mastoid air cells
		Medial pterygoid nerve	Motor nerve to medial pterygoid muscle

→

Table 6-2 *(cont)* **Branches of the sensory root of the trigeminal nerve**

BRANCH	ANATOMICAL REFERENCE	NERVES IT GIVES OFF	INNERVATION
Branches of the anterior division	The anterior division gives off branches that intersperse the muscles of mastication.	Buccal nerve	Skin of the cheeks, retromolar triangle, buccal gingiva of the mandibular molars, and mucobuccal fold in that region; the buccal nerve does not innervate the buccinator muscle (the innervation is made through the facial nerve), nor does it provide innervation to the lower lip or the corner of the mouth
Branches of the posterior division	It descends for a short distance downward and medially to the lateral pterygoid muscle.	Auriculotemporal nerve	Skin over the areas of innervation to the motor of the facial nerve: zygomatic, buccal and mandibular, parotid gland, helix and tragus of the ear, external auditory meatus and tympanic membrane, and temporomandibular joint
		Lingual nerve	Anterior two-thirds of the tongue, mucous membranes of the floor of the mouth, and the gingiva on the lingual side of the mandible; lateral aspect of the nose
		Inferior alveolar nerve (mylohyoid, incisive, and mental nerves)	Pulpal innervation of the mandibular teeth, periodontal tissues, skin of the chin, and skin and mucous membrane of the lower lip, including the corner of the mouth*

*It is thought that the mylohyoid nerve contains sensory fibers that supply the skin on the inferior and anterior surfaces of the mental protuberance. Therefore, anesthesia may be required when the clinician works on the lower lip vermilion. The mylohyoid nerve runs downward and forward in the mylohyoid groove on the medial surface of the ramus and along the body of the mandible to reach the mylohyoid muscle. Besides the mental block, the incisive block can also be necessary in order to fully anesthetize the lower lip.[1]

The **zygomatic nerve** is a branch of the maxillary nerve and is divided into the zygomaticofacial and zygomaticotemporal nerves. The zygomaticotemporal nerve is not described here because it is not relevant for procedures involving facial fillers. The zygomaticotemporal nerve runs along the lower outer aspect of the orbit. It then passes through a small canal in the zygomatic bone and arrives into the temporal fossa. It passes superiorly between the bone and the temporalis muscle. It then goes through the temporal fascia just a couple of centimeters superior to the zygomatic arch and primarily innervates the scalp above the temporal region, and this area is not important when injecting fillers. The zygomaticofacial nerve, on the other hand, emerges to the face through the zygomaticofacial foramen and should be addressed for innervating the skin of the malar region.

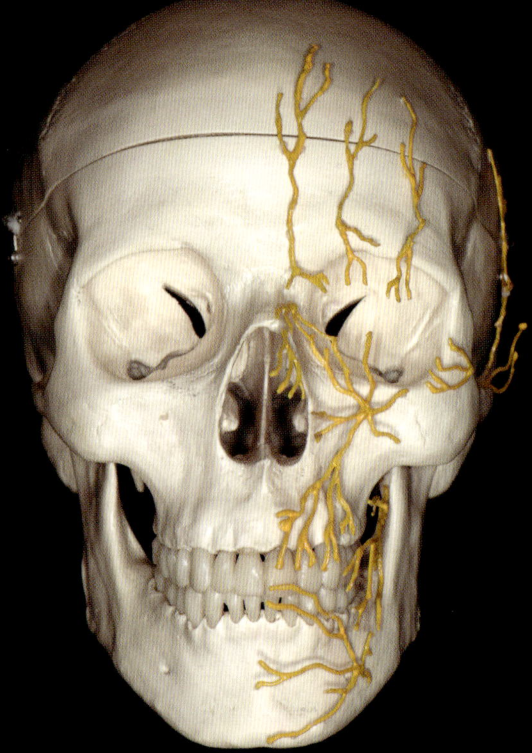

c

Fig 6-3 *(a and b)* Drawing of nerves in resin on the patient's face. *(c)* After polymerization, the resin nerves were removed from the face, painted yellow, and glued onto a skull model in their appropriate locations.

A useful practice to gain confidence in understanding the innervation of the face is to draw the nerves onto a patient's face with resin and then mount the polymerized resin nerves onto a skull model (Fig 6-3).

Important Considerations for Anesthesia Administered in the Lip Area

The buccal branch of the facial nerve, or cranial nerve VII, provides motor innervation to the orbicularis oris and elevators of the lip and lip angle. The majority of muscles responsible for depression of the lip are supplied via the marginal mandibular branch of the facial nerve. The platysma, which is also involved in depression of the lower lip, receives its innervation via the cervical branch of the facial nerve.

The various branches of the trigeminal nerve, or cranial nerve V, provide sensory innervation to the lips. The infraorbital branch of the maxillary division of the trigeminal nerve (cranial nerve V2) supplies the upper lip. The mental nerve derived from the mandibular division of the trigeminal nerve (cranial nerve V3) allows for sensation from the lower lip.[2]

Nerve blocks are useful for achieving anesthesia to a regional area of the body. Regional nerve blocks offer many advantages over local tissue infiltration. First, nerve blocks generally require less anesthetic medication to produce the desired effect when compared to local infiltration. They are useful when local infiltration may not be possible or could result in tissue damage or distortion, which could affect cosmetic outcomes. This is especially important for areas such as the face, where cosmetic results are extremely important. Other indications include wound closure, dental procedures, and contraindication to general anesthesia. Nerve blocks are less useful in situations where the wound may extend over an area that is innervated by several nerves. If the injury crosses the midline, it may be beneficial to perform a nerve block on both sides of the face.

The third branch of the facial nerve, the mandibular nerve, splits into two branches: anterior and posterior. The posterior trunk has three branches, one of which is the inferior alveolar nerve, which has sensory-only branches that traverse the mandibular canal to exit via the mental foramen. Another one of those branches is the mental nerve, which supplies sensation to the skin and buccal mucosa of the lip and the skin of the chin. The incisive nerve continues in the mandibular medullary cavity to the premolars, canines, and incisors. The mental nerve exits through the mental foramen bilaterally in the mandible. The mental foramen is typically located halfway between the upper (alveolar crest) and the lower edge of the mandible in direct line with the second premolar (Fig 6-4). However, the exact location of the mental canal can be variable. In edentulous individuals, there is alveolar bone resorption, which makes the location of the mental foramen closer to the alveolar crest in a majority of patients.[3]

Some regions might present additional innervation. Therefore, for procedures performed in the upper lip, especially at the midline, the infraorbital nerve block is performed for anesthesia in the regions of the lower eyelid, the side of the nose, the upper lip, and the maxillary incisor, canine, premolars, and root of the first molar. In some cases, the total blocking of the nasopalatine nerve is also required to totally desensitize the middle area of the upper lip.[4] According to Malamed,[1] the superior anterior alveolar block results in a deep anesthesia of the buccal soft tissues from the central incisors up to the premolars in 72% of cases. This might explain why, in some cases, the block of only the infraorbital nerves will not promote an effective anesthesia of the middle part of the upper lip. In these situations, the anterior superior alveolar nerve should also be anesthetized. An infiltration anesthesia is therefore recommended at the top of the vestibule next to the root of the maxillary central incisor. For procedures in the lower lip, especially close to the midline, according to Bento et al,[5] the failure in blocking the inferior alveolar nerve might be attributed to the supplementary innervation of the mylohyoid nerve in this region (chin and lower lip).

In all anesthetic procedures, negative blood aspiration is performed prior to injecting the study solution.[6]

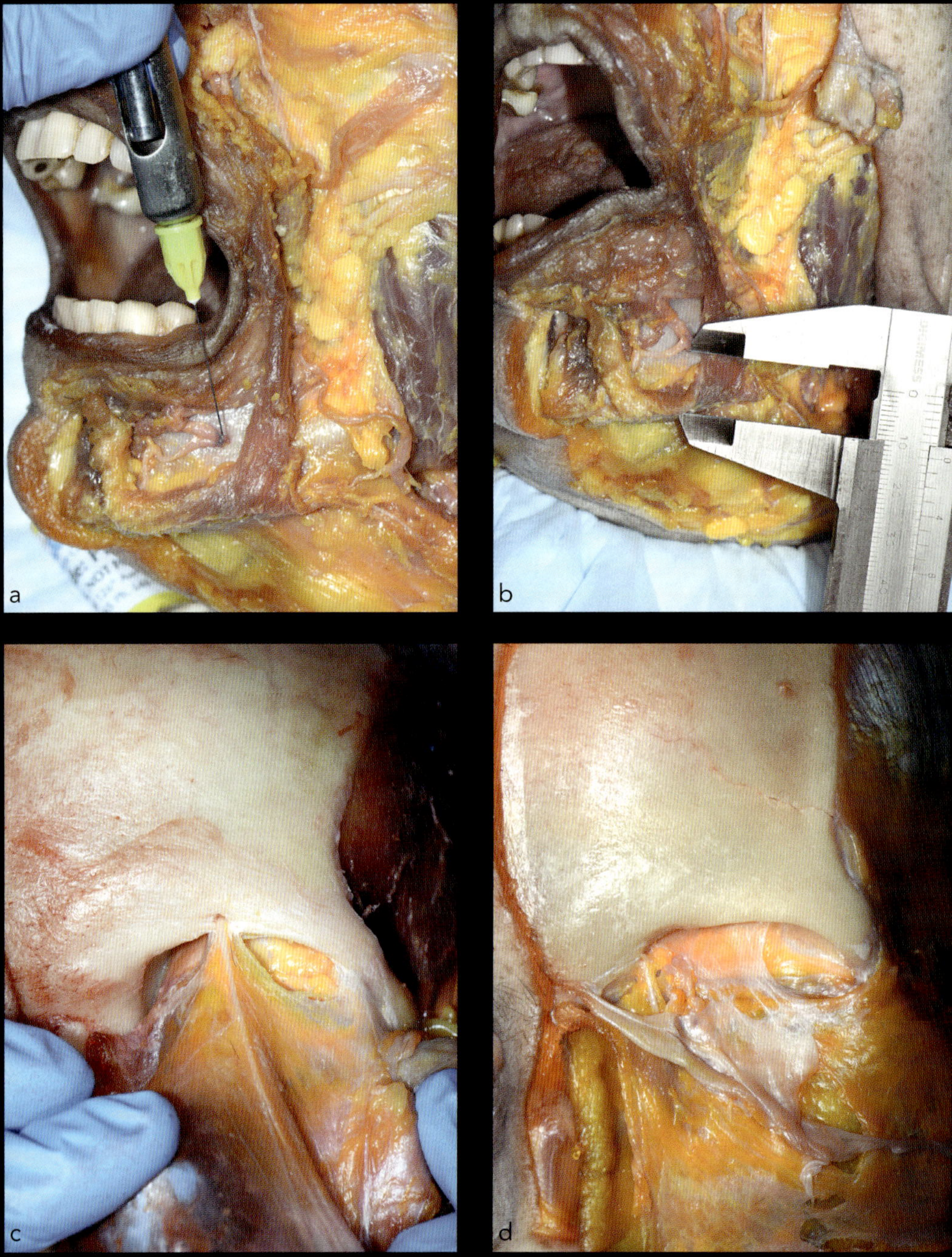

Fig 6-4 *(a)* Mental foramen in a cadaver. This image shows the position of the needle used to block the nerve over the mental foramen. *(b)* Distance from the mental foramen to the mandibular base. *(c)* A visible supraorbital foramen under the muscles of the forehead. *(d)* In some cases, the foramen is not present; instead, there is a fissure as shown here.

In procedures performed in the lower lip, the mental nerve block might be indicated because the mental and incisive nerves supply sensation to the mandibular teeth and skin of the chin and lower lip as well as buccal mucosa. Dentists use the mental/incisive nerve block either alone or in conjunction with the inferior alveolar nerve block. Studies have shown that 47% of patients develop pulp anesthesia in the first molars, 82% to 100% develop pulp anesthesia in the premolars, and 38% of patients develop pulp anesthesia in the lateral incisors. There is a greater chance of success for the incisive nerve block if the injection is given inside the foramen to achieve anesthesia of the second premolar and canine region. There is no difference in anesthetic success of the first premolar if the injection is given inside versus outside of the mental foramen.[7]

Note that a minimal amount of anesthetic should be used when blocking the external nasal nerve to avoid a momentary vascular ischemia. The injection point for this nerve is just below the osseocartilaginous junction, as it grooves the internal surface of the nasal bone and terminates by piercing nasal cartilage to become the external nasal nerve, supplying the skin of the dorsal nose and the nasal apex.[8]

Innervation of the Neck

Understanding the innervation of the neck is also fundamental for esthetic filling procedures because the nerves from the area around the gonial angle, side of the mandible, and base of the chin emerge from the neck.

The cervical plexus is a network of nerve fibers that forms an anastomosis and then splits into cervical spinal nerves (C1, C2, C3, and C4).[9] The trunk of the spinal nerve emerges through the intervertebral foramen and splits into dorsal and ventral rami. The cervical plexus is comprised by the ventral rami of these four upper cervical nerves that emerge from the spine through the intervertebral foramina located on the side of each cervical vertebra and innervate some neck muscles, diaphragm, and areas of the skin at the head, neck, and thorax.

Each ventral ramus connects with the following ramus, forming three loops of lateral convexity (C1 with C2, C2 with C3, and C3 with C4). These three loops and the branches originated by them form the two parts of the cervical plexus (superficial and deep).

The superficial part is composed of fibers essentially sensorial that form a bundle that emerges at the middle of the posterior border of the sternocleidomastoid muscle, where the fibers spread in a fan shape to the neighbor region, external ear, skin of the neck, and region next to the clavicle.[10]

Each ramus, except the first, divides into ascending and descending parts that unite in communicating loops. The first loop (C2 and C3) supplies superficial branches to the head and neck; the second loop (C3 and C4) gives rise to cutaneous nerves supplying the shoulder and thorax. The branches are superficial and deep, where the superficial branches perforate the cervical fascia to innervate the skin and the deep branches innervate the muscles. This chapter does not address the deep part of the cervical plexus.

Table 6-3 Superficial cervical nerves

NERVE	NERVES IT GIVES OFF	INNERVATION
Ascending superficial nerves	Lesser occipital nerve (C2)	It supplies the skin of the posterior surface of the external ear.
	Great auricular nerve (C2 and C3)	The anterior branch supplies the skin of the face over the parotid gland and communicates with the facial nerve. The posterior branch supplies the skin over the mastoid process and on the posterior surface of the auricle.
	Transverse cervical nerve (C2 and C3)	Its ascending branches proceed to the submaxillary region and eventually form a plexus with the cervical branch of the facial nerve below the platysma muscle. The descending branches pierce the platysma muscle and are distributed to the skin over the anterior and lateral aspects of the neck as inferior as the sternum.
Descending superficial nerves	Medial supraclavicular nerve (C3 and C4)	It supplies the skin as far as the median plane, the inferior part of the second rib, and the sternoclavicular joint.
	Intermediate supraclavicular nerve	It supplies the skin over the pectoralis major and deltoid muscles at the level of the second rib.
	Lateral supraclavicular nerve	It supplies the skin of the upper and posterior aspect of the shoulder.

(Based on Netter.[12])

Table 6-4 Important nerves in the neck to be blocked for filling procedures

POINT IN FIG 6-5	NERVE	RAMUS	ACCESS	QUANTITY OF ANESTHETIC
15	Great auricular	C2 and C3	Extraoral	0.6 mL
16	Transverse cervical	C2 and C3	Extraoral	0.6 mL

The superficial branch forms ascending and descending groups. Table 6-3 summarizes the anatomy of these branches. In a superficial cervical plexus block, the anesthesia is given subcutaneously along the posterior border of the sternocleidomastoid muscle.[11]

Because of these anastomoses and ramifications, the author's clinical experience suggests that it is preferable to penetrate the skin, keeping a 3-mm depth with a needle, and deposit anesthetic at posterior and inferior points to those of the areas to be filled. This is possible because the innervation that comes from the neck to the jaw travels superiorly and anteriorly. This approach can also be used if the operator does not want to anesthetize a very large area in cases of small-area fillings.

Table 6-4 summarizes the anesthetic technique for two superficial cervical nerves involved in esthetic filling procedures, and Fig 6-5 illustrates the innervation.

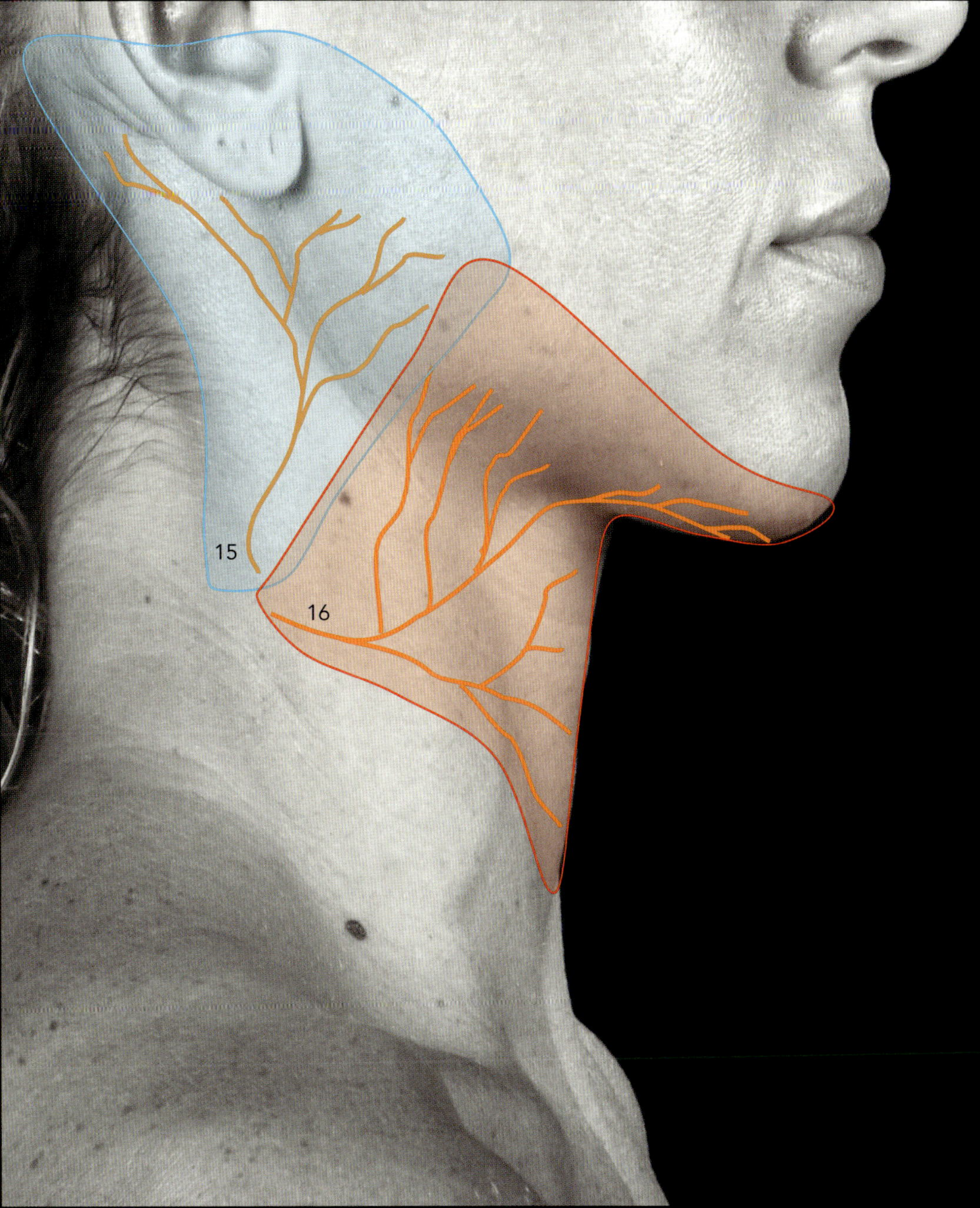

Fig 6-5 General view of important sensory nerve pathways to be blocked for filling procedures at the mandibular area close to the neck. These nerves are described in Table 6-4. In case the operator does not want to block a very extensive area, a needle can be inserted at a depth of 3 mm to deposit the anesthetic in posterior and inferior points in the areas that will be filled. This is possible because the innervation that emerges from the neck to the jaw travels superiorly and anteriorly.

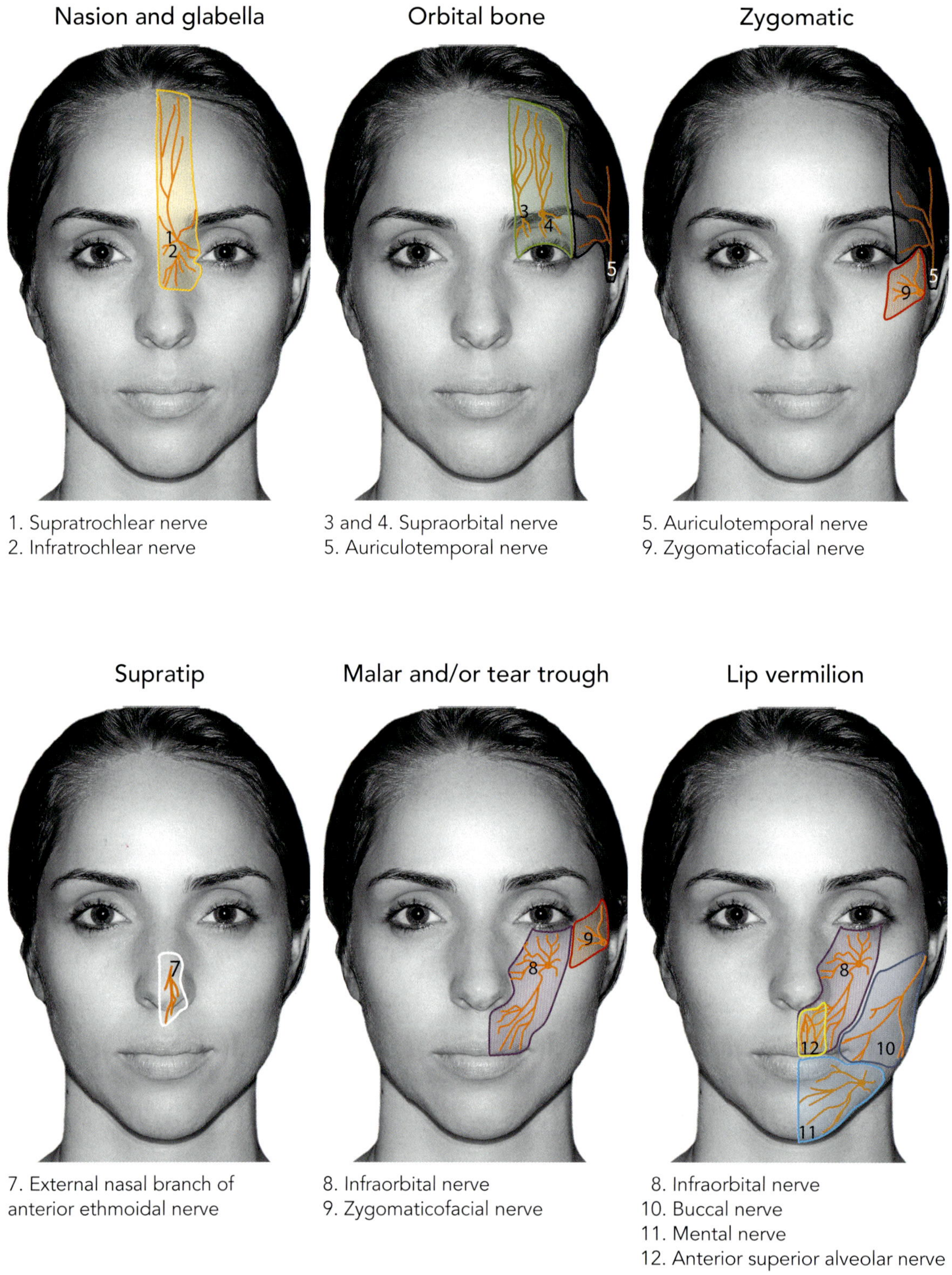

Filling Procedures and Target Nerves

Figure 6-6 illustrates the target nerves and resulting anesthetized areas for various locations on the face to be filled.

Marionettes and vermilion of the lower lip

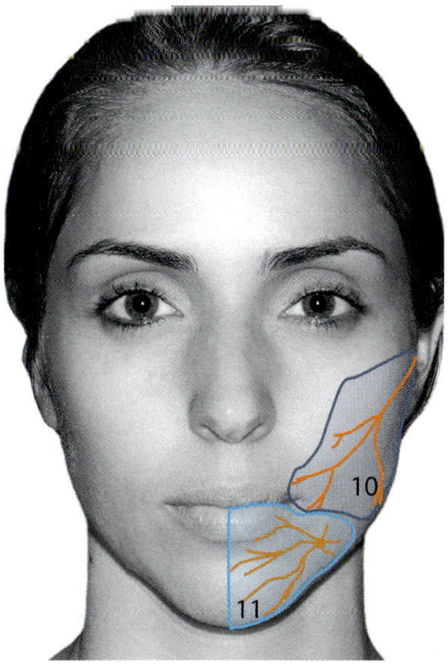

10. Buccal nerve
11. Mental nerve

Chin: mentolabial sulcus, lateral advancement, and base

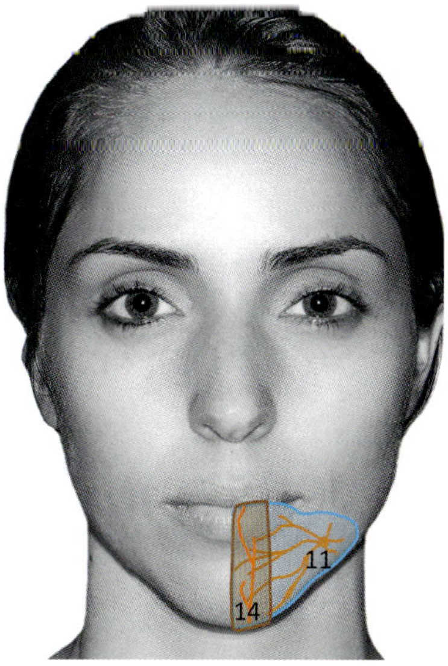

11. Mental nerve
14. Mylohyoid nerve

Note: In order to numb the base of the chin, the transverse cervical nerve and eventually the mylohyoid nerve should also be numbed.

Philtrum

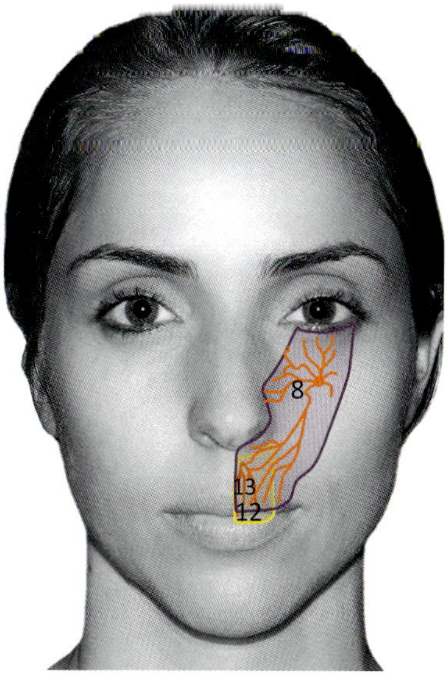

8. Infraorbital nerve
12. Anterior superior alveolar nerve
13. Nasopalatine nerve

Nasolabial fold/upper lip (vermilion)

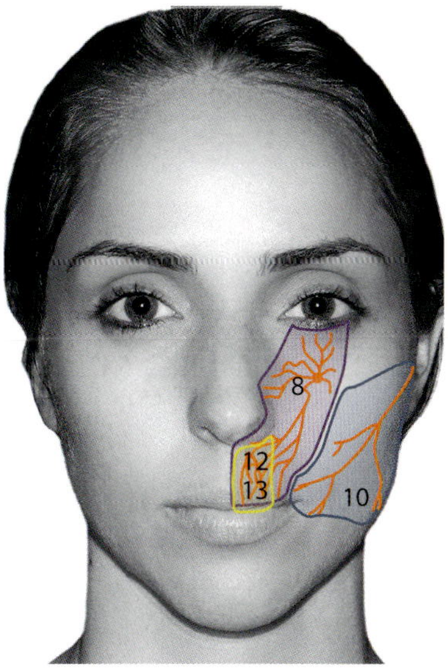

8. Infraorbital nerve
10. Buccal nerve
12. Anterior superior alveolar nerve
13. Nasopalatine nerve

Fig 6-6 The figures above and at left list the areas to be filled, the extent of anesthetic area obtained (colored areas), and the nerves to be anesthetized (numbers below the figures).

HINT: To increase the efficacy of the anesthesia, the operator can penetrate the needle up to the target point and inject 80% of the recommended dosage. The remaining 20% is then injected during the removal of the needle. This will promote a longer anesthesia because the target point will have been considered in three dimensions (right and left, upper and lower, and depth and superficiality). This will result in a more effective and wider anesthesia. However, the patient should be advised that he or she will feel something like a small electric shock during the removal of the needle. This happens when the more superficial branch comes into contact with the anesthetic liquid.

Table 6-5 Anesthetics and maximum dosage by body weight

LOCAL ANESTHETIC	MAXIMUM DOSE (PER BODY WEIGHT IN KG)	NUMBER OF CARTRIDGES (1.8 ML) PER 60-KG ADULT	ABSOLUTE MAXIMUM (REGARDLESS OF THE WEIGHT)
2% lidocaine	4.4 mg	7	300 mg
3% lidocaine	4.4 mg	4.5	300 mg
2% mepivacaine	4.4 mg	7	300 mg
3% mepivacaine	4.4 mg	4.5	300 mg
Articaine	7 mg	5.5	500 mg
3% prilocaine	6 mg	6.5	400 mg
0.5% bupivacaine	1.3 mg	8.5	90 mg

(Based on Andrade.[13])

Caution on Dosage

Calculating the maximum dose of anesthetic considered safe in each consultation does not depend on the number of areas to be injected. It is important to consider the sum of the anesthetic amounts being used per session. The calculation should be made considering the following factors:

- *Anesthetic concentration:* Recommended by the manufacturer in the package insert (2% means 20 mg/mL and 3% means 30 mg/mL).
- *Amount of anesthetic:* Each cartridge for carpule syringes contains 1.8 mL.
- *Patient's body weight:* The patient should inform the operator of his or her weight or should be weighed.
- *Maximum dose by body weight (in kg):* See Table 6-5. Doses greater than the ones described might affect the central nervous system and cardiac conditions.

Vasoconstrictors

It is also important to consider whether or not to use vasoconstrictors. There are no randomized clinical trials in the literature that demonstrate and evaluate the effects of vasoconstrictors on the dermis and epidermis in humans. While the author uses anesthetics with vasoconstrictors (always in small amounts) in his clinical practice, caution is recommended.

References

1. Malamed SF. Manual de Anestesia Local. Rio de Janeiro: Elsevier, 2013.
2. Piccinin MA, Zito PM. Anatomy, Head, Lips. Treasure Island, FL: StatPearls, 2018.
3. Nardi NM, Schaefer TJ. Nerve Block, Infraorbital. Treasure Island, FL: StatPearls, 2018.
4. Meyer TN, Lemos LL, Nascimento CNM, Lellis WRR. Effectiveness of nasopalatine nerve block for anesthesia of maxillary central incisors after failure of the anterior superior alveolar nerve block technique. Braz Dent J 2007;18:69–73.
5. Bento LFA, Carvalho ASO, Santos EGF, Ávila EC, Mora K, Lima FJC. Inervação sensitiva dos dentes inferiores pelo nervo milohióide. https://even3storage.blob.core.windows.net/anais/79738.pdf Accessed 18 August 2018.
6. Mostafa MF, Herdan R, Elshazly M. Comparative study of levobupivacaine and bupivacaine for bilateral maxillary nerve block during pediatric primary cleft palate surgery: A randomized double-blind controlled study. Korean J Anesthesiol 2018;71:135–140.
7. Betz D, Fane K. Nerve Block, Mental. Treasure Island, FL: StatPearls, 2018.
8. Radiopedia. https://radiopaedia.org/articles/anterior-ethmoidal-nerve. Accessed 10 June 2018.
9. Dermatologia. https://books.google.com/books?isbn=8535269746. Accessed 10 June 2018.
10. Machado A. Neuroanatomia funcional, ed 2. São Paulo: Editora Atheneu, 2004.
11. Perisanidis C, Saranteas T, Kostopanagiotou G. Ultrasound-guided combined intermediate and deep cervical plexus nerve block for regional anaesthesia in oral and maxillofacial surgery. Dentomaxillofac Radiol 2013;2:29945724.
12. Netter FH. Atlas de Anatomia Humana, ed 2. Porto Alegre: Artmed, 2000.
13. Andrade ED. Terapêutica medicamentosa em odontologia, ed 3. São Paulo: Artes Médicas, 2014.

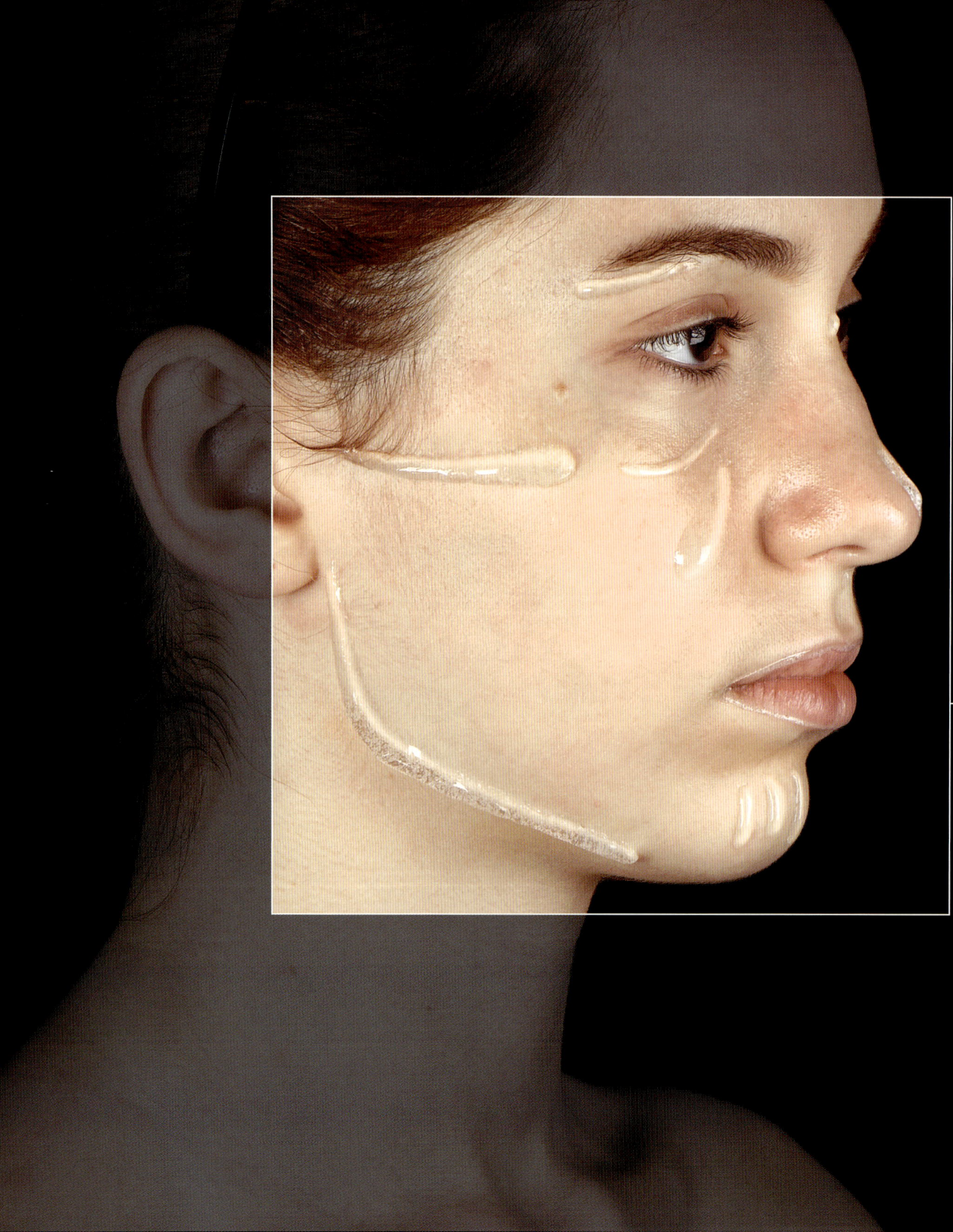

CHAPTER

07

Facial Regions and Possible Filler Therapies

Swelling

The application of a good-quality hyaluronic acid (HA) filler is very safe because of its biocompatibility. However, swelling can be a problem and is associated with all fillers, especially in the tear trough area. Swelling occurs because of the hydrophilic nature of the gels and also the inherent disruption of normal vascular and lymphatic dynamics.[1]

The risk of persistent swelling can be minimized in a variety of ways. Firstly, careful thought must be applied when considering the type of filler material to be used around the eyes. There is a range of products available, and the choice of filler should match the location being injected. If you are using the same filler for all parts of the face, you are likely doing something wrong. Highly cross-linked HA gels are excellent for larger-volume and deeper fills such as the nasolabial folds or lateral cheeks. However, these gels are more prone to swelling and should be avoided around the eyes in favor of less cross-linked preparations or blends.[2] In addition, remember that when treating the tear troughs, small volumes are the key. If you are used to treating areas where large injection volumes are used, you will find the volume requirements around the tear trough very different, as often 0.05 to 0.2 mL is more than sufficient for each tear trough deformity.

Injection Location

Figures 7-1 to 7-18 show the approximate location of the injected product for various regions of the face. The recommended products, as well as the instruments to be used during injection, are described in order of priority (first, second, third choice). Please note that the first choice is preferred but the other choices are acceptable. The volumes to be used might also vary in each case. The suggested route of administration is subcutaneous, that is, approximately 3 mm below the epidermis, except for the tear trough and palpebromalar groove, where the juxtaperiosteal injection is recommended. The skin is very thin in these two regions, which helps to visualize the volume of filler right below it, and thus small amounts of the filler should be injected. Large quantities can still partially block the lymphatic system, leading to recurrent swelling. The use of very hydrophilic fillers in this area should be avoided. Additionally, it is important to observe that at the tear trough and palpebromalar groove, juxtaperiosteal injections should be made so that the fibers of the orbicularis oculi muscle can hide undesirable volumes.

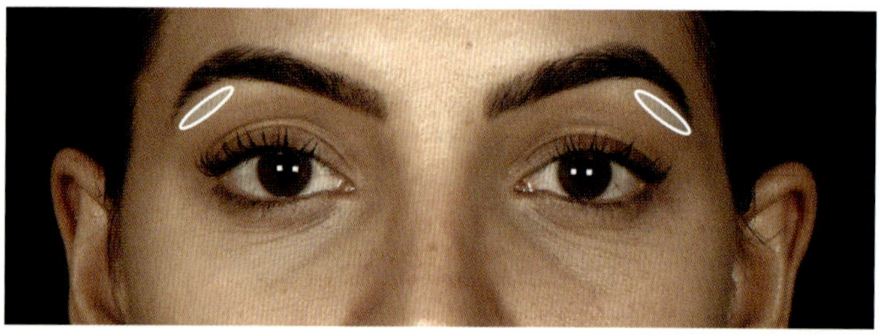

PRODUCT	INSTRUMENT	QUANTITY
Restylane Defyne or Kysse	22G, 23G, or 25G cannula or needle	0.1–0.2 mL

Fig 7-1 Injection location for orbit structuring.

- The filament should have a bone background, but this procedure does not require juxtaperiosteal injection.
- Inject to a 3-mm depth.
- Massage the area, curving the lateral part of the filament.
- This therapy projects the lateral of the orbit in a horizontal plane.

Fig 7-2 Injection location for eversion of the lip vermilion.

- Use a needle to make short filaments and a 25G cannula for long filaments.
- The filaments should be more superficial so they will become evident.
- Always inject at the vermilion.
- For better definition, do not massage the area.
- This therapy rejuvenates the mouth.

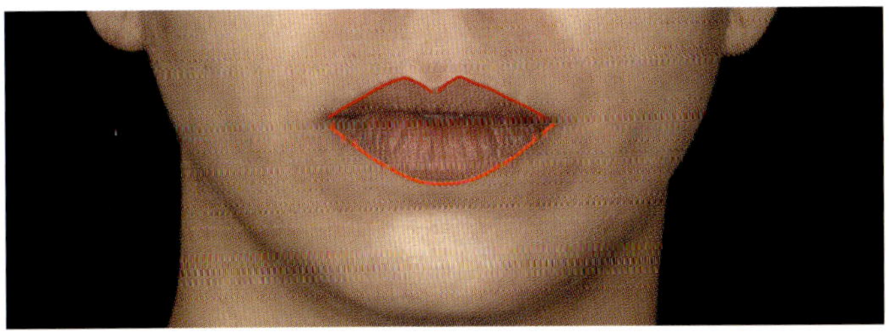

PRODUCT	INSTRUMENT	QUANTITY
Restylane Kysse	25G cannula	0.05–0.1 mL in each long filament

Fig 7-3 Injection location for the lip tubercle.

- The needle should stop at 3 mm.
- The injection should follow the midline.

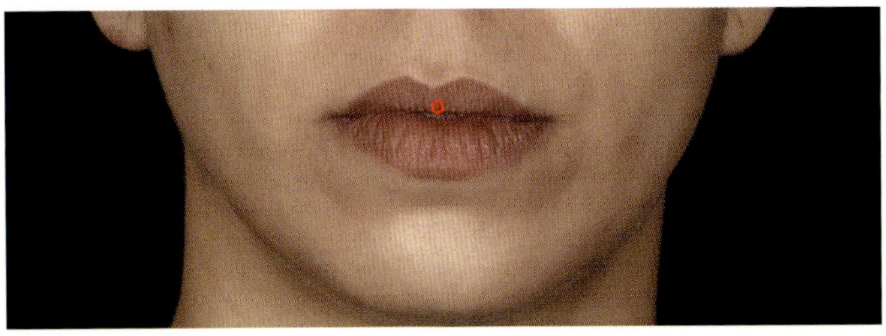

PRODUCT	INSTRUMENT	QUANTITY
Restylane Kysse	Needle	0.05–0.1 mL

Fig 7-4 Injection location for volumization of the lip vermilion.

- If you notice that the lips are flat, evaluate a possible decrease of the occlusal vertical dimension as a possible cause.
- For better definition, do not massage the area and make a deeper injection (3 mm).
- The lower filaments can be interrupted in the width of the philtrum sulcus in order to cause a depression at the midline to fit the upper lip tubercle.

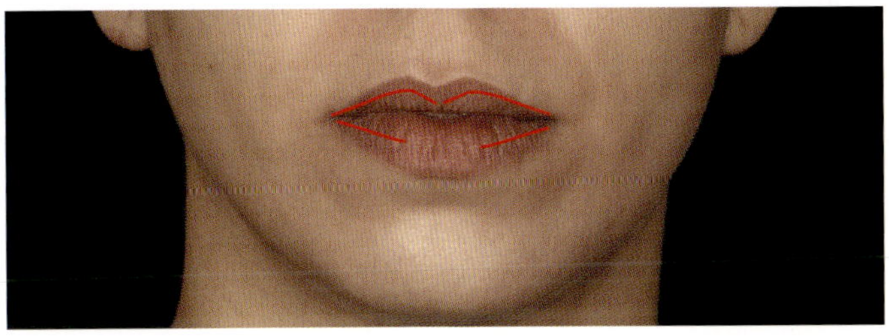

PRODUCT	INSTRUMENT	QUANTITY
Restylane Kysse	25G cannula	0.1 mL in each long filament

Fig 7-5 Injection location for philtrum columns.

- The injection should be performed close to the dermis (never in the dermis but more superficial).
- The bevel should be turned downward.
- Inject the filler in the philtrum before the eversion filament in the Cupid's bow, because the philtrum already contributes to that. Only then analyze if there is still a need to create the Cupid's bow near the midline.

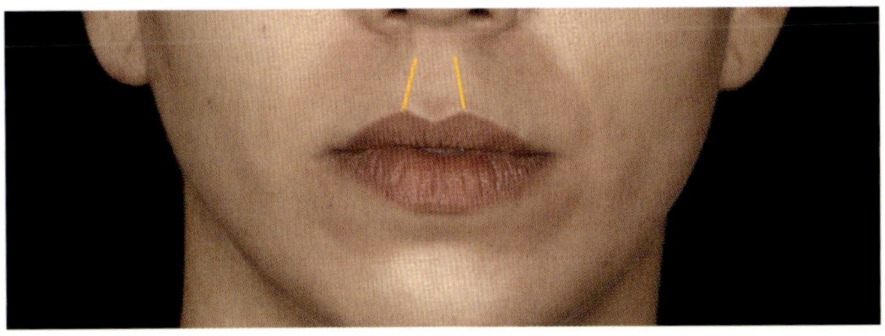

PRODUCT	INSTRUMENT	QUANTITY
Restylane Kysse	Needle	0.05 mL in each column

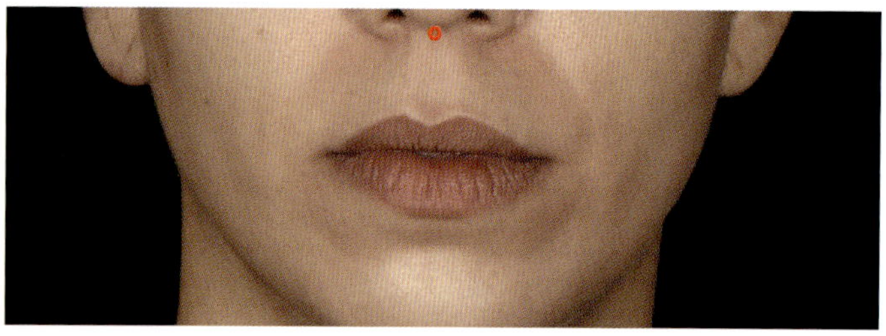

PRODUCT	INSTRUMENT	QUANTITY
Restylane Defyne or Kysse	22G, 23G, or 25G cannula or needle	Min. 0.2 mL Max. 0.3 mL

Fig 7-6 Injection location for the subnasale point.

- The injection should be made 3 mm deep.
- Do not inject inside the columella.
- Do not inject at the anterior nasal spine. Deeper injections of fillers demand larger amounts of material and are dangerous because the blood vessels are larger than in the more superficial layers.

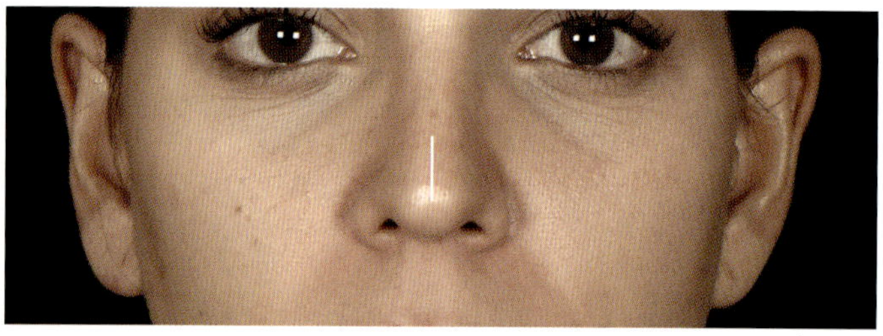

PRODUCT	INSTRUMENT	QUANTITY
Restylane Kysse	25G or 23G cannula	0.1+0.1+0.1 mL injected in 30-day intervals

Fig 7-7 Injection location at the supratip.

- Caution should be taken in patients who previously underwent rhinoplasty because of necrosis concerns.
- This therapy is contraindicated for Asian patients because they do not show enough skin elasticity in this area.
- The length of the filament is equal to the height of the alar cartilage plus 1 mm.
- Redness in the tip of the nose for more than 7 days can mean an excess of the product was used. In that case, future injections should have a reduced amount of filler.

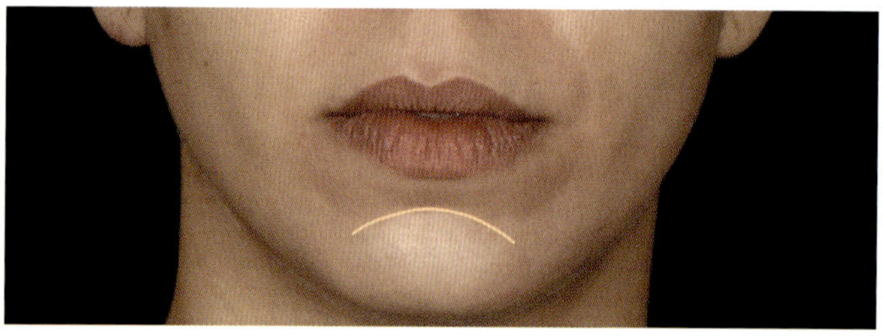

PRODUCT	INSTRUMENT	QUANTITY
Restylane Defyne or Kysse if the skin is thin	22G or 23G curved cannula	0.1–0.5 mL

Fig 7-8 Injection location at the mentolabial sulcus.

- The depth of the cannula should be 3 mm.
- This therapy increases the length of the lower lip. It also corrects the inclined lip (Class II).
- This therapy makes the person's face more dolichofacial and balances the ratio between the measurement of the upper lip and lower lip.
- This therapy lifts the lower lip and helps with passive sealing of the lips.
- It also promotes the chin-face integration.

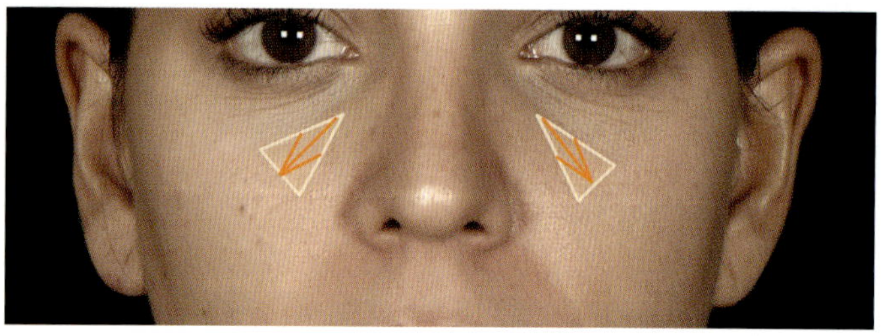

PRODUCT	INSTRUMENT	QUANTITY
Restylane Defyne or Kysse	22G or 23G cannula	0.5–1.0 mL in each side

Fig 7-9 Injection location for malar deficiency.

- Draw a triangle. The injection should be 3 to 4 mm deep.
- Avoid a deep plane because of the infraorbital foramen and the risk of internal bleeding.
- This therapy may worsen the infraorbital depressions. Thus, inform the patient that these depressions might also need filler injections.

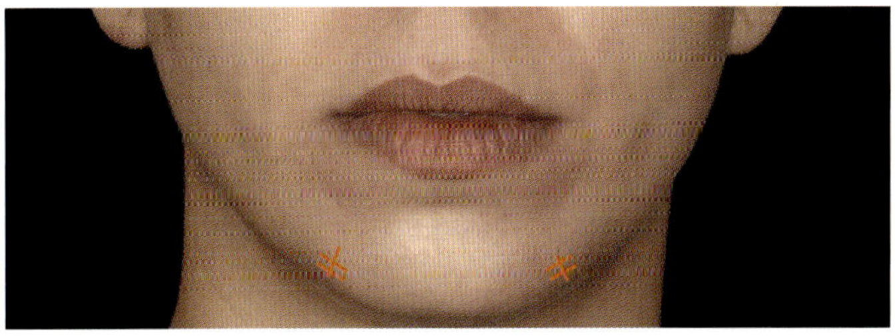

Fig 7-10 Injection location for the prejowl sulcus.

- The cannula should be 3 mm deep.
- Extraoral access is recommended.
- This therapy promotes the chin-face integration.
- Inform the patient that at the end of the therapy, the filling will be noticeable to the touch and that this is normal.

PRODUCT	INSTRUMENT	QUANTITY
Restylane Defyne or Kysse	22G, 23G, or 25G cannula	0.5 mL in each side

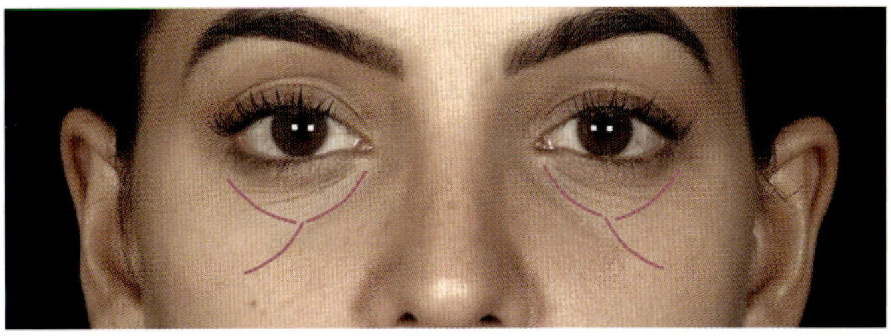

Fig 7-11 Injection location for infraorbital depressions.

- CAUTION: Dark circles are a result of darkening of the skin and should not be treated with facial fillers. Fillers should only be injected in case of infrapalpebral depression.
- This is the only filling procedure that should be done using a juxtaperiosteal injection.
- Maintain a distance of 5 mm from the plica semilunaris.

PRODUCT	INSTRUMENT	QUANTITY
Restylane Fynesse	25G, 23G, or 22G curved cannula	0.5 mL in each side

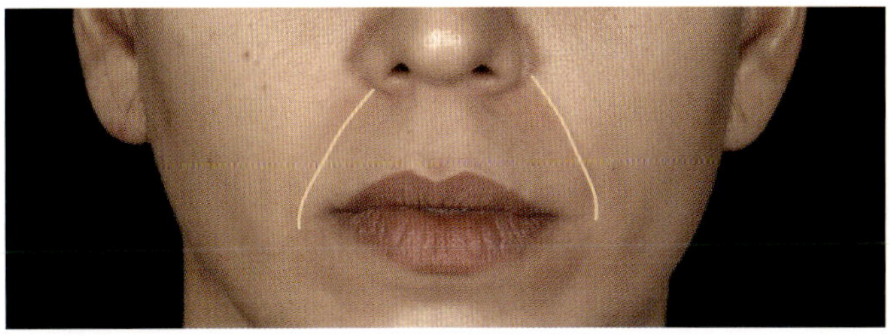

Fig 7-12 Injection location at the nasolabial folds.

- After using the cannula to make the filament, use the needle to make a filling just like the shape of a zipper (only in a more pronounced sulcus). Do not extend it to the ala nasi.
- This is the preferred site for beginners, although it is less important than other sites such as the marionette lines, except in cases of maxillary deficiency.
- The marionette lines are the priority.
- Before injecting, enter and remove the cannula at least four times against the dermis, following the sulcus. It will make the subcutaneous tissue thinner in order to achieve a better result.
- Inject a uniform amount of the filler, but do not inject a larger volume in the superior border of the groove to avoid blocking the vessels.

PRODUCT	INSTRUMENT	QUANTITY
Restylane Defyne or Kysse	22G or 23G cannula	0.5–1.0 mL in each side

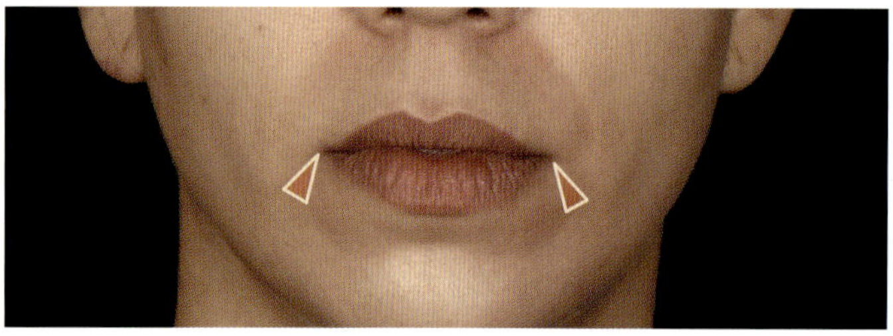

PRODUCT	INSTRUMENT	QUANTITY
Restylane Defyne or Kysse	22G or 23G cannula or needle	0.3–0.5 mL in each side

Fig 7-13 Injection location for marionette lines.

- In some cases, the drawing in this area will be a filament, in others a filament with small perpendicular dashes (similar to the shape of a zipper), and in others a triangle.
- The fan technique can be used to inject the filler inside the triangle area.
- This therapy promotes the chin-face integration.

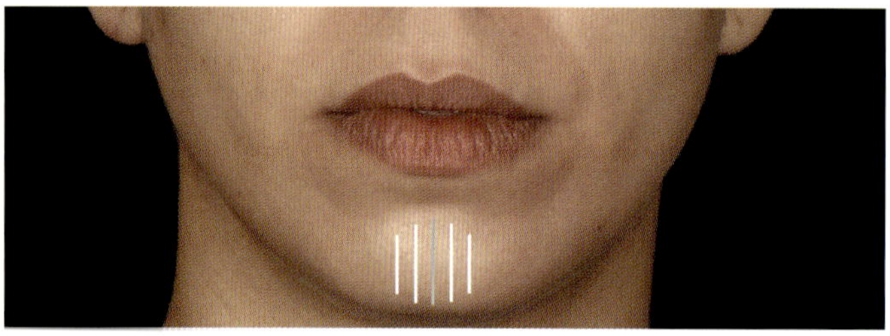

PRODUCT	INSTRUMENT	QUANTITY
Restylane Volyme, Defyne, or Kysse	22G or 23G cannula	1.0–4.0 mL

Fig 7-14 Injection location for chin volumization.

- Preoperative botulinum toxin should be injected in cases of wrinkled skin.
- Injecting the filament at the midline will result in a more feminine face. It is also a more effective technique to volumize the chin in terms of the profile. When the filler is not injected at the midline, the face in frontal view will be improved.
- This therapy better defines the jawline.
- However, it makes the mentolabial grooves worse.

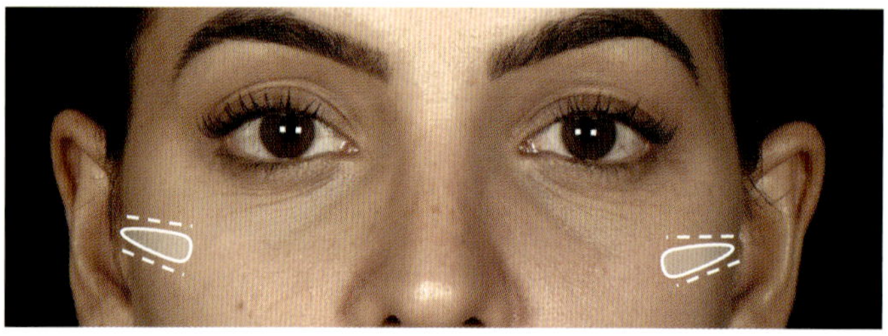

PRODUCT	INSTRUMENT	QUANTITY
Restylane Defyne or Kysse	22G or 23G cannula ×50 mm	0.5 mL in each side

Fig 7-15 Injection location at the zygomatic arch.

- Mark the lower bony ridge of the zygomatic arch by palpation.
- To mark the upper bony ridge, follow the horizontal level of the ceiling of the acoustic meatus and the floor of the orbit.
- This area is wider in its anterior portion, and therefore a larger amount should be injected in this region, as the drawing suggests.

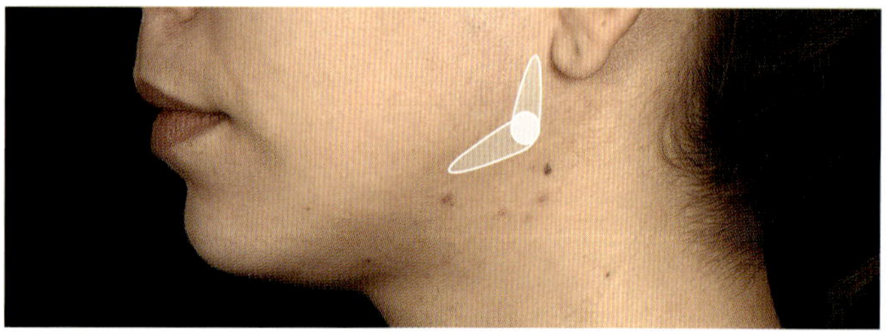

PRODUCT	INSTRUMENT	QUANTITY
Restylane Defyne or Kysse	22G straight cannula	0.5–1 mL in each angle

Fig 7-16 Injection location at the gonial angle.

- To draw the patient's gonial angle: Use the tips of the fingers (four fingers of a hand at the same time) to find the limits. Two fingers will touch the ramus and two fingers the base of the jaw. The goal is to locate the bone and also to measure the angle. Then the second drawing will have a bone background.

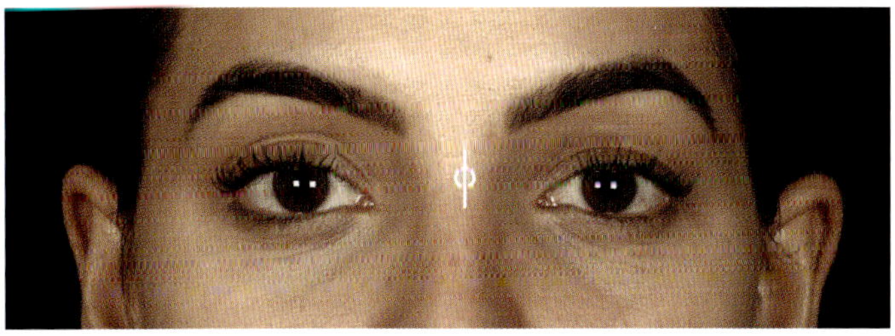

Fig 7-17 Injection location at the nasion.

- This therapy decreases the appearance of the hooked nose.
- It also increases the femininity of the face.
- CAUTION: There is a risk of blindness with this procedure. Do not make lateral filaments to the midline; this increases the risk of vessel compression.
- The cannula should penetrate 3 mm deep, inside the glabella fat pad.

PRODUCT	INSTRUMENT	QUANTITY
Restylane Kysse or Defyne	22G, 23G, or 25G cannula	0.05–0.1 mL

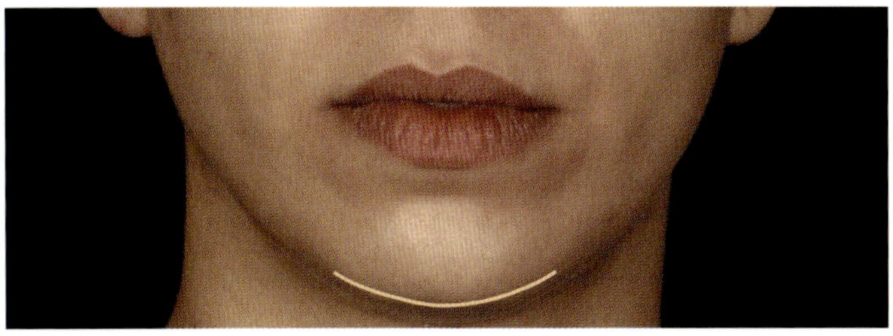

Fig 7-18 Injection location in the submental area.

- This therapy makes the person's face more dolichofacial and balances the ratio between the measurement of the upper lip and the lower lip.
- The total length (skin and vermilion) of the upper lip multiplied by two must equal that of the lower lip plus 1, 2, 3, or 4 mm.
- Inject the filler against the bone support in the jaw at 3 mm deep.
- This therapy decreases the view of the submentalis region from the frontal perspective.

PRODUCT	INSTRUMENT	QUANTITY
Restylane Defyne or Kysse	22G or 23G curved cannula	0.5–1 mL

Perception of Facial Anatomy

A good esthetics treatment depends on a good diagnosis. An accurate diagnosis is made when the clinician understands three principles of facial anatomy: dominance, 3D vision, and image composition.

Dominance

According to this principle, a large anatomical structure close to a regular-sized anatomical structure causes the latter to be perceived as smaller than it really is. The opposite is also true; that is, a small anatomical structure next to a regular-sized anatomical structure causes the latter to be seen as larger. A simple comparison would be, for instance, a picture of a medium-sized car parked next to a large truck. Because the truck is larger than the average-size car, it makes the average-size car look even smaller. In this case, it can then be said that the truck is the dominant object of the scene, decreasing the impact or importance of the car.

This concept is important when it comes to facial anatomy perception. Take, for example, an individual with large and long teeth and thin lips analyzed in frontal view. At first, it is necessary to diagnose if the ideal approach would be to reduce the size of the teeth or to increase the labial volume. When the size of the teeth is harmonious, injecting fillers in the lips can be one possible procedure. This would balance the dominance between the teeth and lips, as a bulging lip would decrease the perception of dominant teeth without changing their size. This procedure will result in facial harmony. Another example, now in profile view, would be an individual who has a nose of a regular size but a deficient chin. This deficiency changes the perception of the size of the nose, making it look too long, that is, dominant in the face of this patient.

3D vision

The skill to make a good diagnosis is directly associated with the ability to see an object in depth. A lot of individuals observe an object by considering only two dimensions (ie, its height and width). However, it is fundamental to also perceive the third dimension—its depth. Only then will the perception of the object be complete. This gives the clinician the chance to better calculate the volume of filler to be used.

Take, for example, a patient with malar deficiency. When drawing the area to be treated, some clinicians misjudge the amount of material to be injected. If the volume of material used is less than required, a depression can be observed. On the other hand, if the volume is larger than required, this will result in an overfill. A useful way to think about facial features is to avoid classifying individual anatomical structures as "too big" or "too small" but instead classifying them as large or narrow, long or short, and concave, leveled, or convex.

Image composition

A facial analysis should be based on the same principles as the perception of a geometric form. By doing so, the face will be perceived as a set of points, line segments, planes, edges, circumferences (curved lines), and angles. To better diagnose the need for possible procedures using fillers, the clinician should look for these geometric forms.

For example, generally rounded faces (with circumferences, curved lines, few straight lines, undefined angles, and few planes) in adults are perceived as more childlike. Fillers can be injected to make the lines of the face look straighter and the angles more defined and to create planes. All of these geometric changes will give the face a more defined look.

A good way to think about the geometry of the face and dermal fillers is in terms of light. When you inject a filler in an area, the volume is increased, and the region will therefore get more light. The use of fillers therefore transforms shadows into light. Several mathematical rules can be used for image composition analysis, and they are described in chapter 5.

Diagram for Treatment with Fillers

Planning is a fundamental part of treatment with fillers. The clinician must record the target sites to be injected, and Fig 7-19 shows a template that can used. This template can also be useful during the treatment presentation to help patients understand the planning of the areas to be filled.

How to use it:

1. Open the diagram available via QR code.
2. Delete the underlying photograph of the model.
3. Copy and paste the photograph of the patient to be analyzed.
4. Right-click on the photograph and then click "Arrange" and "Send to Back."
5. Delete any treatments that will not be performed in that specific patient.
6. Slightly adjust the position and length of each site, as different faces can be larger, shorter, longer, or wider. To make these adjustments, first left-click on the area to be injected. While keeping the control key pressed, use the keyboard arrows to change the position of the area.

Table 7-1 lists the appropriate doses/volumes and recommended products for the various sites in the face.

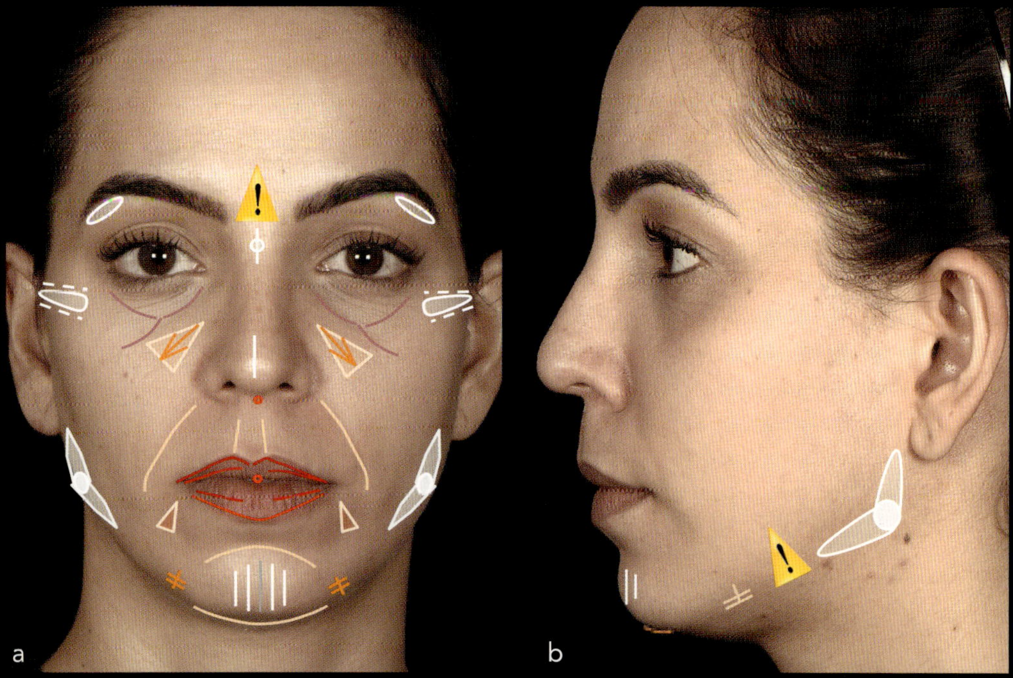

Fig 7-19 *(a)* Diagram for using fillers in frontal view showing several treatments that could be performed in the face. The triangle highlights the glabella, an area to be avoided because of the risk of necrosis and blindness. *(b)* Diagram for using fillers in profile view showing possible treatments to improve the jawline definition. The triangle highlights the lower jaw fat area, which should be avoided because it is naturally large. These diagrams are available via QR code.

Table 7-1 Recommended filler doses/volumes and products for various regions of the face

SITE	DOSE/VOLUME	PRODUCT
Nasion	0.05–0.1 mL of a syringe	Restylane Kysse or Juvéderm Volift
Columella base	0.2–0.3 mL of a syringe	Restylane Defyne or Kysse or Juvéderm Volift
Supratip	0.05–0.1 mL of a syringe	Restylane Kysse or Defyne or Juvéderm Volift
Philtrum	0.05 mL of a syringe for each column	Restylane Kysse or Juvéderm Volift
Lip vermilion	A maximum of 1 syringe	Restylane Kysse or Juvéderm Volbella or Volift
Mentalis (chin)	1–4 syringes	Restylane Volyme or Defyne or Juvéderm Voluma
Nasolabial sulcus	0.5 mL to 1 syringe for each sulcus	Restylane Defyne or Kysse or Juvéderm Volift
Tear trough	0.05 mL of a syringe for each eye	Restylane Fynesse or Juvéderm Volbella
Prejowls	0.5 mL of a syringe for each side	Restylane Defyne or Kysse or Juvéderm Volift
Marionette lines	0.3–0.5 mL of a syringe for each side	Restylane Defyne or Kysse or Juvéderm Volift
Malar deficiency	0.5–1.0 mL of a syringe for each side	Restylane Defyne or Kysse or Juvéderm Volift
Gonial angle	0.5 mL to 1 syringe for each side	Restylane Defyne or Kysse or Juvéderm Volift
Orbit restructuring	0.1–0.2 mL for each orbit	Restylane Defyne or Kysse
Zygomatic bone definition	0.5 mL of a syringe for each side	Restylane Defyne or Kysse or Juvéderm Volift
Submentalis	0.5 mL to 1 syringe	Restylane Defyne or Kysse or Juvéderm Volift
Fine perioral wrinkles	0.5 mL of a syringe for each side	Restylane Skinbooster or Fynesse or Juvéderm Hydrate
Mentolabial sulcus	0.1 mL to 0.5 of a syringe for each sulcus	Restylane Defyne

Restructuring the Orbit

Anatomy

The definitive adult male and female facial shape is present following puberty,[3] where the male skull is on average 8.5% larger than the female skull[4] and men have approximately 15% greater body mass than women.[5] The nasal, cranial, and facial dimorphism are also observed at puberty, showing that adult male faces are larger and characterized locally by more prominent nasal and chin regions and less prominent infraorbital and malar regions.[6]

The human ocular globe is located inside a bone cavity. The bony ridges of this cavity are relatively regular except on its upper side, where there is a noticeable volume that stands out from the regular contour of the orbit. This volume is greater in women. The result is a slight bowing that is characteristic of younger people. With aging, a certain degree of flattening at this prominent part of the orbit might occur, and it is initially observed around the age of 35 years.

The brow ridge (superciliary arch) and glabella are prominent in males, while females show a flat brow ridge and glabella and a more obvious superior and lateral surface of the orbit. The lowest part of the female's forehead is protruded in its lateral portion and in males in its medial portion.

Visual interpretation

Orbits that are flat in their upper lateral portion suggest aging in female faces as well as masculinity. On the other hand, prominent orbits in their superior lateral portion suggest joviality in female faces.

Diagnosis

The decision to use fillers in the orbit can be made by observing the patient's face in frontal and profile views. Observe the vertical distance between the lower part of the lateral third of the eyebrow and the upper part of the eyelid. This distance should be markedly greater in women than in men.

Technique

Draw a straight line immediately below the hairy area of the eyebrow, including the caudal third. Through palpation, check if the drawing matches the bone. If not, move the horizontal level of the drawing upward until there is bone to support the filler; otherwise, the result will be barely visible. Use a 22G cannula to deposit the filler 2 to 3 mm deep.

Clinical case

Figure 7-20 illustrates orbit restructuring in conjunction with other dermal filler treatments. The following volumes were used at the sites listed:

- *Orbit restructuring:* Two 0.1-mL filaments of Emervel Lips HA (corresponds to Restylane Kysse) in the left eyebrow and 0.1 mL in the right eyebrow, delivered with a 22G cannula
- *Skinbooster in jugal area:* 1 mL of Restylane Vital (corresponds to Restylane Skinbooster) in each side of the face, delivered with a filler needle
- *Nasolabial folds:* 0.5 mL of Emervel Deep (corresponds to Restylane Defyne) in each side, delivered with a 22G cannula
- *Lip vermilion:* 0.8 mL of Emervel Lips, delivered with a 25G cannula

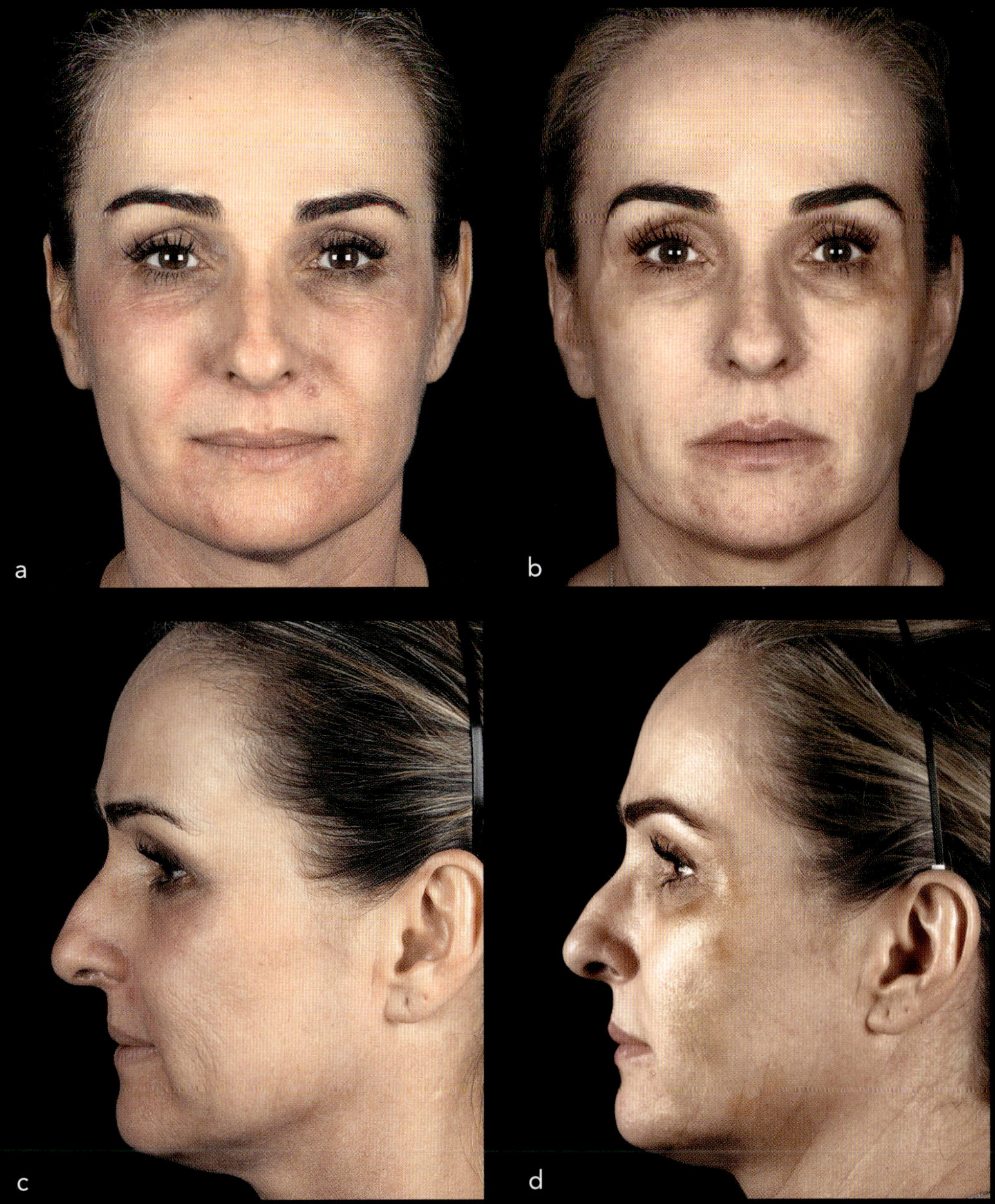

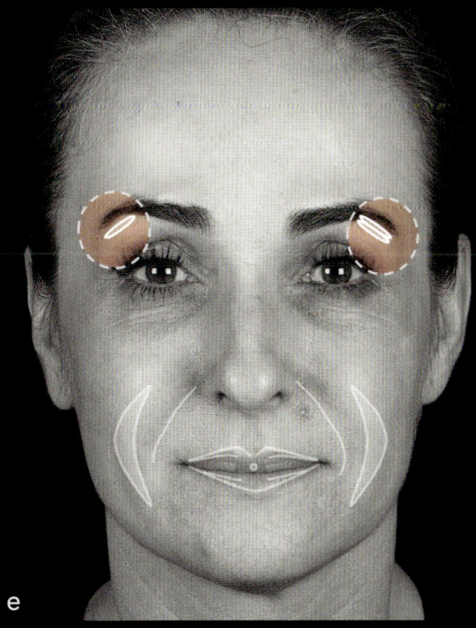

Fig 7-20 Orbit restructuring. *(a)* Pretreatment frontal view. *(b)* Posttreatment frontal view. *(c)* Pretreatment profile. *(d)* Posttreatment profile. *(e)* Injection sites marked.

Nasion

Anatomy

Nasion is the deepest part of the nasal root. Although the use of fillers in this region has a nice effect, caution should be taken when injecting a filler in the nasion because of its complex vascularization and anastomosis. In case there is a vascular compression caused by an excess of product injected, a decrease or complete blockage of the venous supply might occur. To avoid this devastating complication, do not inject fillers in the lateral part of the midline where there is a greater concentration of larger vessels. Large amounts of fillers should also be avoided as well as very dense fillers. Intravascular injections can also affect the blood supply. Thus, the use of a cannula instead of a needle is preferred to decrease the chance of this type of accident. Both compression and embolization of vessels of the face may result in necrosis, but in this area there is also the risk of compromising the vascularization of the eye with possible irreversible blindness.

Risk of blindness

Although the risk of blindness from fillers is rare, it is critical for clinicians using dermal fillers to have a firm knowledge of the vascular anatomy and to understand key prevention and management strategies. Beleznay et al[7] reported 98 cases of vision changes resulting from filler injection. The sites that were high risk for complications were glabella (38.8%), the nasal region (25.5%), the nasolabial fold (13.3%), and the forehead (12.2%). Autologous fat (47.9%) was the most common filler type to cause this complication, followed by HA (23.5%). The most common symptoms were immediate vision loss and pain. Most cases of vision loss did not recover. Central nervous system complications were seen in 23.5% of the cases. No treatments were found to be consistently successful in treating this blindness.

Visual impairment stands as a rare yet catastrophic adverse event associated with intravascular embolization of injected material to the retina or other areas of the central nervous system, potentially leading to permanent vision loss.[8] Iatrogenic retinal artery occlusion (IRAO) can be caused by anterograde or retrograde embolism. Anterograde thromboembolism, as a cause of IRAO, is related to major vascular procedures such as carotid artery stenting or cerebral aneurysm coil embolization.[9,10] It seems to have more additional risk than the known thromboembolic risk for retinal artery occlusion. Further, a substance accidentally injected into arterioles during cosmetic procedures can migrate to the proximal site of the arterial system against the arterial flow resulting from the great injecting force and subsequently can move distally to obstruct the ophthalmic or retinal artery, or any cerebral artery branching from the internal carotid artery. Preconditions, including local increase in pressure and well-vascularized tissue, have been proposed for the intravasation of subcutaneously injected fat materials, resulting in fat embolism.[9,11] Figure 7-21 shows the mechanism of IRAO caused by fillers.

The possible inlet of retrograde flow differs depending on the injection site. Below are the arteries involved in each region[9] (Fig 7-22):

1. *Glabellar region*: Supratrochlear artery, supraorbital artery
2. *Nasolabial fold*: Anastomosis of the dorsal nasal artery from the ophthalmic artery and the angular artery and lateral nasal artery from the facial artery[12]
3. *Temple*: Superficial temporal artery and its branches
4. *Eyelid*: Anastomoses between the internal and external carotid arteries and between the medial and lateral palpebral arteries

Prevention

Several points are critical for prevention[7,13]:

- Know the location and depth of facial vessels.
- Place the cannula superficially and medially to avoid injecting the filler into vessels and their anastomosing branches.
- Use a 22G to 25G cannula.

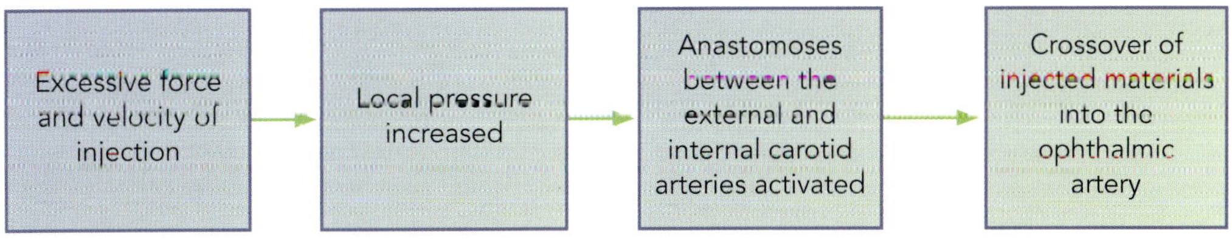

Fig 7-21 Mechanism of IRAO caused by fillers.

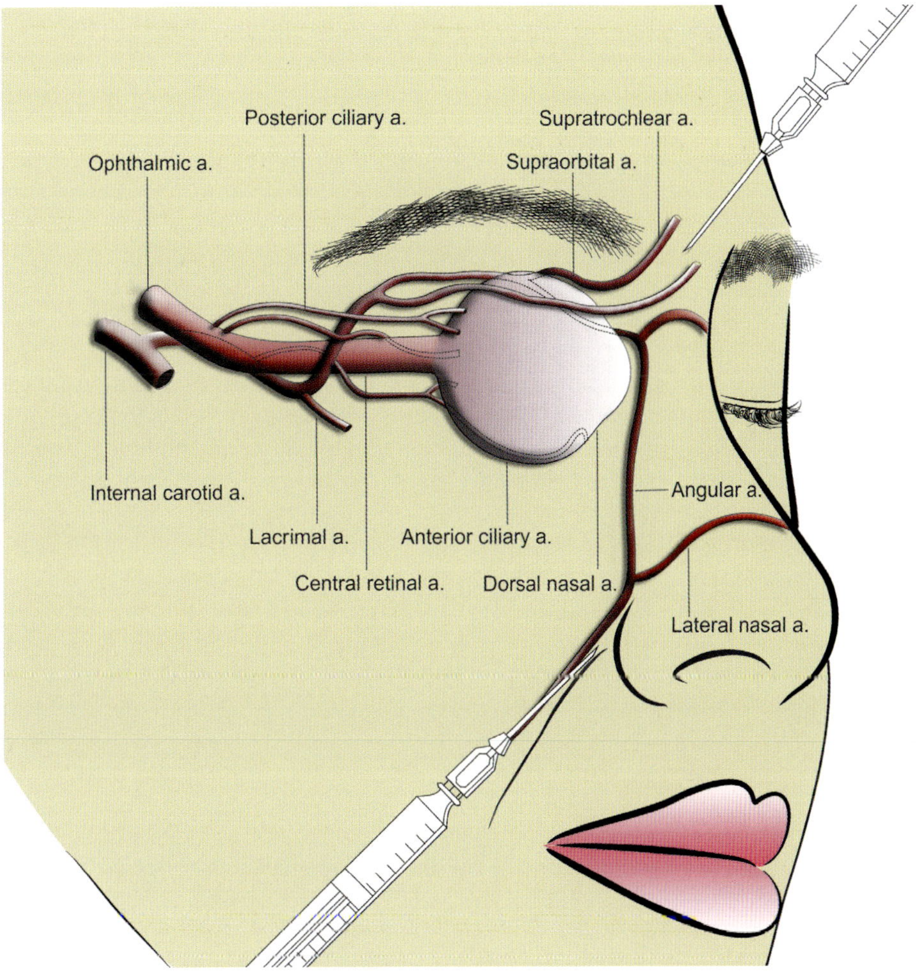

Fig 7-22 Scheme of the blood supply of the face and eye in relation to the sites of cosmetic facial filler injections. The supratrochlear and supraorbital arteries are the possible inlets for retrograde flow in the glabellar region. The anastomosis of the dorsal nasal artery from the ophthalmic artery and the angular artery and lateral nasal artery from the facial artery is the possible inlet for retrograde flow in the nasolabial fold. a., artery. (Reprinted with permission from Park et al.[9])

- Inject slowly and with minimal pressure.
- Consider using a cannula because they are less likely to pierce a blood vessel.
- Avoid overcorrection because higher volumes in small areas can cause compression of adjacent vessels by exceeding the intravascular pressure.

Management strategies

The following strategies can help with case management[7,13]:

- If a patient complains of ocular pain or vision changes, stop the injection at once. Immediately contact an ophthalmologist or oculoplastic colleague and urgently transfer the patient directly there.
- Consider treating the injected area and surrounding location with hyaluronidase if HA filler is used.
- Consider retrobulbar injection of 300 to 600 units (2–4 mL) of hyaluronidase if HA filler is used.
- Reduction of intraocular pressure should be considered. Mechanisms to achieve this include ocular massage, anterior chamber paracentesis, intravenous mannitol, and acetazolamide.
- Given the relatively high prevalence of central nervous system complications that accompany blindness, it is important to monitor the patient's neurologic status and consider imaging studies of the brain if visual complications occur.

Visual interpretation of the nasion

The deeper the nasion, the more pronounced the glabella will look. As previously described, men have a more evident glabella horizontal projection than women. For this reason, fillers can be used in the nasion to decrease the evidence of the glabella, which would add femininity to the face. The injection of fillers in the nasion will also minimize the perception of a hook-shaped nose (see Fig 7-23).

In males, a very deep nasion gives the face an appearance of austerity, which is known as a *Lombrosian profile*. This kind of profile can be smoothed with fillers injected in the nasion. When the glabella has a lot of horizontal projection, a discrete line can occur between the glabella and the forehead (ophryon line). Because men have a more evident glabella, it is natural that their ophryon is more noticeable in profile view than in females. Although this is a male feature, the author does not recommend the injection of fillers in the glabella in order to make it more evident because of the high risk of blindness and necrosis.

Diagnosis

Observe the photograph of the patient in profile. It is not advisable to make a diagnosis without a previous photographic evaluation.

Technique

Draw a short vertical straight line over the nasion. The middle of this line should be at the deepest part of the nasal root. Confirm the marking by observing the patient in frontal and profile views. If after the removal of the initial needle any abundant or throbbing bleeding is noticed, interrupt the application and do not insert the cannula. The patient should be scheduled for the next day. The next injection should be administered at the opposite end of the marking, therefore not entering the same point tried previously but rather at the opposite end.

Use a 22G cannula to insert the filler 2 to 3 mm deep. Inject into the glabella fat pad, which is able to accommodate the filler without causing too much pressure on the irrigation. Do not exceed 0.1 mL of filler per session. If the area demands more than 0.1 mL, wait 30 days to add more fillers.

Clinical case

Figure 7-23 illustrates dermal filler treatment at the nasion and lip vermilion. The following volumes were used:

- *Nasion:* One 0.05-mL filament of Emervel Lips, delivered with a 22G cannula
- *Lip vermilion:* 0.9 mL of Emervel Lips, delivered with a 25G cannula

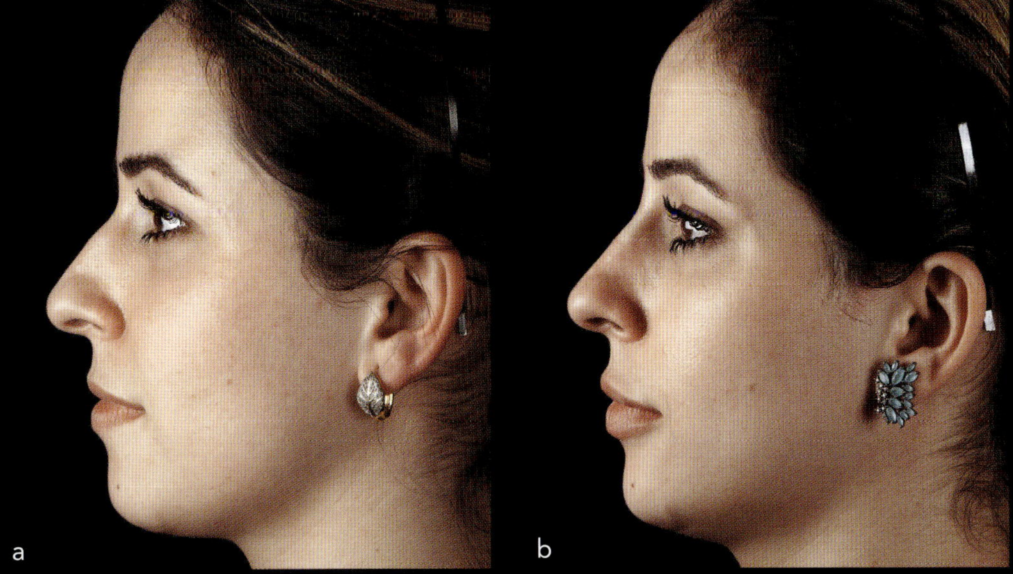

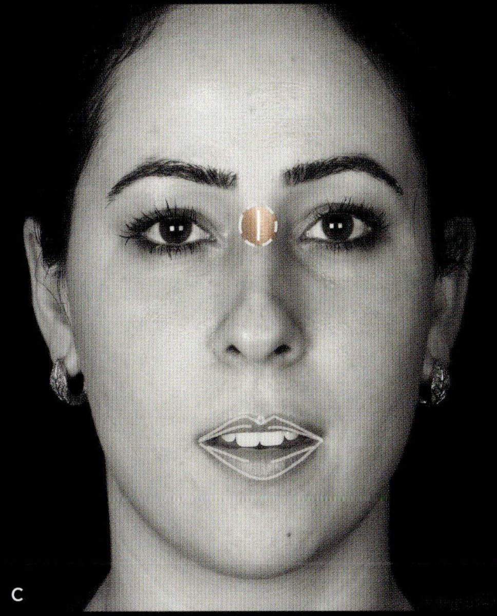

Fig 7-23 Filler treatment at the nasion. *(a)* Pretreatment profile. *(b)* Posttreatment profile. Note the reduction in the hook shape of the nose. *(c)* Injection sites marked (on posttreatment photograph).

Zygomatic Arch Restructuring

Anatomy

The zygomatic bone lies in the middle third of the face. It is connected to the face via the maxilla and frontal, sphenoid, and temporal bones. It has two parts: *(1)* The posterior part is in the shape of an arch (zygomatic arch). *(2)* Anteriorly, the zygomatic bone supports the lateral part of the orbit and is shaped like an arrow pointing downward. The presence of the arch causes a lateralization of the facial tissues that is characteristic of younger people.

Visual interpretation

The zygomatic bone is anatomically important for facial esthetics because it helps to define the face in frontal and profile views. In a frontal view, a prominent zygomatic arch increases the width of the middle third of the face. As it pushes the soft tissues from side to side, there is a slight depression above it in the temporal region and another slight depression below in the buccal mucosa region. The depression above the zygomatic bone is shallower and shorter, while the depression located below is deeper and longer. In a profile view, this prominence created by the zygomatic bone creates a shadow over the buccal mucosa area, which is located over the thinnest part of the masseter muscle. It is a teardrop-shaped muscle, narrower (about 10 mm thick) at the region close to the zygomatic bone and wider (about 20 mm thick) next to the mandible in a frontal view.

Considerations

- The greater the bizygomatic distance is in relation to the bigonial distance, the greater the perception that the face is triangular, which is a female feature. Males tend to have more square faces.
- Visible prominences in the face at the zygomatic arch suggest joviality and also give the idea that the individual is thin. The use of facial fillers at the right points will make the patient look thinner.
- Rounded faces where the lateral prominence of the zygomatic arch is not perceived are viewed as more childlike.
- Flat faces where the lateral prominence of the zygomatic arch is not perceived suggest aging and may look too long.
- According to Arnett and Bergman,[14] the bizygomatic distance in females is 5% larger than in males, proportionally to the length of face (see chapter 5). Therefore, the use of fillers in the zygomatic area is important to reinforce the femininity of a face.

Diagnosis

The jugal depression can be obtained by using fillers over the zygomatic arch, removing the buccal fat pad (bichectomy), or both. Before deciding on this approach, the clinician should ascertain the need to surgically remove the buccal fat pad, which has rare indications. In most of the patients submitted for buccal fat removal, the result is poor because the buccal fat pad is deep to the masseter muscle; this means that when the fat pad is removed, the masseter muscle continues to support the buccal mucosa region, and the result is not very noticeable.

When the buccal fat pad is very bulky, it occupies an area that goes beyond the masseter and buccinator muscles. It presents an expressive buccal extension, anterior to the anterior border of the masseter muscle. To make a diagnosis, the patient should be asked to keep his or her teeth closed without smiling while the practitioner taps the index finger several times on the patient's face. If there is a ripple under the skin, the patient may benefit from the surgical removal of this fat pad. However, an intrabuccal inspection should still be performed, because a bulky fat pad will cause a slight bulging of the jugal mucosa region as it lateralizes the buccinator muscle laterally to the mandibular ramus. This contributes to the formation of a white line in the jugal mucosa called an *alba line* at the level of the occlusion.

Another issue to consider is that in cases where the masseter muscle is very bulky, often associated with bruxism, it compresses the buccal fat pad, increasing its buccal extension. When this occurs, the muscle should be kept within the correct dimensions with the application of botulinum toxin.

The decision to use a filler at the zygomatic arch should be made by observing the patient's face in frontal and profile views in photographs. Ideally, the bizygomatic distance should be larger than the bigonial distance. The use of fillers over the zygomatic arch region will make it more prominent and will also increase the bizygomatic distance.

Technique

Ask the patient to keep his or her mouth slightly open to keep the masseter muscle relaxed. Put the index finger immediately below the inferior bony ridge of the zygomatic arch. Use the finger as a ruler and draw the lower limit of the zygomatic arch on one side of the face. Repeat the same pro-

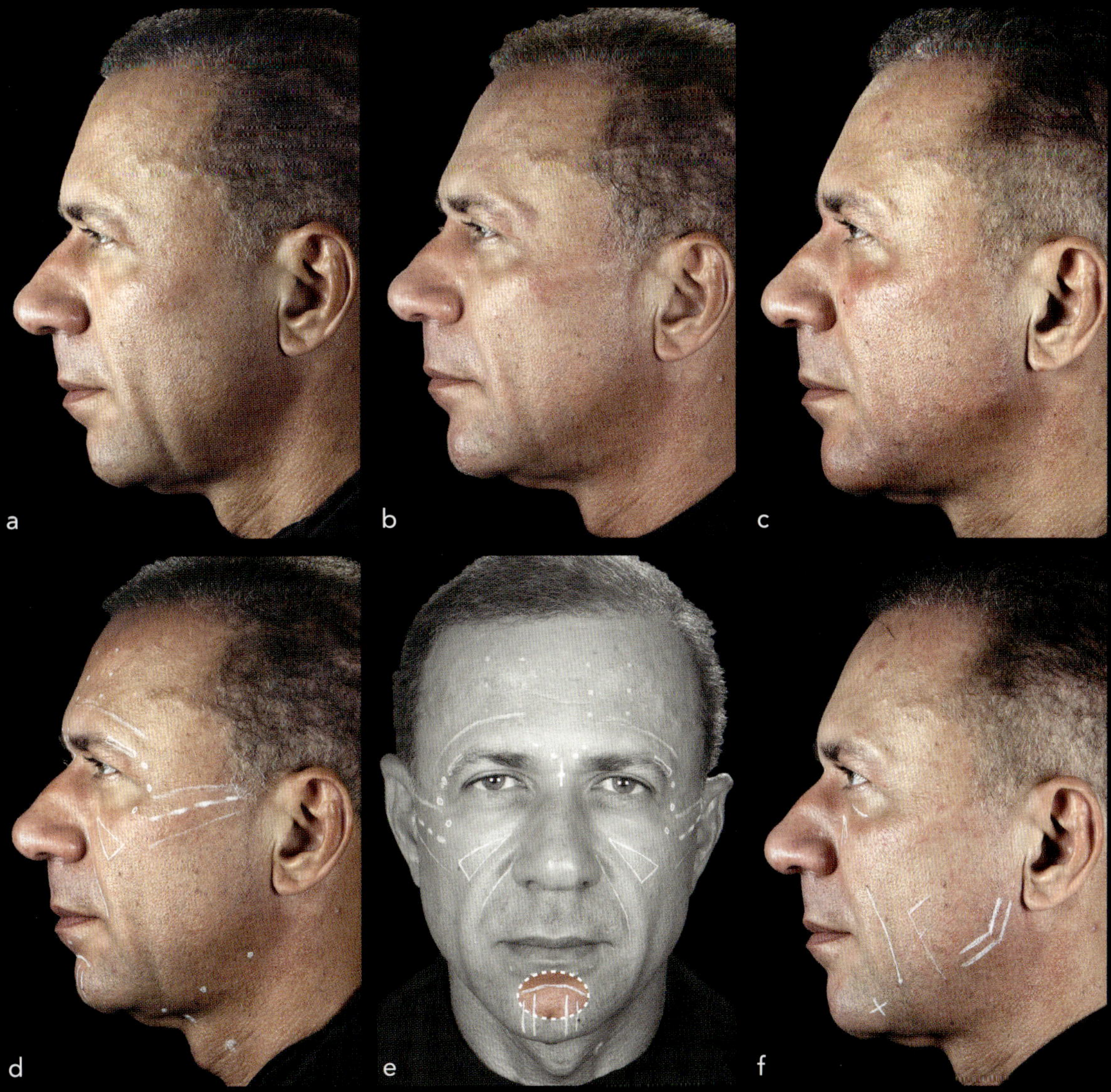

Fig 7-24 Zygomatic arch and mentolabial fold restructuring. *(a)* Pretreatment profile. *(b)* Profile after the first phase of treatment. *(c)* Profile after the second phase of treatment. *(d and e)* Injection sites marked for the first phase of treatment. The small circles correspond to the botulinum toxin injections. Note the correct mark in the mentolabial fold. *(f)* Injection sites marked for the second phase of treatment. The letter F drawn on the face of the patient corresponds to the route of the vein and facial artery; caution should be observed here.

cedure on the opposite side. Check if the horizontal level is correct in both sides by positioning the nail of the right index finger over the drawing on the left side. Then position the other index finger nail over the other side of the face and observe both levels from a frontal view. This drawing of the inferior limit of the arch only works as a reference to draw the filler line. After that, draw a line parallel to the first, in the largest lateral prominence of the zygomatic arch. In frontal and lateral views, verify if this second line is correctly positioned. Then erase the first line. Use a 22G cannula (50 mm long) to deposit the filler 3 mm deep.

Clinical case

Figure 7-24 illustrates dermal filler treatment for zygomatic arch and mentolabial fold restructuring. Treatment was divided into two phases. In the first phase of treatment, filler injections were performed in conjunction with botulinum toxin injections. The following volumes were used at the sites listed:

- *Zygomatic arch:* One 0.3-mL filament of Restylane Defyne in each side, delivered with a 22G cannula
- *Nasion:* 0.15 mL of Restylane Defyne, delivered with a 22G cannula
- *Orbit:* 0.15 mL of Restylane Defyne in each side, delivered with a 22G cannula
- *Malar:* 0.5 mL of Restylane Defyne in each side
- *Chin:* 1 mL of Restylane Defyne, delivered with a 22G cannula
- *Mentolabial fold (subcision made using a cannula):* 0.5 mL of Restylane Defyne, delivered with a 22G cannula
- *Nasolabial fold:* 1 mL of Restylane Defyne in each side, delivered with a 22G cannula

The second phase of filler treatment focused primarily on the cheeks and chin area:

- *Malar:* 0.3 mL of Restylane Defyne in each side, delivered with a 22G cannula
- *Nasion:* 0.2 mL of Restylane Defyne, delivered with a 22G cannula
- *Jugal fold:* 0.5 mL of Restylane Defyne in each side, delivered with a 22G cannula
- *Gonial:* 1 mL of Restylane Defyne in each side
- *Prejowl sulcus:* 0.3 mL of Restylane Defyne, delivered with a 22G cannula
- *Infrapalpebral depression:* 0.2 mL of Restylane Fynesse, delivered with a 25G cannula

Mentolabial fold

The mentolabial fold is a sulcus that defines the limit between the chin and lower lip. It is horizontal and curved. In cases like this one, where the patient presents with a deep mentolabial fold and will undergo chin augmentation with fillers, fillers must also be injected at the mentolabial fold because the chin treatment will make the sulcus even deeper. In this patient, a previous 3-mm-deep subcision with a 22G needle (0.70 × 25 mm) was made. The needle's oscillation should be minimal to avoid gel accumulation laterally in the sulcus. After the subcision, a curved 22G cannula in the shape of the drawing was introduced, and a 0.5-mL filament was injected. As a result, the fold was made shallower, and its shape became smoother.

The use of fillers in this groove leads to the visual integration between the chin and mandible. In Class II patients showing little horizontal projection of the chin, the lower lip tends to become hypotonic, inclined, and anteriorly advanced. The use of a filler in this groove helps to flatten the lower lip when it is too inclined.

Infraorbital Hollowness

Anatomy

Clarification is needed regarding the definitions and classification of *grooves* and *hollowness* of the infraorbital region depending on the cause, anatomical characteristics, and appearance. A *groove* in the infraorbital region (GIR) refers to a narrow furrow around the infraorbital rim at the lid-cheek junction, and *hollowness* of the infraorbital region (HIR) refers to a sunken space in the infraorbital area.[15] It is possible to observe patients with both GIRs and HIR.

GIRs can be classified as nasojugal grooves (or folds), tear trough deformities, and palpebromalar grooves; these can be differentiated based on anatomical characteristics[15–19] (Fig 7-25):

- A tear trough deformity is considered to be located 2 to 3 mm inferior to the orbital rim at the lid-cheek junction; it is present at the junction between the palpebral and orbital parts of the orbicularis oculi muscle, and this junction also corresponds precisely to the superior border of the malar fat pad.
- A palpebromalar groove is located at the lateral lid-cheek junction based on the midpupillary line, whereas the tear trough deformity should be defined as the groove that exists medial to the midpupillary line.
- A nasojugal groove corresponds to the location of the inferior border of the orbicularis oculi muscle.

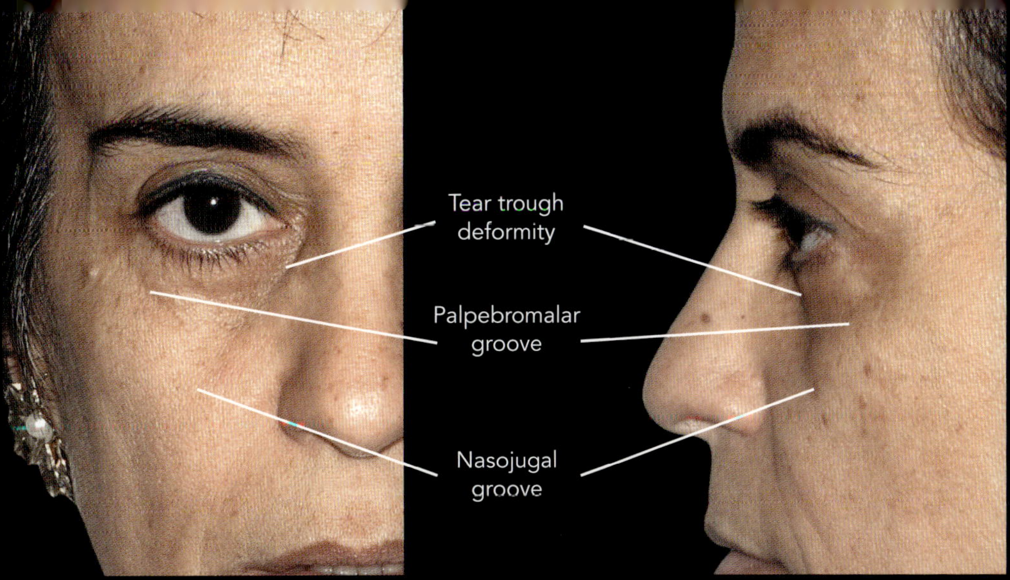

Fig 7-25 Identification of a tear trough deformity, palpebromalar groove, and nasojugal groove.

All of these GIRs are caused by the herniation of intraorbital or infraorbital fat, atrophy of the skin and subcutaneous fat, contraction of the orbital part of the orbicularis oculi muscle, and malar bone resorption.[15]

Visual interpretation

Infraorbital hollowness is part of a set of features concerning facial skeletonization because it resembles the hollow of the eye in the bony skull, giving the patient an aged look. The deeper the hollowness, the less light it gets; therefore, when pushed back out, the skin begins to receive more light and shows a lighter aspect.

Diagnosis

The best evaluation of infraorbital hollowness is made by observing the face and frontal and profile photographs with the light source above the patient's head (the "shower technique"; see chapter 2 of the author's companion book, *Botulinum Toxin for Facial Harmony*). Avoid performing the clinical examination soon after the patient wakes up, as some individuals wake up with some swelling under their eyes. It is important to understand the difference between dark circles and hollowness. It is a mistake to use fillers for dark circles when there is no groove or hollowness. The use of fillers in this case will not lighten the skin and will result in an undesirable volume under the eyes. The nasojugal groove in particular can benefit from the use of fillers at the malar region.

Technique

Observe which of the three grooves is present, and draw each one of them in the patient's face in order to mark the area to be injected. Check via palpation if the drawing matches the bone underneath. If not, the result may not be good. As the skin below the eyes is very thin, this is the only region where it is advisable to inject the filler deep under the muscular plane, that is, to fill in

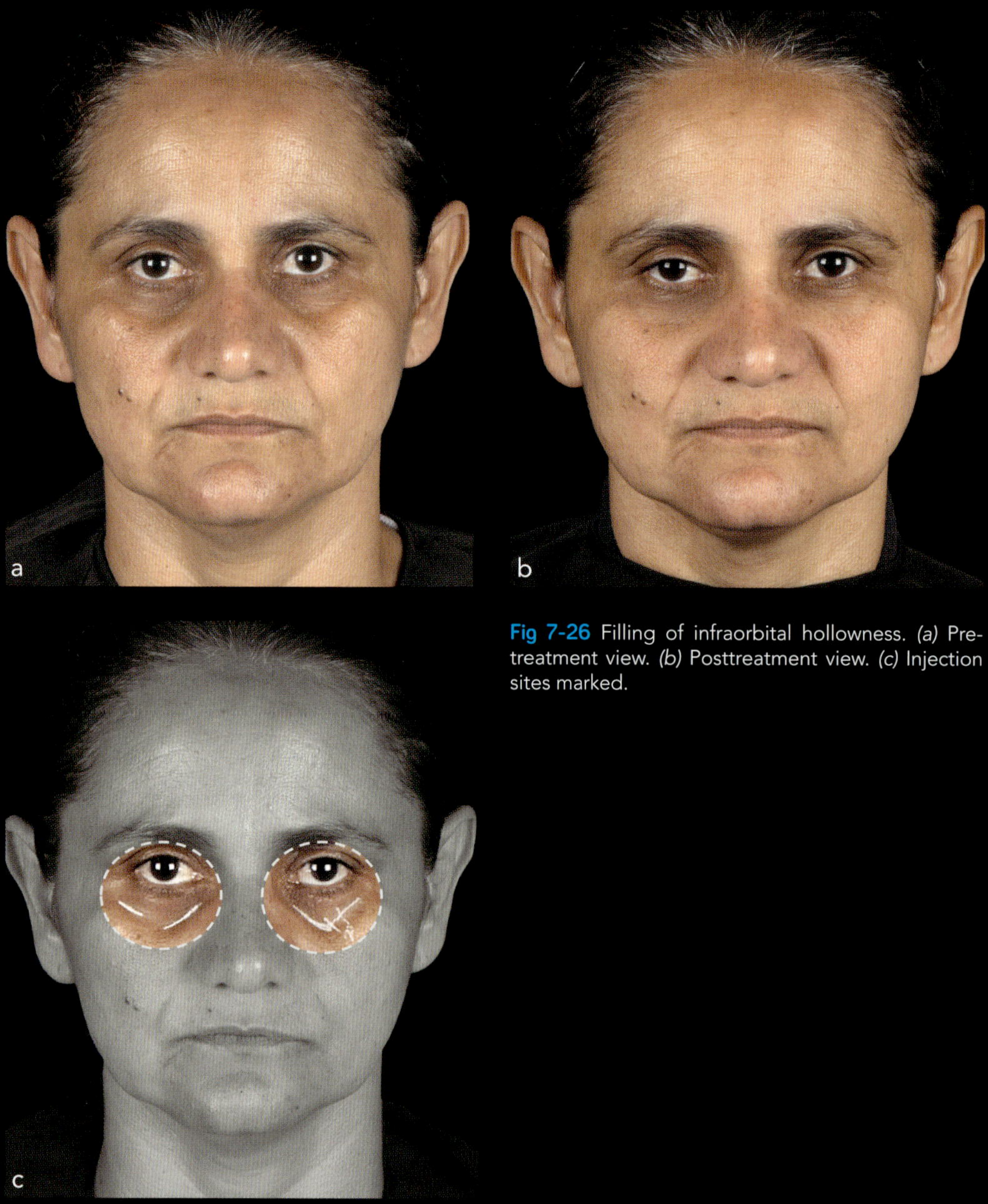

Fig 7-26 Filling of infraorbital hollowness. *(a)* Pretreatment view. *(b)* Posttreatment view. *(c)* Injection sites marked.

contact with the periosteum. Through this technique, the orbicularis oculi muscle is used to hide the filler, avoiding bumps.

The filler is injected in the juxtaperiosteal plane using a 25G cannula. It is also advisable to use fillers that do not attract too much water. If the operator uses a filler that attracts water to the infraorbital depressions, it may result in swelling.

Clinical case

Figure 7-26 shows filler treatment in a patient with infraorbital hollowness. The tear trough deformities and palpebromalar grooves were treated as follows:

- *Tear trough deformity:* One 0.05-mL filament of Renova Fill in each side of the face, delivered with a 25G cannula
- *Palpebromalar groove:* One 0.05-mL filament of Renova Fill, delivered with a 25G cannula

Malar Depression

Anatomy

The human eyeball is located inside a bony cavity. The bony edges of this malar region are in the jawbone laterally to the piriform opening of the nose, medially to the zygomatic bone, and below the infraorbital edge. In this region, the maxilla presents a depression that accommodates the insertion of the levator labii superioris muscle and the levator anguli oris muscle (just below the infraorbital foramen). The perception of this depression on the surface of the skin is not esthetically pleasing. The distance from the alveolar process above the second premolar to the infraorbital margin was found to be between 30 and 49 mm, the average being 39.2 mm.[20]

Visual interpretation

This depression can become visible with aging as subcutaneous volume decreases. A depressed malar region suggests aging, excessive loss of weight, and a "tired face." On the other hand, a regular and slightly convex malar region suggests joviality. Women show more volume in this region than men.

For patients with horizontal maxillary deficiency whose profile is concave, the use of fillers in the malar region decreases the visual dominance of the chin. Advancing the malar region with fillers may change the profile from concave to convex. The filler should be injected in the philtrum columns, subnasale point (nasolabial angle), upper lip (eversion), and nasolabial fold. By following this technique, the entire middle third of the face is advanced. The eversion of the lower lip and use of fillers in the chin are not recommended because they would accentuate the appearance of a concave face.

Diagnosis

Malar deficiencies may appear as a result of facial aging but may also be associated with horizontal maxillary deficiency unrelated to age. In these cases, an evaluation by the oral and maxillofacial surgeon is recommended. If the patient does not want surgery or cannot tolerate it, the maxilla area can be advanced with fillers.

The need to fill the malar region can be better analyzed by observing profile photographs. If the malar region is flat or even depressed, there will be less light reflection and this region will appear darker.

Technique

The area where the filler will be injected can be marked by drawing an isosceles triangle (ie, a triangle with two sides of equal length) with an inclination of 45 degrees. The two equal sides of the triangle should be positioned in the lateral limits of the depressed area and should not be treated with fillers (see Fig 7-27e). The base of the triangle should not be drawn at the continuation of the inferior bony ridge level of the zygomatic bone. The apex of the triangle should point to the medial palpebral fissure. Use a 22G to inject filler filaments 3 mm deep inside the triangle.

A variation of this technique would be to use an intraoral access, depositing the filler deeply next to the periosteum. However, this technique is not recommended for three reasons: *(1)* Intraoral access could take bacteria from the mouth to the subcutaneous tissue. Skin asepsis is more predictable. *(2)* The cannula or needle could damage vessels and nerves that emerge from the infraorbital foramen, causing morbidity and/or postoperative complications. *(3)* Deep fillers require a larger volume to be injected, because the gel must push the layer of deep fat, the musculature, and the layer of superficial fat to the dermis and epidermis. For superficial injection of fillers at the fat layer, only the dermis and epidermis have to be lifted.

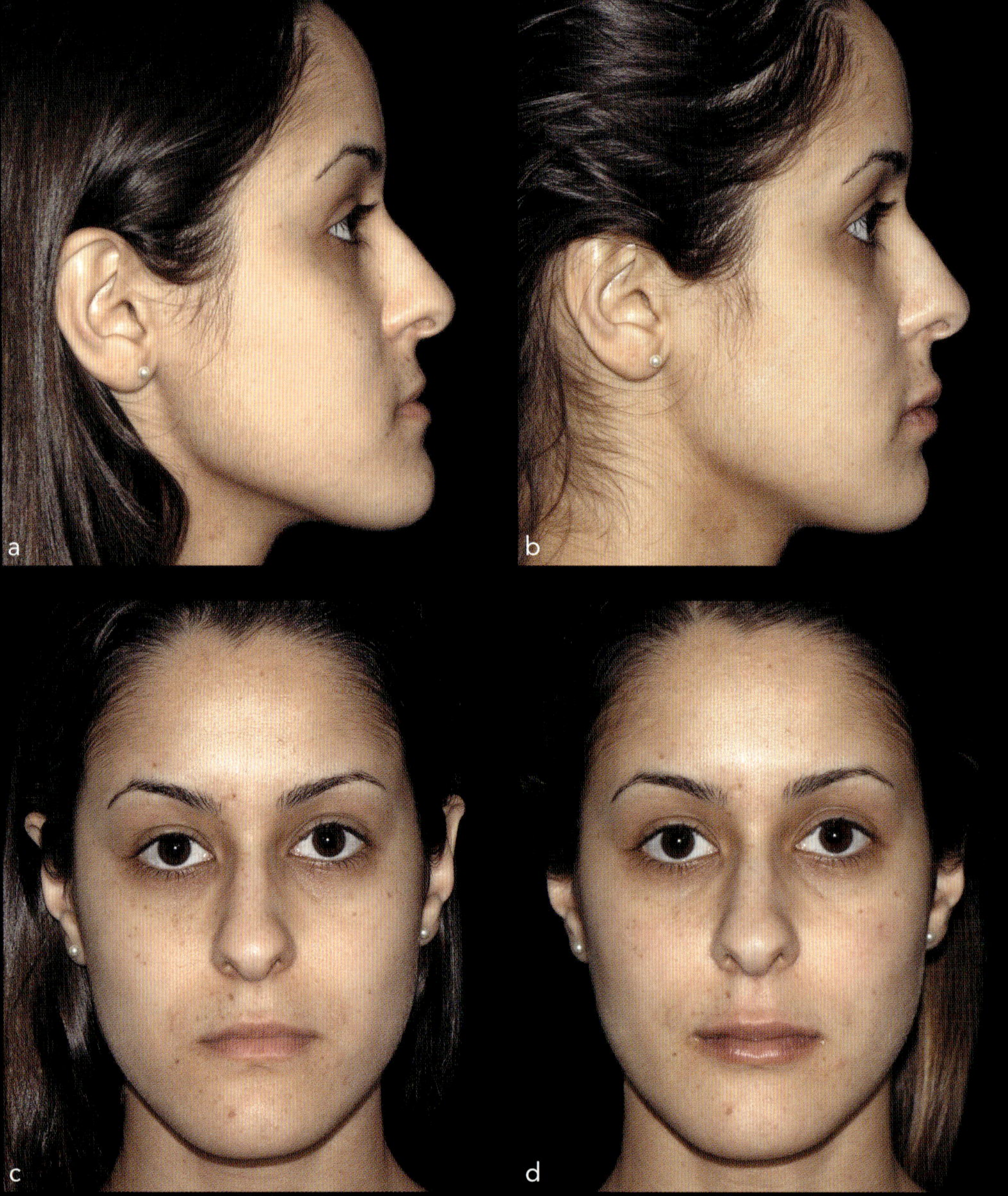

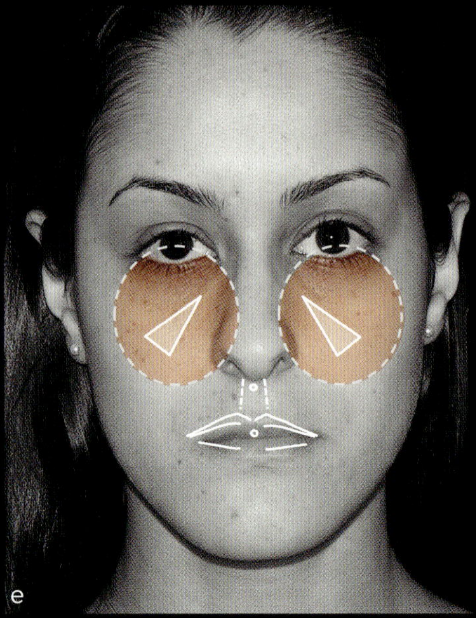

Fig 7-27 Malar depression treated with fillers. *(a)* Pretreatment profile. *(b)* Posttreatment profile. *(c)* Pretreatment frontal view. *(d)* Posttreatment frontal view. *(e)* Injection sites marked. In this case, the malar depression was not related to age but rather associated with maxillary horizontal deficiency. The filler increased the definition of the malar region.

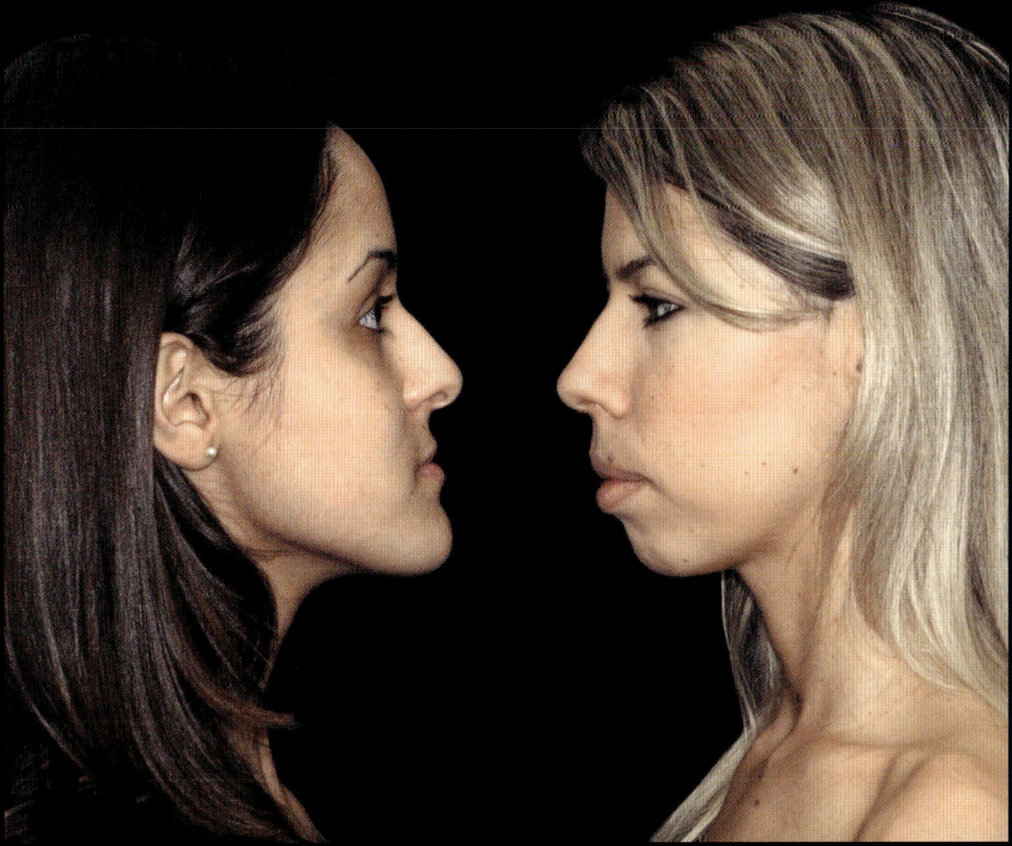

Fig 7-28 Photograph showing two patients in profile looking at each other. The patient on the left has a horizontal maxillary deficiency—that is, a concave profile. The patient on the right has a horizontal chin deficiency—that is, a convex profile.

Clinical case

Figure 7-27 illustrates a case of malar depression treated with HA fillers at multiple sites:

- *Malar:* 1.0 mL of Restylane Perlane (corresponds to Restylane Defyne) in each side, delivered with a 22G cannula
- *Philtrum column:* 0.05 mL of Restylane Perlane in each side, delivered with a filler needle
- *Lip vermilion:* 0.6 mL of Restylane, delivered with a 25G cannula

The effect of malar depression on the profile is highlighted in Fig 7-28, which compares this patient's profile with that of a patient with horizontal chin deficiency.

Chin Augmentation

Anatomy

The chin is located in the most anterior and resistant mobile bone of the face, the mandible. The upper limit of the chin is the mentolabial fold in the skin, which coincides with point B' (B point). Its lower limit in a frontal or profile view is the menton point (ME'). Its lateral border is the lateral menton (MEL'), which coincides with the mental tubercle.

The largest lateral protuberance in the mandible is the gonion point, and the largest lateral protuberance at the anterior aspect is the mental tubercle.

Visual interpretation

The mental tubercle is a noticeable bone protuberance that pushes the skin of the chin anteriorly to cause a discrete elevation; this is an important point of balance for facial esthetics, especially in a frontal view. With age, the chin rotates in an anterosuperior direction, and this can be caused by a decrease in occlusal vertical dimension. In these cases, it is important to recover this dimension and use fillers in the lip contour to decrease the aspect of a projected menton. Injecting fillers in the submental region is also suggested to increase the chin volume downward, hiding the horizontal projection. On the other hand, some patients might show structural problems (eg, a horizontal deficiency of the chin) that is not related to age. In these patients, the chin is not able to balance the horizontal projection of the nose, making the nose appear longer than it actually is. This is best evaluated in a profile photograph where the true vertical line is drawn (see chapter 5).

A low-volume chin suggests fragility, an excessively long nose, and a childish face. On the other hand, a regular chin with a normal convexity suggests strength and balances the nose dominance. Advancing the chin with the use of fillers can decrease the perception of a long nose. In addition to correcting deficiencies of the horizontal projection in this area, fillers can also improve the definition of the jawline.

Diagnosis

Horizontal deficiencies of the chin are generally inherited structural deficiencies. In these cases, an evaluation by an oral and maxillofacial surgeon is recommended. Surgery should be considered especially in cases of functional problems, such as malocclusion and insufficient airway. However, if the patient declines surgical treatment, if surgery is contraindicated, or if there are no functional problems associated, chin advancement with fillers is possible. The need to perform a chin advancement can best be analyzed by looking at photographs of the patient in profile. If the chin is deficient, the skin of the neck may have less support, resulting in an esthetically unpleasant submental volume. The filler in this case helps to stretch the skin of this region and smooth excessive volume.

Technique

The limits of the area to be injected with a filler should be marked by drawing a line over the mentolabial fold, which is the superior limit of the chin. The width of the area to be injected should be wider than the nose and narrower than the mouth. This lateral limit coincides with the metal tubercle. The inferior limit should be the mentalis insertion in the skin and should always go beyond this superficial insertion.

Several vertical lines should be drawn: The first line should match the midline, followed by four other lines on each side of the chin that decrease in size (see Fig 7-29c). Injecting the filler in the midline increases the projection of the chin, which will give it a rounded look. On the other hand, the filler can be injected only in the side lines, which will provide a more squared look to the chin that results in a slight sinking of the midline. These are two possible sculpture procedures of the chin through fillers.

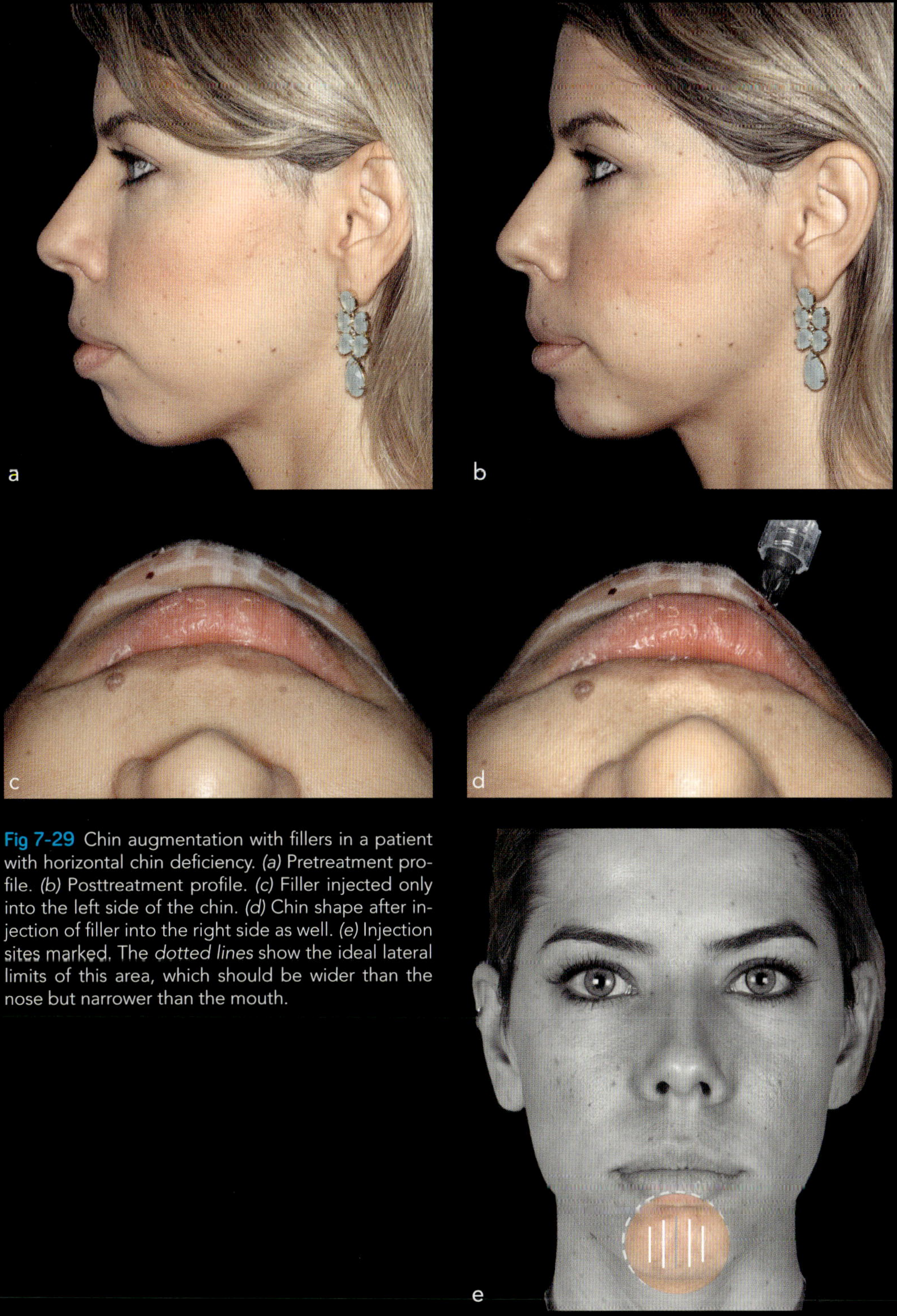

Fig 7-29 Chin augmentation with fillers in a patient with horizontal chin deficiency. *(a)* Pretreatment profile. *(b)* Posttreatment profile. *(c)* Filler injected only into the left side of the chin. *(d)* Chin shape after injection of filler into the right side as well. *(e)* Injection sites marked. The *dotted lines* show the ideal lateral limits of this area, which should be wider than the nose but narrower than the mouth.

For this kind of procedure, a 22G or 23G cannula is used to penetrate 3 mm deep, injecting filaments that follow the drawn lines. One variation of this technique would be to use an intraoral access, but this technique is not recommended for the same reasons outlined previously under "Malar Depression."

Clinical case

Figure 7-29 illustrates chin augmentation with fillers in a patient with horizontal chin deficiency. A 22G needle was used to inject 2.0 mL of Restylane Perlane into the chin.

07

Nasolabial Fold

Anatomy

The nasolabial fold is a linear depression that starts at the level of the alar cartilage and descends in a diagonal plane, ending in a horizontal level of the buccal commissure. At this point, it becomes a curved line. In young people, this fold is usually only observed during the smile; however, it becomes static as we age (around 28 years). That is, it becomes visible depending on the muscle action and because of the natural decrease in fat volume of the subcutaneous tissue. Lipodystrophy resulting from diabetes or antiretroviral drugs[21] can also cause this fold to become more visible.

Visual interpretation

Static grooves increase the perception of aging. The nasolabial fold is among the most common complaints of older patients seeking filler treatment. However, because this groove is very common, it is not often a treatment priority when compared to marionette grooves or malar depressions, which develop at more advanced ages. While the nasolabial fold is not considered a priority for the clinician, patients are often very concerned about it in terms of esthetics, possibly because it is generally the longest of all grooves. This groove decreases the visual dominance of the lip vermilion and becomes deeper during the smile due to the action of muscles involved in facial expression. When fillers are injected to smooth the fold, it rejuvenates the face.

Diagnosis

A nasolabial fold can be diagnosed early or late. The ideal is to treat it early, at the first sign of the fold, when the face is observed without any muscular action preventing it from becoming static. A magnifying glass can be used for this diagnosis. Early treatment can be offered to the patient and should be very well explained, because the patient will not see a noticeable difference from the preventive treatment. In cases of late diagnosis, where the groove is already static, it is necessary to diagnose the depth of this groove and classify it as shallow or deep. This diagnosis can be done by pressing the skin of the groove with the index finger and thumb perpendicularly to the direction of the groove. If the groove disappears, it is considered as shallow and easy to treat, but if the groove remains, it is classified as deep, requiring a more complex approach with worse results. The patient should be informed about this aspect of the treatment.

The need to use fillers in the nasolabial fold can best be analyzed by looking at the patient's frontal view photographs, preferably using the technique in which the flash is positioned above the patient's head and pointed at his or her face (the "shower technique"; see chapter 2 of the author's companion book, *Botulinum Toxin for Facial Harmony*). The evaluation can also be done in person, but the photographic analysis is always recommended.

Technique

Shallow grooves can be treated by depositing fillers about 3 mm deep in the form of longitudinal filaments over the groove. Deep grooves may need additional transverse short filaments or even a subcision. If a subcision is required, it should be made at the same depth (3 mm) and preferably with a 22G cannula, which may also be used for filling. It is very important to avoid a high oscillation of the cannula or needle to prevent a lateral space from being opened at the groove and filler accumulating out of the groove, which would lead to an undesired result. The subcision, when poorly executed, leaves the skin very loose, which leads to a large volumizing action of the filler and results in excessive volume.

In general, deep nasolabial folds do not disappear after filling but become milder. It should be explained to the patient beforehand that the intention is to soften the groove rather than eliminate it.

The area to be injected with fillers can be delimited by drawing a longitudinal line that matches the groove. If the groove has curves, the cannula should be equally curved before the filler is injected.

A 22G cannula inserted 3 mm deep is used to deposit a filament that will follow the line drawn over the groove. If the filler is injected lateral to this line, the groove can get deeper.

The deepest part of the nasolabial fold is usually its upper limit. For this reason, many clinicians tend to inject a larger amount of fillers in this area. However, this practice as well as the practice of deep injections should be avoided because of the presence of the angular artery (a branch of the facial artery) located at the border between the nose and the maxillary bone. Embolization and/or compression of the angular artery could lead to necrosis of the nasal skin by obstruction of its lateral nasal branch, which irrigates the ala nasi. Because it anastomoses with the nasal dorsal branches at the level of the medial angle of the eye, it could compromise the irrigation of the dorsum of the nose through a retrograde embolization. Additionally, it is important to consider that even at the level of the medial angle of the eye, the angular artery anastomoses with the ophthalmic artery, which can lead to blindness.

Marionette lines

It is important to consider that treating marionette lines is more important than treating the nasolabial fold, as it is not uncommon to see relatively young people showing the nasolabial groove early, around the age of 30 years. On the other hand, marionette lines are usually present in patients over 50 years of age. Thus, laypeople consider marionette lines to be a much more obvious sign of aging than the nasolabial fold. Marionette lines can be treated in much the same way as the nasolabial fold.

Clinical case

Figure 7-30 shows the case of a woman with a deepened nasolabial fold and marionette lines appropriate for her age. Prior to filler treatment, botulinum toxin was injected to correct asymmetries in the lower lip and eyebrows and to address aging of the face that could not be corrected with fillers (see Figs 7-30a to 7-30c). Botulinum toxin was injected at the following sites:

- *Occipitofrontalis:* 2U at six points of the left occipitofrontalis and seven points of the right occipitofrontalis
- *Orbicularis oculi:* 2U at one point on each side of the face
- *Glabella:* 3U at three points
- *Orbicularis oris:* 1U at four points
- *Depressor labii inferioris:* 2U at one point on the left side and 1U at one point on the right side

Once the facial asymmetry was corrected, the following volumes of fillers were injected at the sites listed (see Fig 7-30f):

- *Nasolabial fold:* 1.0 mL of Restylane Perlane in each side of the face, delivered with a filler needle
- *Lip vermilion:* 0.6 mL of Restylane Perlane in the whole area, delivered with a filler needle
- *Mentolabial fold:* 0.4 mL of Restylane Perlane in the whole area, delivered with a filler needle
- *Nasolabial angle (subnasale point):* 0.4 mL of Restylane, delivered with a filler needle
- *Infrapalpebral depression:* 0.05 mL of Restylane in each side of the eye, delivered with a filler needle
- *Marionette lines:* 0.3 mL of Restylane Perlane in each side, delivered with a 25G cannula

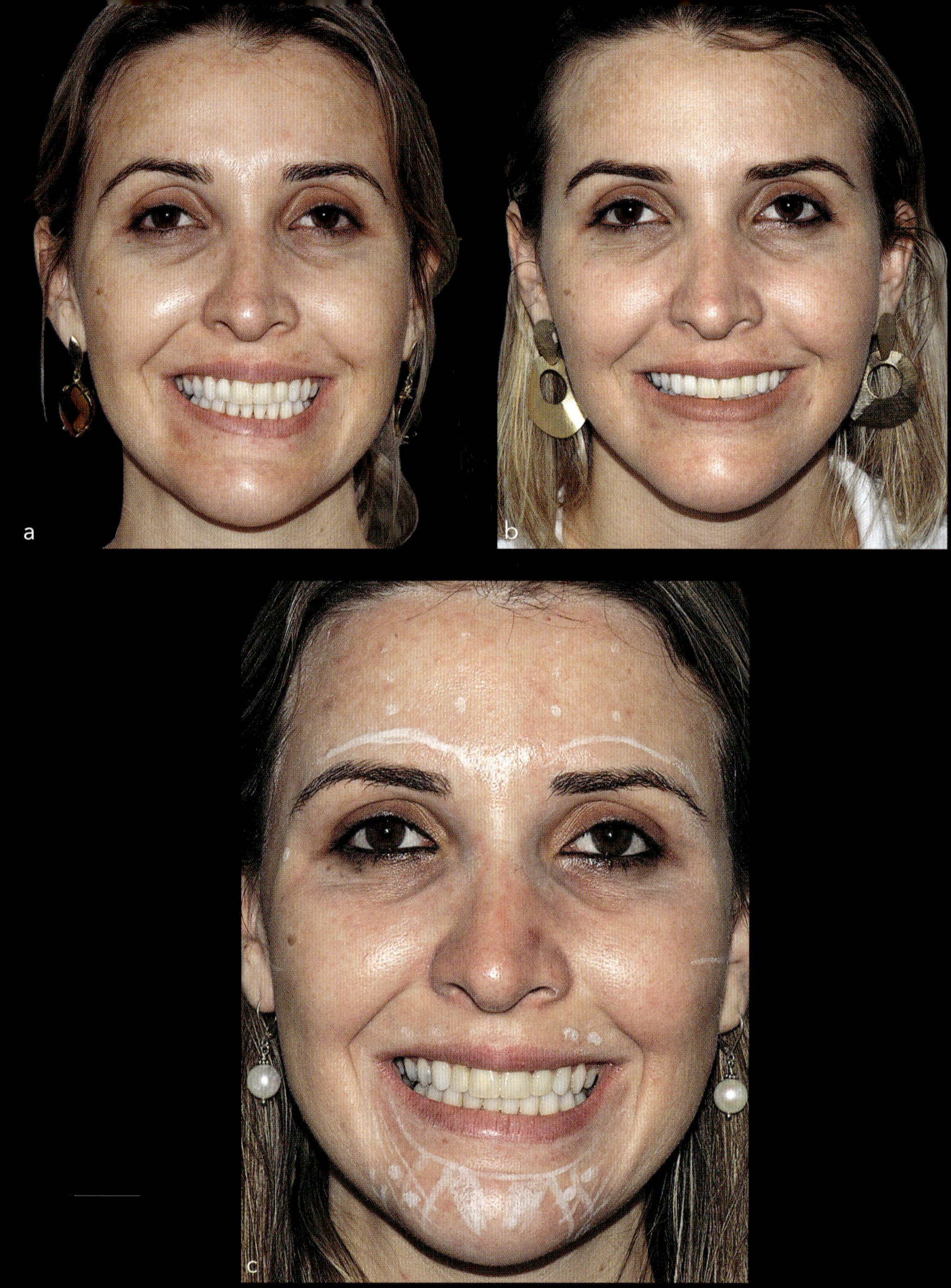

Fig 7-30 Filler treatment for nasolabial fold and marionette lines. *(a)* Pretreatment smile. Notice the lower lip asymmetry, lower gummy smile, and eyebrow asymmetry. *(b)* Posttreatment smile after botulinum toxin injection to correct the asymmetries and gummy smile. *(c)* Injection sites marked. *(d)* Frontal view after botulinum toxin treatment but before filler treatment. *(e)* Frontal view after filler treatment. *(f)* Injection sites marked. *(g and h)* Profile views before and after filler treatment. The use of filler made the nasolabial fold smoother and eliminated the marionette lines. *(i)* Demarcation of areas around the marionette lines. The filler should be injected using a 22G or 23G cannula with one single filament or several filaments. The ideal depth is 3 mm. If a good result is not observed at the end of the treatment, a subcision followed by the injection of a filler may be used. The patient should be informed that subcisions usually cause bruising.

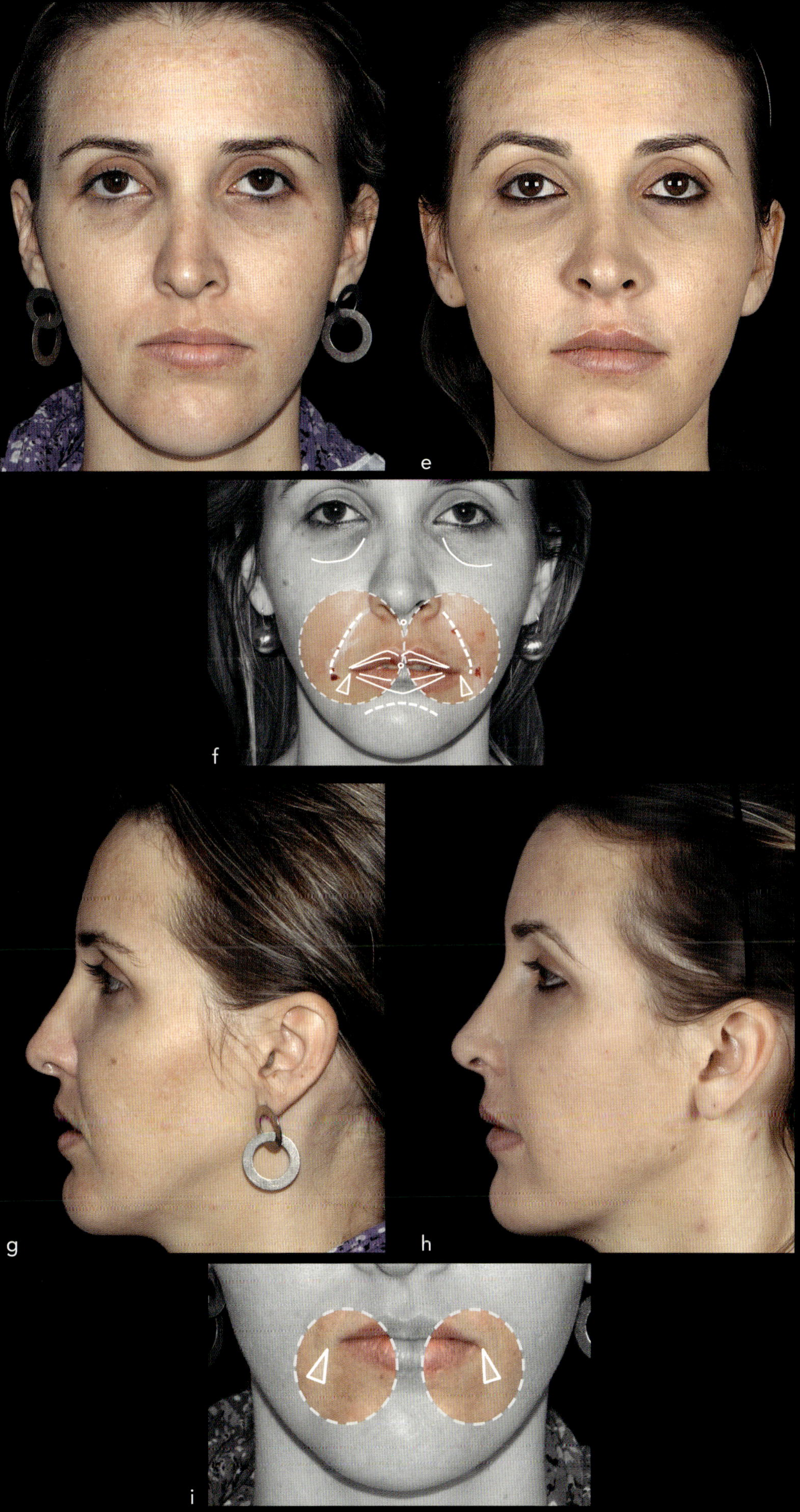

d e f g h i

Subnasale Point

Anatomy

The subnasale point is where the nasal septum and upper lip meet. It is where the columella of the nose ends and the groove of the philtrum begins. Considering the columella and the philtrum as straight in a profile view, one can observe an angle formed in the junction of these two lines, the nasolabial angle. Asian people and black people have a more closed nasolabial angle when compared to white people.[22]

The columella is the part of skin and cartilage that supports the tip of the nose, passing between the nostrils. It should be visible in a frontal view and primarily visible in a profile view. Also, it should ideally occupy a position 2 to 3 mm lower than the inferior border of the ala nasi to be esthetically pleasing.[23] In cases where it is not visible, it is called a *retracted* or *hidden columella*. The use of fillers at the subnasale point can lower the horizontal level of the columella, making it more visible and thus more esthetically pleasing.

The philtrum's arterial supply is carried out by the arch formed by the central artery of the philtrum, the left and right lateral ascendant arteries of the philtrum, and the left and right accessory arteries of the philtrum.[24] It is important to note that the arteries that make up this arch in the philtrum are located above the orbicularis oris muscle. The superior labial artery is located deep to the orbicular oris muscle, emitting perforating branches to reach the skin. An anatomical study conducted in cadavers by Garcia de Mitchell et al demonstrated the existence of a fat compartment superficial to the orbicularis oris muscle.[25] This fat compartment is the target injection site.

Visual interpretation

One of the subtle differences between the profiles of males and females is the nasolabial angle. The average nasolabial angle in women is 95 to 105 degrees, while in men it ranges from 90 to 95 degrees.[26] Therefore, one of the methods to give more femininity to a face is to inject fillers in the nasolabial angle to make it more open. A retracted columella visually makes the nose look wider and sagging, whereas a visible columella makes the nose look narrower and steeper and offers a better view of the upper lip.

The clinician should consider that the main objective of the use of fillers in the subnasale point is not to elevate the nasal tip but rather to open the nasolabial angle. If the main objective *is* to lift up the nose, it is also necessary to inject fillers in the supratip. This approach in the supratip is more dangerous than in the subnasale point.

Diagnosis

The nasolabial angle may be less than average in the following cases:

- As a person ages, this angle tends to decrease because of the retrusion of the anterior wall of the maxilla.[26]
- In patients with horizontal maxillary deficiency, the nasolabial angle tends to be more closed, because the anterior nasal spine shows a retracted position, providing less support to the columella. An oral and maxillofacial surgeon would be able to study the case and see if the best treatment would be surgery or the use of fillers in this area.
- Horizontal projection of the maxillary anterior teeth can also close the nasolabial angle. This can be diagnosed by analyzing a profile photograph and another photograph of the entire face with the patient smiling.
- If, during the smile, the tip of the nose descends a lot, this can be caused by the action of the depressor septi nasi muscle when it is hyperkinetic. In this case, the ideal treatment would be botulinum toxin injection to relax the muscle.

The volume injected at the nasolabial angle should be limited. This angle should not be projected to the point that it is positioned at the same level as the vermilion of the upper lip. In a profile view, the nasolabial angle should be posterior to the upper lip vermilion. The nasolabial angle can be

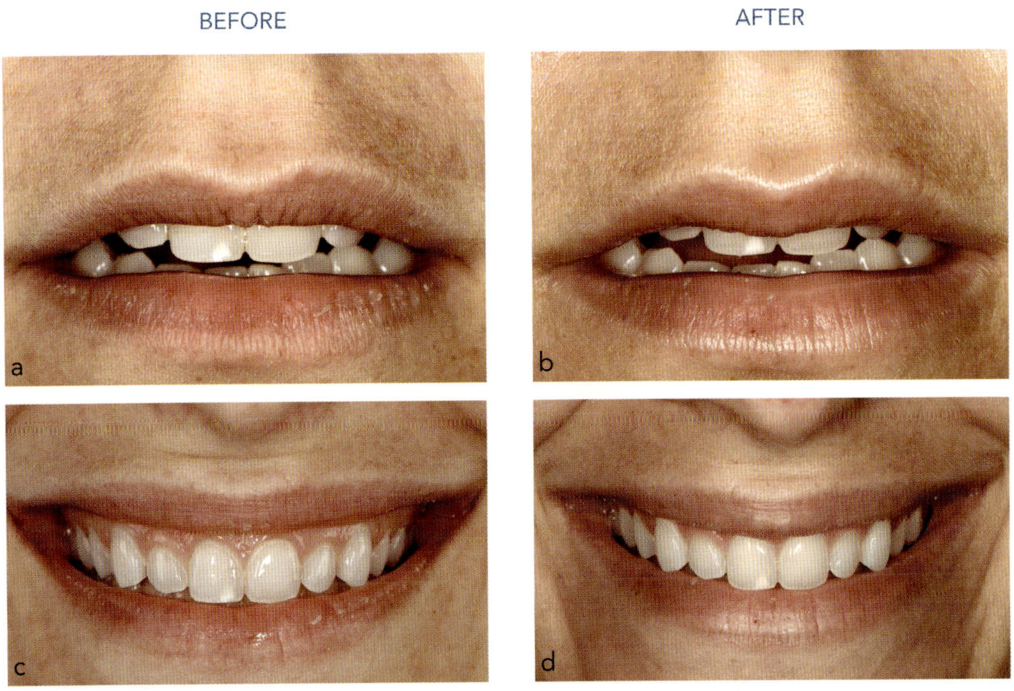

Fig 7-31 Horizontal level of the upper lip before *(a and c)* and after *(b and d)* filler treatment at the subnasale point. *(a and b)* Horizontal level of the upper lip at rest without sealing and in the absence of muscular activity. *(c and d)* Horizontal level of the upper lip during the smile. Note the reduced horizontal level of the upper lip at rest and during the smile after filler treatment. Also note the smoothing of the horizontal nasolabial fold.

measured in a digital photograph of the face in profile, where tangential lines are drawn to the columella and the skin of the upper lip, using programs such as PowerPoint or Keynote.

Opening of the nasolabial angle, in addition to pushing the skin from the subnasale point to the anterior aspect, slightly lifts the nose up and lowers the horizontal level of the upper lip. This approach decreases the display of maxillary anterior teeth during rest and smile (Fig 7-31). Thus, this procedure is only indicated when the patient displays a little gingival tissue when smiling.

Patients with a deep vestibule may develop a horizontal fold in the skin of the upper lip at the level of the philtrum groove and transverse to it. This occurs because, during the smile, the lip is drawn against this bone concavity and the skin is folded. A filler injected in the nasion point can soften this fold or even prevent its formation, also stopping it from becoming a static wrinkle.

Technique

The use of fillers in the horizontal fold in the skin of the upper lip, at the level of the philtrum groove and transverse to it, is not necessary. The application of fillers at the nasion point would slightly limit the movement of the upper lip during smile, preventing the skin of the philtrum from creasing.

The filler can be injected deeply in the subnasale point along the periosteum or superficially (3 mm deep). The superficial injection of fillers provides the following advantages:

- It does not affect the function of the orbicularis oris and depressor septi nasi muscles, because the filler stays above these muscles.
- A smaller volume of the filler is required because at this depth the filler does not have to push the muscle to the surface, only the dermis and the epidermis.
- The filler is injected in a superficial level in relation to the larger blood vessels. The deep vessels are usually larger in all regions of the face. In this depth, the superior labial artery, a branch of the facial artery, ramifies in a septal branch and alar branch toward the nose.

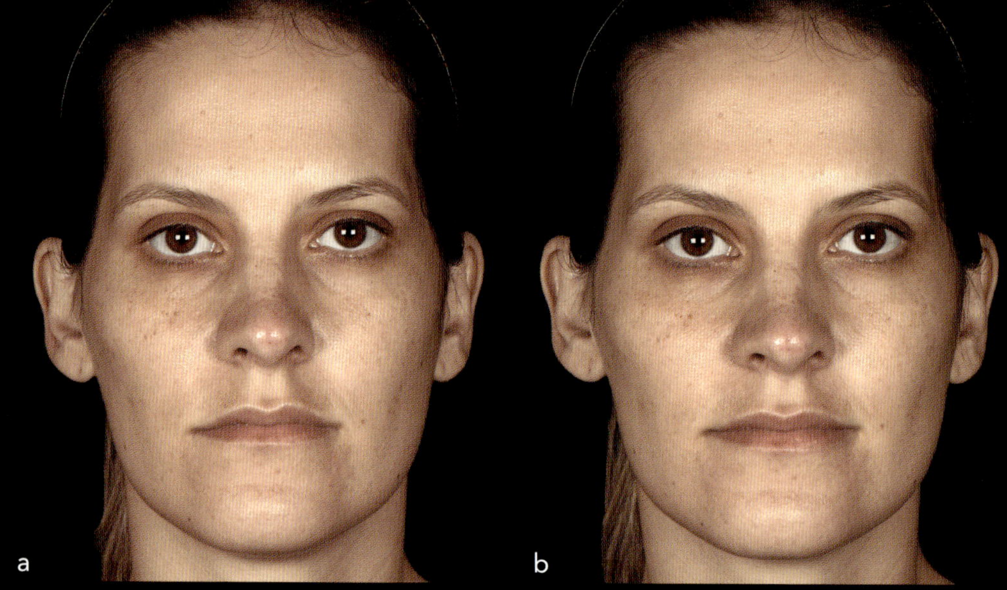

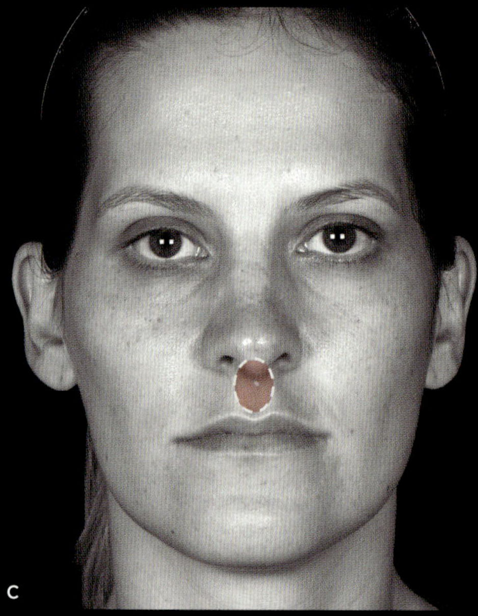

Fig 7-32 Filler treatment at the subnasale point to open the nasolabial angle. *(a)* Pretreatment view. *(b)* Posttreatment view. *(c)* Injection sites marked. *(d and e)* Comparison of nasolabial angles before and after filler treatment. Note that if the upper lip had not been everted with fillers, the nasolabial angle would have been opened even more.

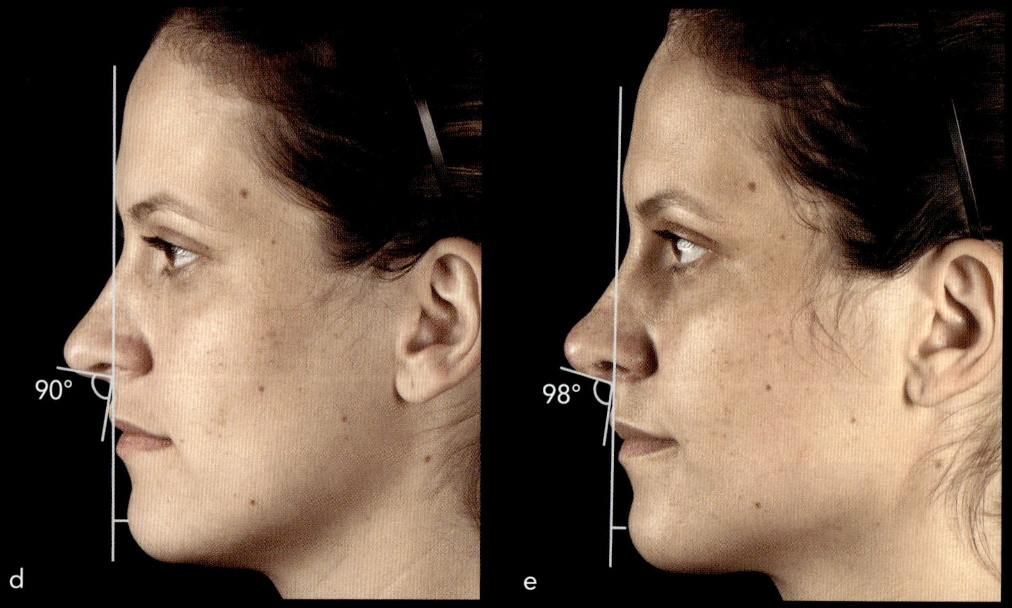

The nasion point can then be treated with fillers by locating the nasolabial angle bisector using a 22G cannula that should be kept steady (3 mm deep). Thus, the risk of necrosis is low. The amount injected should not exceed 0.3 mL.

It should be explained to the patient that when only the nasion point is treated with a filler, the expected result should be the opening of this angle and not the lifting of the nose. In order to lift the nose, the filler should also be injected in the supratip. The area to be treated can be delimited by drawing a point in the lip-columella limit.

Clinical case

Figure 7-32 illustrates filler treatment at the subnasale point. The following volumes were used at the sites listed:

- *Subnasale point:* 0.3 mL of Emervel Deep, delivered with a 25G cannula
- *Lip vermilion:* 0.3 mL of Emervel Lips, delivered with a 25G cannula

Supratip

Anatomy

The *supratip* is the name given to the area of the nose just above the nasal tip along the facial midline. The lateral limits are formed by the supra-alar crease. This part of the nose is movable to palpation and is supported by the major alar cartilage and lateral cartilage of the nose. These two cartilages together form the upper limit of the supratip. When the major alar cartilage has a larger horizontal projection than the lateral cartilage of the nose, a step is formed between these parts called a *supratip break* (a small depression, when present). This gives the perception that the tip of the nose is lifted up, which is esthetically pleasing.

Visual interpretation

One of the parameters observed when considering a nose as esthetically pleasing is an upward tip. In a nose considered well defined, its anatomical sites should be easily identified. This definition will result in a sculpted nose with a less monotonous anatomy. One of the approaches to benefit the nose is to use fillers in the supratip, making it more prominent than the other parts of the dorsum. The filler can also cause the formation of a supratip break, giving more definition to the nose. A low supratip suggests aging, whereas a lifted supratip suggests joviality and femininity.

Diagnosis

By observing the patient's face and profile and frontal photographs, the clinician can decide if the use of fillers in the supratip is needed. It is common for the patient to ask for this approach. In a profile view, observe if the supratip is aligned with the dorsum of the nose or if it is inclined slightly upward. The treatment with filler is recommended in cases where the supratip is low.

Technique

By observing the patient in profile, mark the point of greatest projection of the nose. This will be the lower limit of the filament. Draw a line that matches the facial midline. The length of the filament should be the vertical measurement of the ala nasi in lateral view (the average is 12 mL) plus 1 mm. This is the ideal length of the filament. With this method, at the end of the filler injection it will be easy to observe that the supratip break is on a higher horizontal level than the upper limit of the wing of the nose. Use a 25G cannula (2 to 3 mm deep). Never use needles in this area due to

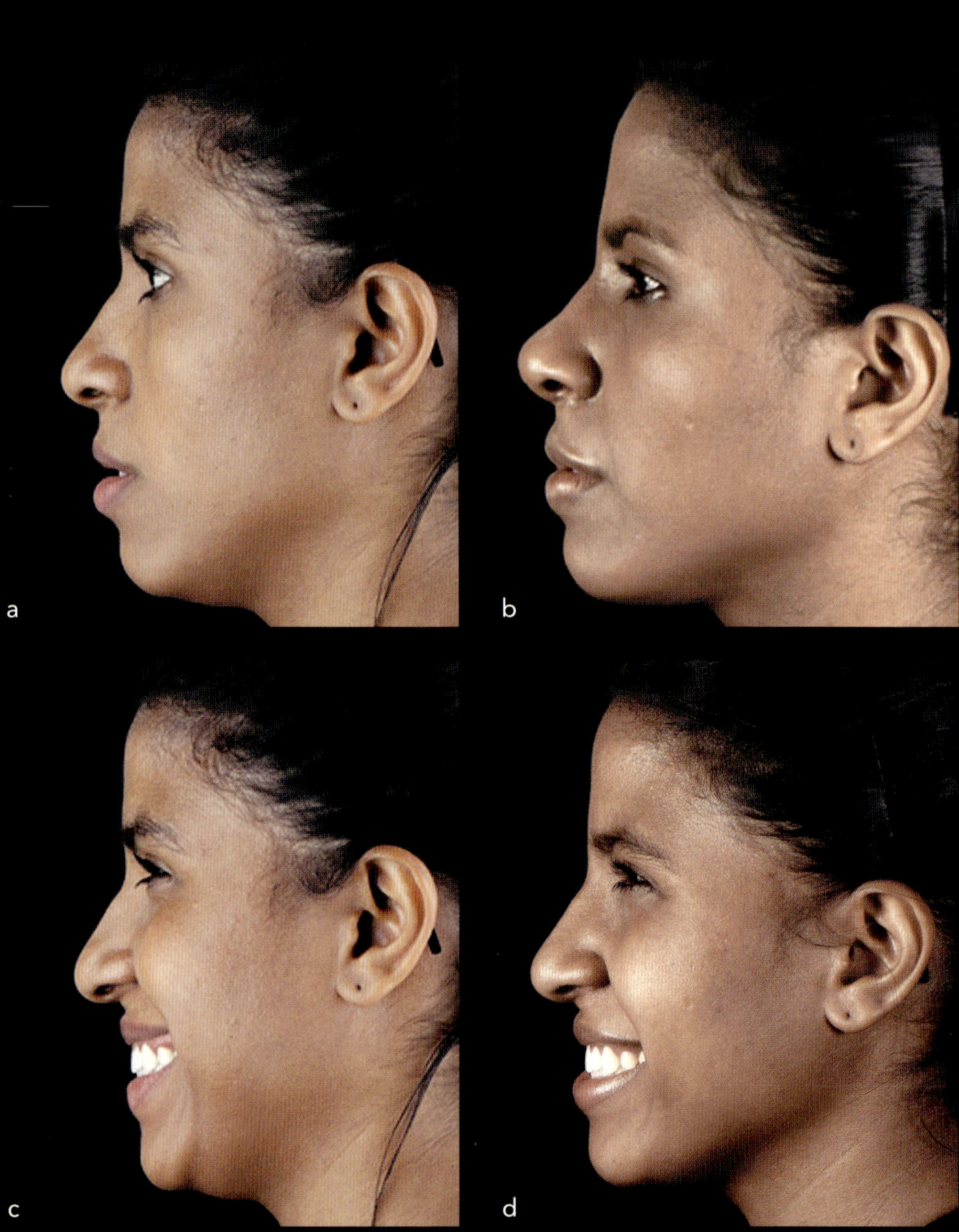

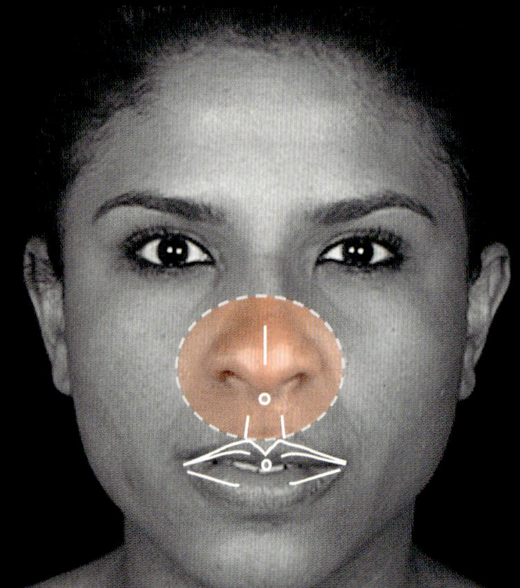

Fig 7-33 Filler treatment at the supratip. *(a)* Pretreatment profile at rest. *(b)* Posttreatment profile at rest. *(c)* Pretreatment profile while smiling. Note the gummy smile and low supratip. *(d)* Posttreatment profile while smiling. Note that even while smiling, the patient's nasal tip is inclined upward. The gummy smile was treated with a botulinum toxin injection in the levator labii superioris alaeque nasi and depressor septi nasi muscles. *(e)* Injection sites marked.

the risk of embolization; aspiration before injection gives the practitioner a false sense of safety, because after the needle is filled with the filler, the blood no longer flows back into the syringe.

Never inject more than 0.1 mL in the supratip to prevent the vessels from being compressed, which would compromise the blood supply in this region. Patients who have undergone previous rhinoplasty and are still not satisfied with the result can have their supratip treated with fillers but only after reading and signing an informed consent that advises them about the risk of a vascular compression. Patients with previous rhinoplasty surgery show a higher risk of necrosis because the postsurgical tissue tends to develop a certain degree of fibrosis, making it less elastic. If, after injecting 0.1 mL, the desired effect has not yet been achieved, a further injection can be made after 30 days, a period that should be observed for the tissue accommodation.

Clinical case

Figure 7-33 shows the case of a patient with a low supratip. Fillers were injected with the following volumes at the sites listed:

- *Supratip:* 0.1 mL of Restylane Defyne in the midline, delivered with a 25G cannula
- *Nasolabial angle:* 0.3 mL of Restylane Defyne, delivered with a 25G cannula
- *Philtrum columns:* 0.05 mL of Restylane Kysse in each side, delivered with a 13-mm needle
- *Lip vermilion:* 0.9 mL of Restylane Kysse, delivered with a 25G cannula

Prejowl Sulcus

Anatomy

The prejowl is located between the chin and the mandible body. When present, it is a depressed area whose beginning matches a vertical line tangent to the oral commissure in a frontal view of the patient at rest and not smiling. It extends a few millimeters posteriorly. Its lower limit is the base of the jaw, from where it extends superiorly a few millimeters. If present, this depression is caused by the strong insertion of the mandibular cutaneous ligament and the gravitational ptosis of the fat tissues in the face (jowl fat).

Visual interpretation

Some patients do not show a depression in this region. Thus, the chin is visually integrated with the mandible, giving a perception that the mandible and the chin are a harmonious single body. However, when present, the prejowl sulcus causes a lack of harmony because visually the chin is not perfectly integrated with the mandible. The more depressed this region is, the more evident the visualization of the inferior jaw fat will be.

Deepening of the prejowl sulcus suggests aging and lack of harmony and makes the presence of the inferior jaw fat more evident. On the other hand, the absence of a deep menton lateral region suggests strength, youth, and harmony in the jawline.

Diagnosis

The need to have fillers injected in the prejowl sulcus might be evaluated by looking at the patient's face and also analyzing frontal and profile photographs. The ideal is to have a continuous jawline with no interruption in this region.

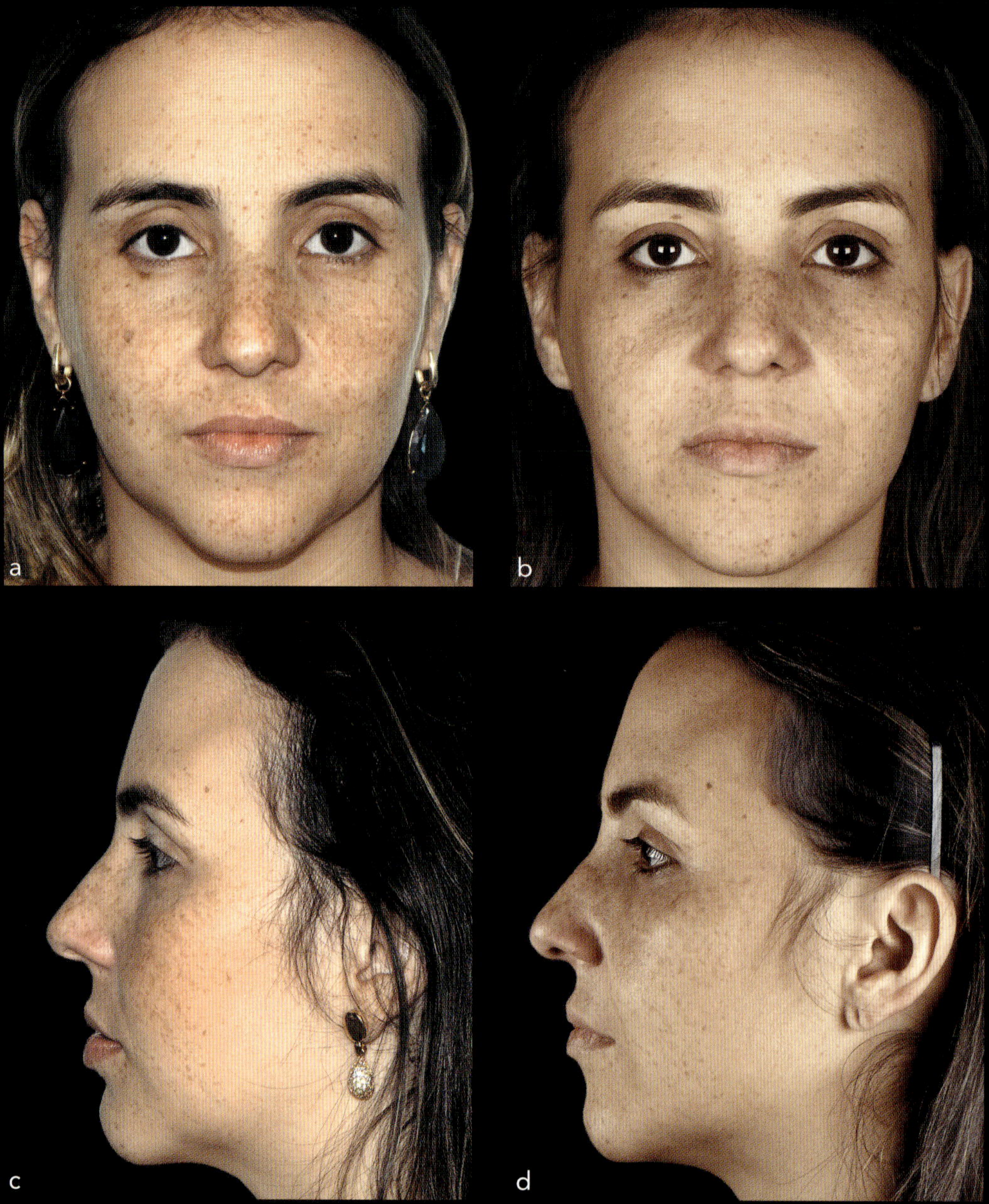

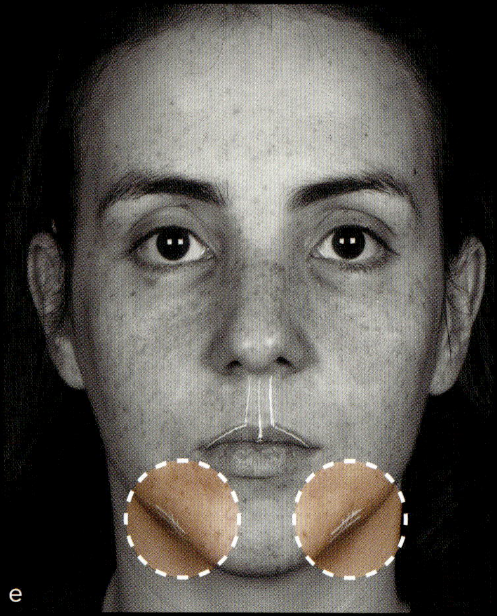

Fig 7-34 Filler treatment for a prejowl sulcus. *(a)* Pretreatment frontal view. *(b)* Posttreatment frontal view. *(c)* Pretreatment profile. *(d)* Posttreatment profile. Note that the skin of the neck is more stretched, decreasing the visualization of the submental fat. The major esthetic deficiency in this face was the prejowl sulcus. The upper lip also had to be everted so that it had a horizontal projection higher than that of the lower lip. *(e)* Injection sites marked.

Technique

Before injecting the filler, draw over the skin the accurate position of the filler filaments that will be subcutaneously inserted. With the patient sitting in a chair and the operator standing in front, observe the deepest point in the prejowl sulcus.

Draw in this point a vertical line following the depression. Then draw two horizontal lines that follow the side of the jaw along the depressed area. The embossed areas should not be marked, only the depressed areas.

Use a 22G or 23G cannula and inject the filler 3 mm deep. The volume to be injected is proportional to the depth of the sulcus, but an average of 0.5 mL of filler might be used in each side of the face. To ensure a more effective treatment, a subcision in the mandibular cutaneous ligament can be performed. However, this is a high-risk procedure because this ligament helps to maintain the position of the inferior jaw fat.

Clinical case

Figure 7-34 illustrates the treatment of a prejowl sulcus with fillers. The following volumes of fillers were injected at the sites listed:

- *Prejowl sulcus:* Three filaments of Emervel Deep (0.15 mL each) following the drawing, delivered with a 22G cannula
- *Philtrum columns:* 0.05 mL of Emervel Lips, delivered with a 13-mm needle
- *Eversion of the upper lip:* 0.1 mL of Emervel Lips in each side, delivered with a 25G cannula

Submental Lengthening

Anatomy

The submental region is located under the mandible in its most anterior part, and it laterally extends to the midline until it reaches the mouth width during the muscle rest. This region is supplied both by the submental artery, a branch of the facial artery, and the mental branches. They are both located deep to the platysma muscle. Therefore, the juxtaperiosteal filling procedure should be avoided in this area.

Visual interpretation

When the most anterior part of the submental region of an individual's face in frontal view is in a lower level compared to its posterior portion, it is considered esthetically pleasing. Some patients show a double chin, where the most posterior part of the submental region occupies a lower level than its anterior region. In general, this feature is considered esthetically unpleasant.

The presence of this volume decreases both the dominance of the mandible and the definition of the jawline, suggesting that the patient is overweight and/or in the process of aging. On the other hand, a flat posterior part of the submental region with no volume suggests youthfulness, strength, healthy body weight, and good definition of the jawline.

Diagnosis

The presence of a double chin can be an indication for the use of fillers in the submental region. This treatment is also indicated in patients with a decreased lower lip length in relation to the upper lip. It can also be used to increase the perception that the individual is dolichofacial (see the esthetic references for this region described in chapter 5).

Technique

Ask the patient to look at the horizon without inclining his or her head. Then draw a curved filament in the most anterior part of the submental region that matches the disposition of the inferior border of the mandible. It is important to have a bone support for a better effect of the filler. The width of the filament should not exceed the width of the mouth during muscle rest. The next step is to bend the 22G or 23G cannula by copying the shape of the drawing. The puncture can be done in one side, and when inserting the cannula, the midline can be crossed and a single filament inserted 3 mm deep, that is, superficially to the platysma muscle. Another easier possibility is to do two separate filaments, one to the left and the other to the right.

The volume to be injected is proportional to the amount of elongation desired for this area, but on average a total of 0.5 to 1 mL of the filler can be injected. For a more effective procedure when indicated, botulinum toxin can be injected in the mentalis muscle and anterior bands of the platysma prior to filler treatment.

Clinical case

Figure 7-35 shows filler treatment for submental lengthening. The following volumes of filler were used at the sites listed:

- *Submental region (elongation):* One 0.15-mL filament of Emervel Defyne, following the drawing and delivered with a 22G curved cannula
- *Prejowl sulcus:* Three 0.15-mL filaments of Emervel Deep, following the drawing and delivered with a 22G cannula
- *Philtrum columns:* 0.05 mL of Emervel Lips, delivered with a 13-mm needle
- *Eversion of the upper and lower lip:* 0.1 mL of Emervel Lips in each side of each lip (0.4 mL total), delivered with a 25G cannula

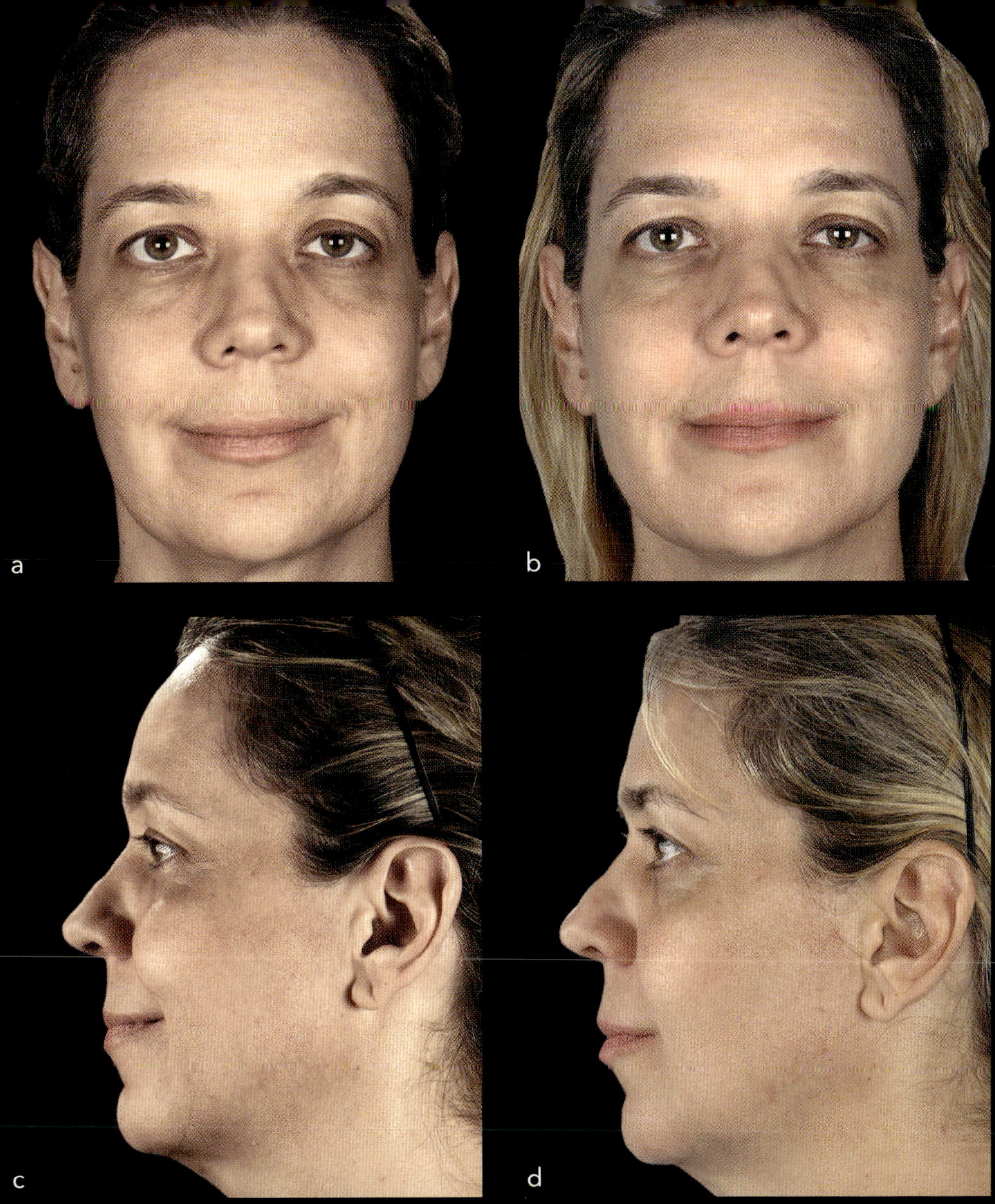

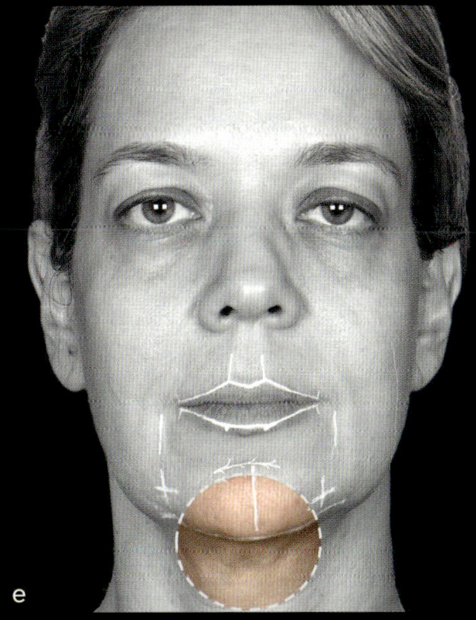

Fig 7-35 Filler treatment for submental lengthening. *(a)* Pretreatment frontal view. *(b)* Posttreatment frontal view. *(c)* Pretreatment profile. *(d)* Posttreatment profile. Note that there was an improvement in the contour of the chin, which was shorter before the treatment. *(e)* Injection sites marked. A vertical line was drawn in the chin just as a reference for the facial midline. This area was not injected with fillers, nor were the marionette lines. Before the injection of fillers, the platysma bands were treated with botulinum toxin injections.

Gonial Angle

Anatomy

The gonial angle is formed by the junction of the ramus of the mandible (ramus line) with its base (mandibular line) at the most posterior and inferior part of the mandible. Upadhyay et al[27] observed a variation in mandibular angle with age, sex, and even dental status. The study reported a 6-degree increase in gonial angle for edentulous patients. The average measurements for the gonial angle are 120 to 130 degrees up to the time of eruption of the second molars and 120 to 150 degrees in old age. The gonial angle in males is greater than that measured in females. Findings concerning sex differences may also be explained by the fact that, on average, men have greater masticatory force than women.

Visual interpretation

A marked gonial angle helps define the jawline and, consequently, the definition between the head and neck. It is best observed in profile view, but it also influences facial esthetics in frontal view. A marked gonial angle, measuring between 125 and 135 degrees, suggests youthfulness, strength, and healthy body mass. On the other hand, a very open gonial angle between 140 and 150 degrees suggests aging, while a poorly perceptible gonial angle suggests that the patient may be overweight. In a frontal view, the gonial angle has to be the widest part of the mandible. If the frontal observer notes that the widest part is the jowl fat that is anterior to the angle, the gonial filling should be considered.

Diagnosis

Fillers can be injected in this area when the clinician considers that the patient has a poorly defined and/or very open gonial angle. The angle can be measured by drawing it onto the patient's face. In order to do so, position the fingers of the right hand (except the thumb) against the posterior part of the gonial angle so that two fingers touch the posterior edge of the ramus and the other two touch the base of the jaw. Keep your fingers in that position and draw the current angle. The filler should be injected when the angle is unnoticeable or when it is very open (> 135 degrees). The ideal angle is 130 degrees.

Technique

Filler treatment should proceed only after the initial drawing of the gonial angle is accomplished (see previous section). The filler should be injected at a horizontal level slightly above the existing angle, so that the bone at the side of the face will work as a support for the filler gel. The same procedure should be performed on both sides of the face.

The height of the ascending vertical filament should not exceed the lower level of the earlobe. The anterior extension of the horizontal filament should not exceed the posterior limit of the lower jowl fat compartment, as this is already naturally a bulky area. Remember that the facial artery crosses the mandible along the anterior border of the masseter muscle. The insertion holes should be located in the most distant parts of the angle, and the 22G or 23G cannula should be inserted in them and go through the path drawn until it reaches the angle. Right after this, the retroinjection should be performed.

To close the gonial angle, initially make a posterior to anterior insertion hole against the posterior part of the angle, inserting the 22G or 23G cannula 3 mm deep and injecting from 0.1 to 0.3 mL at the angle. After that, follow the same steps as described above.

Clinical case

Figure 7-36 illustrates filler treatment at the gonial angle. First, a 0.3-mL bolus of filler was injected in the new gonial point, and then one ascendant filament and one horizontal filament (0.3 mL of Restylane Defyne) were injected via 22G cannula on each side, following the drawing (see Fig 7-36c).

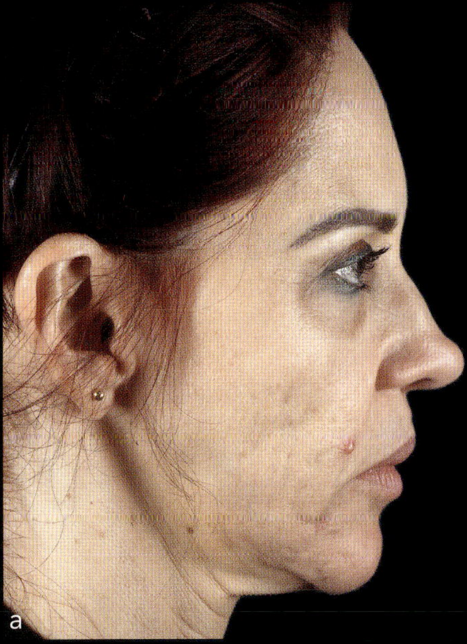
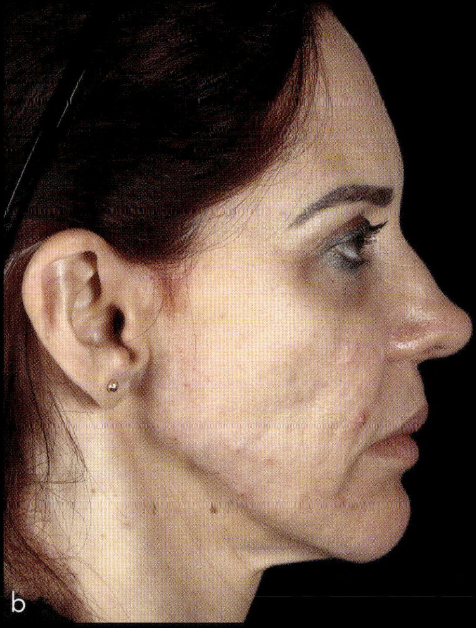

Fig 7-36 Filler treatment at the gonial angle. *(a)* Pretreatment profile. *(b)* Posttreatment profile. *(c)* Injection sites marked. The malar region, while marked, was not injected with fillers. The base of the letter F marks the position where the facial artery crosses the mandibular border. Its pulsation can sometimes be felt. This area should not be treated with fillers. *(d)* The procedure during its execution. Note that after injecting the bolus, there is gel coming out through the orifice, providing an accurate idea of the injection point when you want to close the angle. *(e)* Immediate result after the injection of vertical and horizontal filaments.

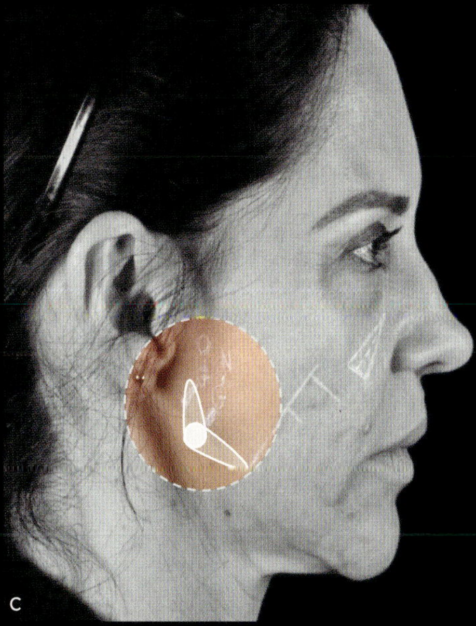

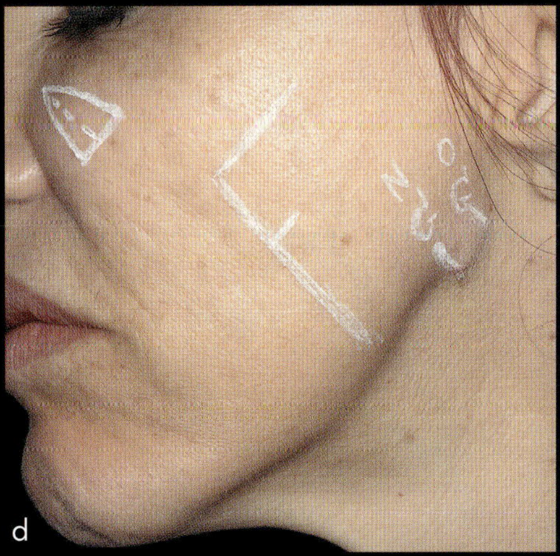
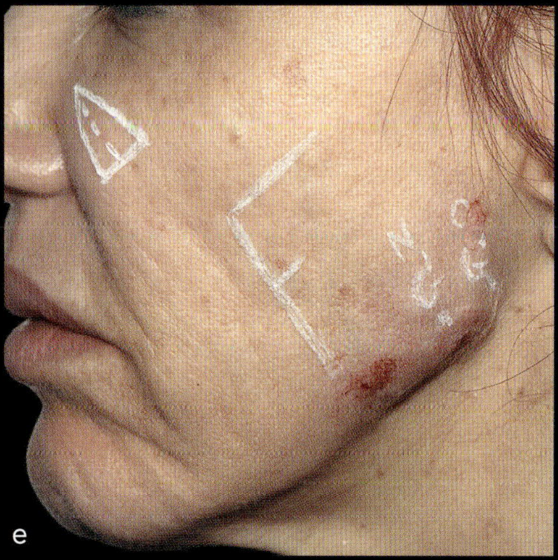

Lip Vermilion

Anatomy

The lip vermilion is the mobile musculofibrous structure that surrounds the most external part of the mouth. Its internal limit is the oral fissure, and its external limit is the skin of the upper and lower lips. It has a thin and translucent epithelial surface coating. This epithelium is keratinized in order to provide protection to the structures covered by it. Deeper in the epithelium is the connective tissue, a thin layer of superficial fat, the orbicularis oris muscle, a very thin layer of deep fat with its labial glands, and the oral mucosa. It is important to emphasize that superficially to the orbicularis oris muscle, the blood vessels are small, while in a deeper layer the vessels are larger, therefore carrying a higher risk during filler treatment.

The lips are related to the teeth when sealed and at rest. Thus, the teeth can influence the horizontal projection of the lips. The main role of the lips is to seal the oral cavity by closing the vestibule of the mouth. Other functions of the lips include speech, suction, and facial expression. They also aid in chewing and swallowing.

Visual interpretation

The lip vermilion stands out on the face by its color and projection just beyond the skin of the lips, thus being a very important structure for facial esthetics. When the volume of the lower lip vermilion is greater than that of the upper lip, and when the upper lip vermilion has a horizontal projection greater than that of the lower lip, the esthetics are considered more pleasant. A bulky vermilion suggests joviality and sensuality. On the other hand, a thin vermilion suggests aging and austerity.

Diagnosis

Some parameters should be observed when the status of a patient's lips is evaluated (see Fig 7-38b):

- *Ideal volume of the lower lip vermilion:* To evaluate this volume, the author uses the measurement of the visible iris in the eye of each patient positioned over the lower lip immediately lateral to the midline.
- *Ideal volume of the upper lip vermilion:* This corresponds to the volume of the lower lip vermilion minus 25%, according to Epker and Stella.[28] It is acceptable to have a lower lip vermilion minus 40%, so the ratio varies from 25% to 40%.
- *Distance between the oral commissures at rest:* According to Suguino et al,[29] this width matches the distance between the irises of the eyes.
- *Distance between the oral commissures during smile:* This width matches the width between the most lateral part of the pupils.
- These references might be verified through a digital photograph in a software program such as PowerPoint or Keynote. In order to accomplish this, the visible iris of the patient can be drawn and transferred to the lower lip so that the volume can be verified. As for the mouth width, it can be verified by tracing perfectly vertical lines tangent to the more medial part of the iris. They should be coincident to the oral commissures during rest. In a photograph where the patient is smiling, a perfect vertical line can be drawn tangent to the most lateral part of the patient's pupil. This line should match the oral commissure.
- The analysis of the horizontal projection of the vermilion can be made by using a true vertical line drawn over a profile photograph of the patient. This line is described in chapter 5.
- The upper lip vermilion stands forward to the lower lip vermilion in the same proportion that the upper eyelid stands forward to the lower eyelid.

Technique

The technique foresees the injection of eversion filaments positioned near the skin/vermilion limit but always tending to the vermilion. These filaments should be very superficially injected with a 25G cannula so that they cause a perceptible linear volume. They should be continuous to the lower lip.

For the upper lip, at the height of each philtrum column, the filaments must change direction, becoming descendant to give the appropriate contour to the Cupid's bow in this region. These shorter filaments can be made with needles.

When the lower lip has a horizontal projection greater than that of the upper lip, only the upper lip should receive the eversion filaments in order to make the profile ideal again.

Volumization filaments to increase the volume of the lips start at the oral commissures just like the eversion filaments so that the same orifices can be used. From the commissure, these filaments should be distant from the eversion filaments in its route in a medial direction but should be injected anteriorly to the wet-dry line of the lips. This line is the maximum limit for the filaments.

In the upper lip vermilion border, at the level of the philtrum columns, these volumization filaments change direction and follow a parallel route to the eversion filaments along the midline. This helps create a convexity along the midline that reinforces the sculpture of the lip tubercle.

As for the lower lip volumization filaments, they should be interrupted at the width of the philtrum column. This helps create larger volumes in the lateral aspects and a small depression in the center of the lower lip where the stomion (lowest part of the inferior limit of the upper lip) should fit. These filaments should be injected 3 mm deep with a 25G cannula. When the upper lip has a volume larger than the lower lip, only the lower lip should be injected with the volumization filaments so that it will have a larger volume than the upper lip.

To inject a bolus in the tubercle of the lip, insert the needle 3 mm deep and deposit 0.05 to 0.1 mL at the stomion to volumize this area so that it will fit in the central depression of the lower lip. This gives the fissure a shape similar to the shape of the Cupid's bow contributing to the desired facial harmony. If the goal is to make the mouth wider, the filler can be injected up to the oral commissures. However, when this is not the goal of treatment, the filler should be injected 3 mm distant from each oral commissure.

Clinical cases

Figure 7-37 illustrates a case of filler treatment at the lip vermilion. The following volumes were used at the sites listed:

- *Lip vermilion:* 1 mL of Restylane Kysse, delivered with a 25G cannula.
- *Philtrum columns:* 0.05 mL of Restylane Kysse in each side, delivered with a 13-mm needle.
- *Prejowl sulcus:* Three 0.15-mL filaments of Emervel Deep, following the drawing and delivered with a 22G cannula.
- *Marionette lines:* 0.3 mL of Emervel Deep in each side, delivered with a 25G cannula.
- *Gonial angle:* One 0.2-mL bolus of Restylane Defyne in the most posterior part of the gonial angle, followed by one 0.3-mL ascendant filament and another 0.5-mL horizontal filament, following the drawing, delivered with a 22G cannula. A total of 1 mL of gel was injected on each side of the face.

Figure 7-38 shows a second case of the use of fillers at the lip vermilion to illustrate the correlation between the facial and labial anatomy. Figure 7-38a shows the patient's face before the use of fillers at the lip vermilion. Figure 7-38b shows how the facial analysis guides the planning for the lip vermilion treatment with fillers:

- The *dotted line* represents the facial midline drawn in an equidistant point between the medial palpebral fissures.
- A *green line* was drawn tangent to the iris of the eye. When drawing this line, three situations might be found: *(1)* When the line coincides with the oral commissure, the mouth has the ideal width for the face and therefore should only be treated if the patient wishes to have a wider mouth to make it more dominant. *(2)* When the oral commissure is short of this green line, the width can be increased by injecting the filler from the oral commissure. In this case, the mouth

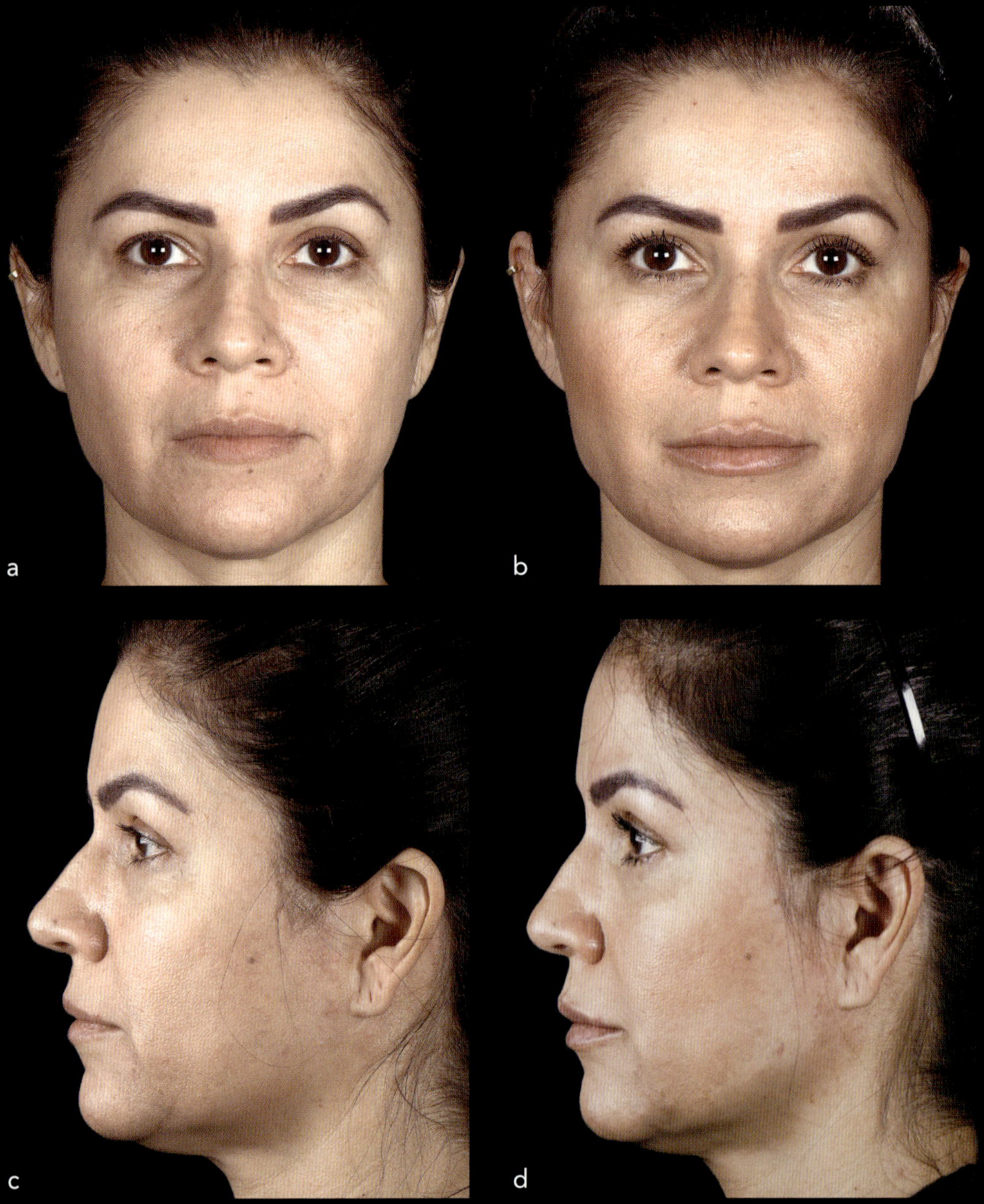

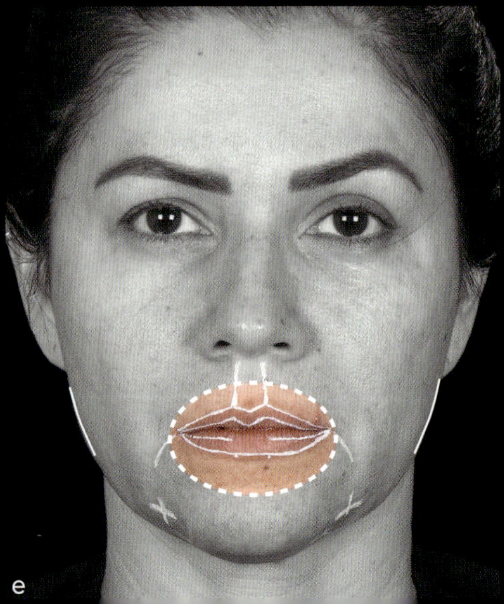

Fig 7-37 Filler treatment at the lip vermilion. *(a)* Pretreatment frontal view. *(b)* Posttreatment frontal view. *(c)* Pretreatment profile. *(d)* Posttreatment profile. Note that there was a greater projection of the lips due to the eversion filaments. If this eversion results in a more closed nasolabial angle, it can be reopened with a filler injected at the subnasale point. *(e)* Injection sites marked.

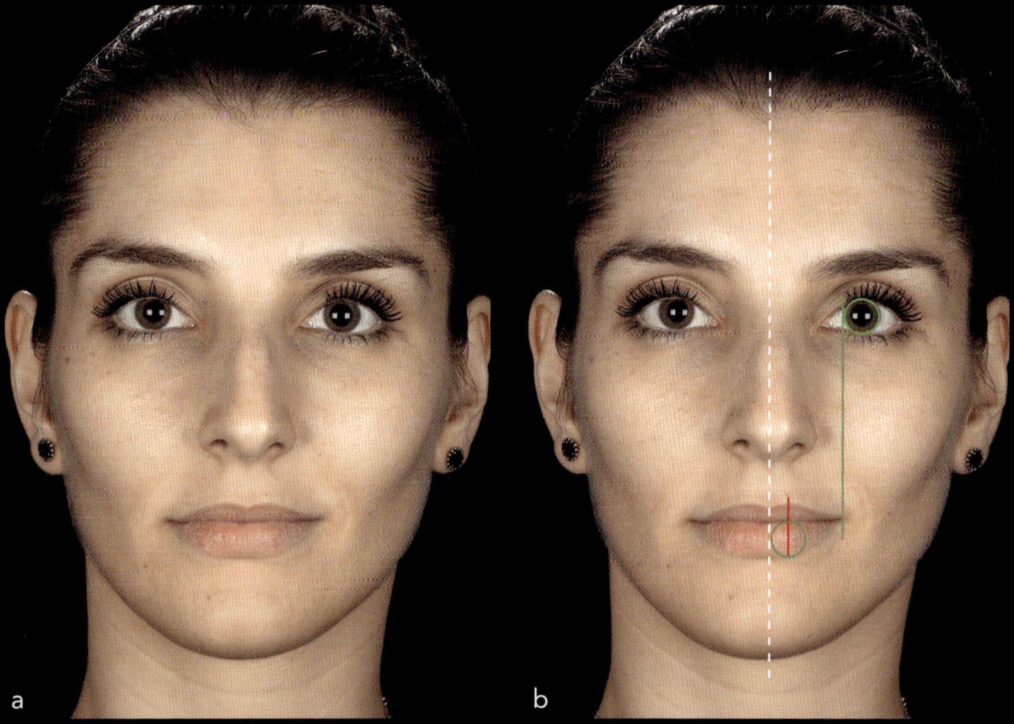

Fig 7-38 *(a)* Pretreatment frontal view of a patient seeking dermal filler treatment at the lip vermilion. *(b)* Facial analysis. See text for details.

width can be increased up to 1.5 mm on each side. *(3)* When this oral commissure is beyond the green line, the mouth is considered wide for the face. Therefore, a volumization might be made but the length of the lip should not be increased. Thus, the filler should be injected at least 3 mm away from each commissure, avoiding any enlargement in a mouth already considered dominant.

- The *green circle* over the eye represents the visible area of the iris that should be the measure for the ideal volume of the lower lip positioned immediately to the midline. The *green circle* over the lower lip vermilion has the same dimension as the circle over the eye, suggesting that the lower lip vermilion already presents an ideal volume and volumization filaments are not necessary.
- The *red line* over the lower lip vermilion represents its ideal volume.
- The *red line* over the upper lip vermilion was obtained by decreasing the length of the red line over the lower lip vermilion by 25%, and it represents the ideal volume for the upper lip. Therefore, in this case, the planning included filaments of volumization to the upper lip so that it would be proportional to the lower lip.

Figure 7-38c shows a close-up view of the lips prior to filler treatment, and Fig 7-38d shows the treatment plan drawn onto the lips with washable ink. This is an indispensable step of filler treatment. The filaments drawn on the contour of the upper lip vermilion represent the demarcation to evert the lip by using fillers, while the inferior filaments drawn under the vermilion of the upper lip represent the demarcation for the lip volumization.

The filaments over the lower lip vermilion represent the position of the filler to evert this lip. The lower lip vermilion was not treated with volumization filaments because it already presented an adequate volume for this particular face.

Figures 7-38e to 7-38h illustrate the outcome of this treatment plan. Because of the forces exerted by the fillers and the shape of the cannula used for application, the lower lip was given an unusual anatomy (see Fig 7-38f).

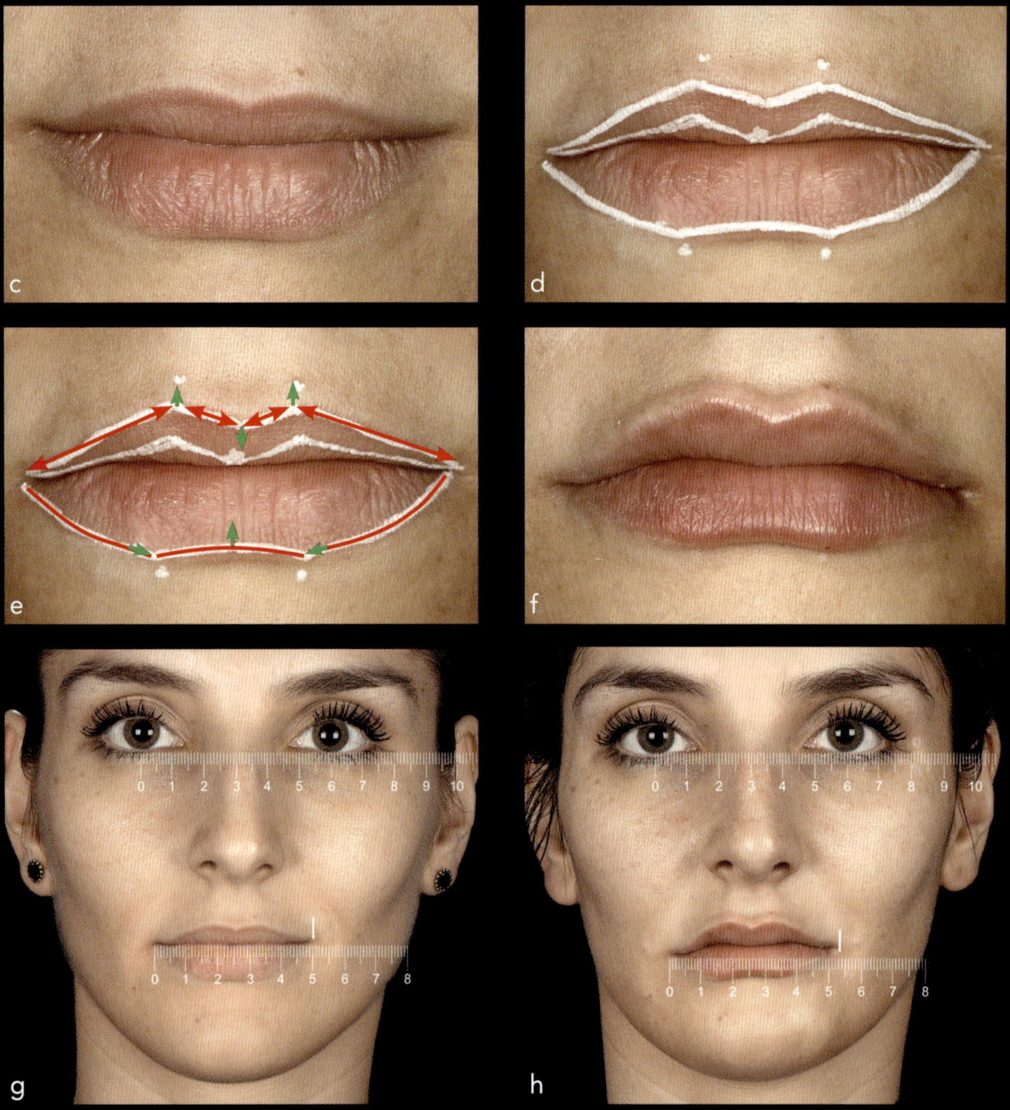

Fig 7-38 *(cont) (c)* Close-up view of lips prior to treatment. *(d)* Treatment plan. See text for details. *(e)* Forces exerted by the filaments *(red lines)* and their resulting vectors *(green arrows)*. These vectors explain why the Cupid's bow becomes more evident after this type of treatment with fillers. *(f)* Immediate result after filling. Note that the curved 25G cannula gave the lower lip an unusual anatomy. *(g and h)* Photographs before and after filling treatment showing the enlargement of the mouth. The measurements of the interpupillary distance confirm that the photographs are the same size, while the measurements of the oral commissures show that the mouth was made 3 mm wider after the filling procedures.

Therapeutic gains of filler treatment

As people age, the teeth become worn, the occlusal vertical dimension is decreased, and the lips become flatter as they approach the teeth. With the lips in contact with the teeth, speech can be impaired and saliva can accumulate in the vestibule. Therefore, it has been postulated that the use of fillers in the lips of some patients, in addition to improving esthetics, may be therapeutic because it can lift the lips away from the teeth, thereby eliminating some of the negative consequences of an aging oral cavity. Figure 7-39 compares an illustration of young lips and teeth (Fig 7-39a) with an illustration of aged lips and teeth (Fig 7-39b). In Fig 7-39a, the small superior *blue circle* suggests the ideal position of the eversion filament, and the inferior *blue circle* suggests the ideal position of the volumization filament. Note that the rounded anatomy of the lips maintains the dry-moist line of the lips away from the teeth, making it ideal for speech. It also distances the lip epithelium of the teeth, preventing saliva from migrating anteriorly and forming accumulations visible during speech.

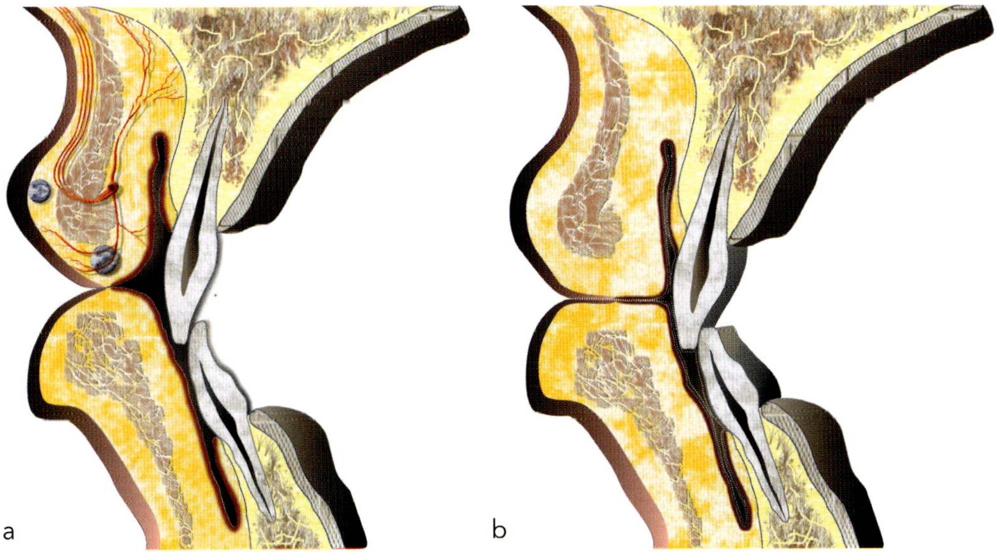

Fig 7-39 Illustration of young lips *(a)* versus aged lips *(b)*. The *blue circles* in *a* show the ideal positions for eversion *(top circle)* and volumization *(bottom circle)* filaments.

Scan this QR code to access videos demonstrating filler treatment.

References

1. Sundaram H, Cassuto D. Biophysical characteristics of hyaluronic acid soft-tissue fillers and their relevance to aesthetic applications. Plast Reconstr Surg 2013;132(4 suppl 2):5S–21S.
2. Yüksel NE, Karabas L, Altintas O, Yildirim Y, Caglar Y. A comparison of the short-term hypotensive effects and side effects of unilateral brimonidine and apraclonidine in patients with elevated intraocular pressure. Opthalmologica 2002;216:45–49.
3. Kesterke MJ, Raffensperger ZD, Heike CL, et al. Using the 3D Facial Norms Database to investigate craniofacial sexual dimorphism in healthy children, adolescents, and adults. Biol Sex Differ 2016;7:23.
4. Zaki ME, Soliman MA, El-Bassyouni HT. A cephalometric study of skulls from the Bahriyah oasis. J Forensic Dent Sci 2012;4:88–92.
5. Weston EM, Friday AE, Liò P. Biometric evidence that sexual selection has shaped the hominin face. PLoS One 2007;2:e710.
6. Castro JCBB. Antropometria óssea e identificação do sexo [dissertation]. São Paulo: Faculdade de Odontologia de Piracicaba da Universidade Estadual de Campinas, Piracicaba, 2017.
7. Beleznay K, Carruthers JDA, Humphrey S, Jones D. Avoiding and treating blindness from fillers: A review of the world literature. Dermatol Surg 2015;41:1097–1117.
8. Lacerda D. Prevention and management of iatrogenic blindness associated with aesthetical filler injections. Dermatol Ther 2018;25:e12722.
9. Park SW, Woo SJ, Park KH, Huh JW, Jung C, Kwon OK. Iatrogenic retinal artery occlusion caused by cosmetic facial filler injections. Am J Ophthalmol 2012;154:653–662.e1.
10. Vos JA, van Werkum MH, Bistervels JH, Ackerstaff RG, Tromp SC, van den Berg JC. Retinal embolization during carotid angioplasty and stenting: Periprocedural data and follow-up. Cardiovasc Intervent Radiol 2010;33:714–719.
11. Müller C, Rahn BA, Pfister U, Meinig RP. The incidence, pathogenesis, diagnosis, and treatment of fat embolism. Orthop Rev 1994;23:107–117.
12. Castillo B Jr, De Alba F, Thornton J, DeBrun G, Pulido J. Retinal artery occlusion following coil embolization of carotid-ophthalmic aneurysms. Arch Ophthalmol 2000;118:851–852.

13. Glaich AS, Cohen JL, Goldberg LH. Injection necrosis of the glabella: Protocol for prevention and treatment after use of dermal fillers. Dermatol Surg 2006;32:276–281.
14. Arnett GW, Bergman RT. Facial keys to orthodontic diagnosis and treatment planning—Part II. Am J Orthod Dentofacial Orthop 1993;103:395–411.
15. Lee JH, Hong G. Definitions of groove and hollowness of the infraorbital region and clinical treatment using soft-tissue filler. Arch Plast Surg 2018;45:214–221.
16. Hwang K. Eponym of naso-jugal fold and tear trough. J Craniofac Surg 2016;27:1350–1353.
17. Yang C, Zhang P, Xing X. Tear trough and palpebromalar groove in young versus elderly adults: A sectional anatomy study. Plast Reconstr Surg 2013;132:796–808.
18. Hwang K, Kim HJ, Kim H, et al. Origin of the lower orbicularis oculi muscle in relation to the nasojugal groove. J Craniofac Surg 2015;26:1389–1393.
19. Wong CH, Hsieh MK, Mendelson B. The tear trough ligament: Anatomical basis for the tear trough deformity. Plast Reconstr Surg 2012;129:1392–1402.
20. William J, Mellinger MD. The canine fossa. Arch Otolaryngol 1940;31:930–937.
21. Diehl LA, Dias JR, Paes ACS, et al. Prevalência da lipodistrofia associada ao HIV em pacientes ambulatoriais brasileiros: Relação com síndrome metabólica e fatores de risco cardiovascular. Arq Bras Endocrinol Metab [online] 2008;52:658–667.
22. Fradeani M. Análise Estética: Uma Abordagem Sistemática para o Tratamento Protético, vol 1. São Paulo: Quintessence, 2006.
23. Ribeiro L, Pessoa MCM, Andrade RM. Tratamento estético da columela nasal: Columela oculta e columela pendente. Rev Bras Cir Plást 2014;29:159–164.
24. Paixão MP. Conheço a anatomia labial? Implicações para o bom preenchimento. Surg Cosmet Dermatol 2015;7:10–16.
25. Garcia de Mitchell CA, Pessa JE, Schaverien MV, Rohrich RJ. The philtrum: Anatomical observations from a new perspective. Plast Reconstr Surg 2008;122:1756–1760.
26. Cardim VLN, Silva ASS, Salomons RL, Dornelles RFV, Blom JOS, Silva AL. Lifting nasolabial com realce do vermelhão. Rev Bras Cir Plást 2011;26:466–471.
27. Upadhyay RB, Upadhyay J, Agrawal P, Rao NN. Analysis of gonial angle in relation to age, gender, and dentition status by radiological and anthropometric methods. J Forensic Dent Sci 2012;4:29–33.
28. Epker BN, Stella JP. Dentofacial Deformities: Integrated Orthodontic and Surgical Correction, vol 1. St Louis: Mosby, 1995.
29. Suguino R, Ramos AL, Terada HH, Furquin LZ, Maeda L, Filho OGS. Análise facial. Rev Dental Press Ortod Ortop Facial 1996;1:86–107.

Index

Page references followed by "f" denote figures; those followed by "b" denote boxes; and those followed by "t" denote tables.

D

E

F

G

H

I

J

K

L

M

N

O

P

R

S

T

U

V

W

Z